Developing children's food products

Related titles:

Food, diet and obesity
(ISBN 978-1-85573-958-1)
Obesity is a global epidemic with large numbers of adults and children overweight or obese in many developed and developing countries. As a result, there is an unprecedented level of interest and research in the complex interactions between our genetic susceptibility, diet and lifestyle in determining individual risk of obesity. With its distinguished editor and international team of contributors, this collection sums up the key themes in weight control research, focusing on their implications and applications for food product development and consumers.

Understanding consumers of food products
(ISBN 978-1-84569-009-0)
It is very important for food businesses, scientists and policy makers to understand consumers of food products: in the case of businesses to develop successful products and in the case of policy makers to gain and retain consumer confidence. Consumers' requirements and desires are affected by issues such as culture, age and gender and issues important to consumers such as diet and health or GM foods will not always be so significant. Therefore food businesses and policy makers need to understand consumers' attitudes and influences upon them to respond effectively. Edited by two distinguished experts, this book is an essential guide for food businesses, food scientists and policy makers.

Food fortification and supplementation
(ISBN 978-1-84569-144-8)
Fortified foods and food supplements remain popular with today's health-conscious consumers and the range of bioactives added to food is increasing. This collection provides a comprehensive summary of the technology of food fortification and supplementation and associated safety and regulatory aspects. The first part covers methods of fortifying foods, not only with vitamins and minerals, but also with other nutraceuticals such as amino acids, polyphenols and fatty acids. Chapters on safe levels for the addition of vitamins and minerals to foods and analysis of polyphenols and antioxidants and other nutraceuticals in fortified foods and supplements are also included. Discussion of regulation concludes the volume.

Details of these books and a complete list of Woodhead's titles can be obtained by:

- visiting our web site at www.woodheadpublishing.com
- contacting Customer Services (e-mail: sales@woodheadpublishing.com; fax: +44 (0) 1223 832819; tel.: +44 (0) 1223 499140 ext. 130; address: Woodhead Publishing Limited, 80 High Street, Sawston, Cambridge CB22 3HJ, UK)

If you would like to receive information on forthcoming titles, please send your address details to: Francis Dodds (address, tel. and fax as above; e-mail: francis.dodds@woodheadpublishing.com). Please confirm which subject areas you are interested in.

Woodhead Publishing Series in Food Science, Technology and Nutrition:
Number 204

Developing children's food products

Edited by
David Kilcast and Fiona Angus

WP
WOODHEAD
PUBLISHING

Oxford Cambridge Philadelphia New Delhi

Published by Woodhead Publishing Limited,
80 High Street, Sawston, Cambridge CB22 3HJ, UK
www.woodheadpublishing.com

Woodhead Publishing, 1518 Walnut Street, Suite 1100, Philadelphia, PA19102-3406, USA

Woodhead Publishing India Private Limited, G-2, Vardaan House, 7/28 Ansari Road, Daryaganj, New Delhi – 110002, India
www.woodheadpublishingindia.com

First published 2011, Woodhead Publishing Limited

British Library Cataloguing in Publication Data
A catalogue record for this book is available from the British Library.

ISBN 978-0-08-101492-9 (print)
ISBN 978-0-85709-113-0 (online)
ISSN 2042-8049 Woodhead Publishing Series in Food Science, Technology and Nutrition (print)
ISSN 2042-8057 Woodhead Publishing Series in Food Science, Technology and Nutrition (online)

The publisher's policy is to use permanent paper from mills that operate a sustainable forestry policy, and which has been manufactured from pulp which is processed using acid-free and elemental chlorine-free practices. Furthermore, the publisher ensures that the text paper and cover board used have met acceptable environmental accreditation standards.

Typeset by Replika Press Pvt Ltd, India

Contents

Part III Design of food and drink products for children

Contributor contact details

(* = main contact)

Editors
D. Kilcast and F. Angus
Leatherhead Food International
Randalls Road
Leatherhead
Surrey KT22 7RY
UK

Email: dkilcast@yahoo.com
fangus@eur.ko.com

Chapter 1
L. R. Marotz
Department of Applied Behavioral Science
1000 Sunnyside
University of Kansas
Lawrence, KS 66045
USA

Email: lrm@ku.edu

Chapter 2
R. Muckelbauer,* L. Libuda and M. Kersting
Research Institute of Child Nutrition
University of Bonn
Heinstueck 11
D-44225 Dortmund
Germany

Email: muckelbauer@fke-do.de
llibuda@gmx.de
kersting@fke-do.de

Chapter 3
G. Rodríguez, J. Fernández and L. A. Moreno*
'Growth, Exercise, Nutrition and Development' (GENUD) Research Group
University of Zaragoza
C/Pedro Cerbuna, 12
50009 Zaragoza
Spain

Email: lmoreno@unizar.es

Chapter 4
D. Benton
Department of Psychology
University of Swansea
Swansea SA2 8PP
Wales
UK

Email: d.benton@swansea.ac.uk

Chapter 5
H. Mackenzie and T. Dean*
School of Health Sciences and Social Work
University of Portsmouth
James Watson West
2 King Richard I Road
Portsmouth
Hampshire PO1 2FR
UK

Email: tara.dean@port.ac.uk

Chapter 6
E. J. Boyland* and J. C. G. Halford
Kissileff Laboratory for the Study of Human Ingestive Behaviour
School of Psychology
Eleanor Rathbone Building
Bedford Street South
University of Liverpool
Liverpool L69 7ZA
UK

Email: e.boyland@liverpool.ac.uk
j.c.g.halford@liverpool.ac.uk

Chapter 7
K. E. Williams
Feeding Program
Penn State Hershey Medical Center
Hershey
PA 17033
USA

Email: feedingprogram@hmc.psu.edu

Chapter 8
H. M. Hendy
Psychology Program
Penn State University, Schuylkill Campus
Schuylkill Haven
PA 17972
USA

Email: hl4@psu.edu

Chapter 9
R. Popper* and J. J. Kroll
Senior Vice President
Peryam and Kroll Research Corporation
3033 West Parker Road, Ste. 217
Plano, TX 75023
USA

Email: richard.popper@pk-research.com

Chapter 10
N. J. Patterson* and C. J. M. Beeren
Sensory and Consumer Science
Leatherhead Food Research
Randalls Road
Leatherhead KT22 7RY
UK

Email: npatterson@leatherheadfood.com
cbeeren@leatherheadfood.com

Chapter 11
Bryan Urbick
Consumer Knowledge Centre Ltd.
Middlesex House
29–45 High Street
Edgware
Middlesex HA8 7UJ
UK

Email: b.urbick@consumer-knowledge.com

Woodhead Publishing Series in Food Science, Technology and Nutrition

1 **Chilled foods: a comprehensive guide** *Edited by C. Dennis and M. Stringer*
2 **Yoghurt: science and technology** *A. Y. Tamime and R. K. Robinson*
3 **Food processing technology: principles and practice** *P. J. Fellows*
4 **Bender's dictionary of nutrition and food technology Sixth edition** *D. A. Bender*
5 **Determination of veterinary residues in food** *Edited by N. T. Crosby*
6 **Food contaminants: sources and surveillance** *Edited by C. Creaser and R. Purchase*
7 **Nitrates and nitrites in food and water** *Edited by M. J. Hill*
8 **Pesticide chemistry and bioscience: the food-environment challenge** *Edited by G. T. Brooks and T. Roberts*
9 **Pesticides: developments, impacts and controls** *Edited by G. A. Best and A. D. Ruthven*
10 **Dietary fibre: chemical and biological aspects** *Edited by D. A. T. Southgate, K. W. Waldron, I. T. Johnson and G. R. Fenwick*
11 **Vitamins and minerals in health and nutrition** *M. Tolonen*
12 **Technology of biscuits, crackers and cookies Second edition** *D. Manley*
13 **Instrumentation and sensors for the food industry** *Edited by E. Kress-Rogers*
14 **Food and cancer prevention: chemical and biological aspects** *Edited by K. W. Waldron, I. T. Johnson and G. R. Fenwick*
15 **Food colloids: proteins, lipids and polysaccharides** *Edited by E. Dickinson and B. Bergenstahl*

16 **Food emulsions and foams** *Edited by E. Dickinson*
17 **Maillard reactions in chemistry, food and health** *Edited by T. P. Labuza, V. Monnier, J. Baynes and J. O'Brien*
18 **The Maillard reaction in foods and medicine** *Edited by J. O'Brien, H. E. Nursten, M. J. Crabbe and J. M. Ames*
19 **Encapsulation and controlled release** *Edited by D. R. Karsa and R. A. Stephenson*
20 **Flavours and fragrances** *Edited by A. D. Swift*
21 **Feta and related cheeses** *Edited by A. Y. Tamime and R. K. Robinson*
22 **Biochemistry of milk products** *Edited by A. T. Andrews and J. R. Varley*
23 **Physical properties of foods and food processing systems** *M. J. Lewis*
24 **Food irradiation: a reference guide** *V. M. Wilkinson and G. Gould*
25 **Kent's technology of cereals: an introduction for students of food science and agriculture Fourth edition** *N. L. Kent and A. D. Evers*
26 **Biosensors for food analysis** *Edited by A. O. Scott*
27 **Separation processes in the food and biotechnology industries: principles and applications** *Edited by A. S. Grandison and M. J. Lewis*
28 **Handbook of indices of food quality and authenticity** *R. S. Singhal, P. K. Kulkarni and D. V. Rege*
29 **Principles and practices for the safe processing of foods** *D. A. Shapton and N. F. Shapton*
30 **Biscuit, cookie and cracker manufacturing manuals Volume 1: ingredients** *D. Manley*
31 **Biscuit, cookie and cracker manufacturing manuals Volume 2: biscuit doughs** *D. Manley*
32 **Biscuit, cookie and cracker manufacturing manuals Volume 3: biscuit dough piece forming** *D. Manley*
33 **Biscuit, cookie and cracker manufacturing manuals Volume 4: baking and cooling of biscuits** *D. Manley*
34 **Biscuit, cookie and cracker manufacturing manuals Volume 5: secondary processing in biscuit manufacturing** *D. Manley*
35 **Biscuit, cookie and cracker manufacturing manuals Volume 6: biscuit packaging and storage** *D. Manley*
36 **Practical dehydration Second edition** *M. Greensmith*
37 **Lawrie's meat science Sixth edition** *R. A. Lawrie*
38 **Yoghurt: science and technology Second edition** *A. Y Tamime and R. K. Robinson*
39 **New ingredients in food processing: biochemistry and agriculture** *G. Linden and D. Lorient*
40 **Benders' dictionary of nutrition and food technology Seventh edition** *D A Bender and A. E. Bender*

41 **Technology of biscuits, crackers and cookies Third edition** *D. Manley*
42 **Food processing technology: principles and practice Second edition** *P. J. Fellows*
43 **Managing frozen foods** *Edited by C. J. Kennedy*
44 **Handbook of hydrocolloids** *Edited by G. O. Phillips and P. A. Williams*
45 **Food labelling** *Edited by J. R. Blanchfield*
46 **Cereal biotechnology** *Edited by P. C. Morris and J. H. Bryce*
47 **Food intolerance and the food industry** *Edited by T. Dean*
48 **The stability and shelf-life of food** *Edited by D. Kilcast and P. Subramaniam*
49 **Functional foods: concept to product** *Edited by G. R. Gibson and C. M. Williams*
50 **Chilled foods: a comprehensive guide Second edition** *Edited by M. Stringer and C. Dennis*
51 **HACCP in the meat industry** *Edited by M. Brown*
52 **Biscuit, cracker and cookie recipes for the food industry** *D. Manley*
53 **Cereals processing technology** *Edited by G. Owens*
54 **Baking problems solved** *S. P. Cauvain and L. S. Young*
55 **Thermal technologies in food processing** *Edited by P. Richardson*
56 **Frying: improving quality** *Edited by J. B. Rossell*
57 **Food chemical safety Volume 1: contaminants** *Edited by D. Watson*
58 **Making the most of HACCP: learning from others' experience** *Edited by T. Mayes and S. Mortimore*
59 **Food process modelling** *Edited by L. M. M. Tijskens, M. L. A. T. M. Hertog and B. M. Nicolaï*
60 **EU food law: a practical guide** *Edited by K. Goodburn*
61 **Extrusion cooking: technologies and applications** *Edited by R. Guy*
62 **Auditing in the food industry: from safety and quality to environmental and other audits** *Edited by M. Dillon and C. Griffith*
63 **Handbook of herbs and spices Volume 1** *Edited by K. V. Peter*
64 **Food product development: maximising success** *M. Earle, R. Earle and A. Anderson*
65 **Instrumentation and sensors for the food industry Second edition** *Edited by E. Kress-Rogers and C. J. B. Brimelow*
66 **Food chemical safety Volume 2: additives** *Edited by D. Watson*
67 **Fruit and vegetable biotechnology** *Edited by V. Valpuesta*
68 **Foodborne pathogens: hazards, risk analysis and control** *Edited by C. de W. Blackburn and P. J. McClure*
69 **Meat refrigeration** *S. J. James and C. James*
70 **Lockhart and Wiseman's crop husbandry Eighth edition** *H. J. S. Finch, A. M. Samuel and G. P. F. Lane*

101 **Poultry meat processing and quality** *Edited by G. Mead*
102 **Functional foods, ageing and degenerative disease** *Edited by C. Remacle and B. Reusens*
103 **Mycotoxins in food: detection and control** *Edited by N. Magan and M. Olsen*
104 **Improving the thermal processing of foods** *Edited by P. Richardson*
105 **Pesticide, veterinary and other residues in food** *Edited by D. Watson*
106 **Starch in food: structure, functions and applications** *Edited by A-C Eliasson*
107 **Functional foods, cardiovascular disease and diabetes** *Edited by A. Arnoldi*
108 **Brewing: science and practice** *D. E. Briggs, P. A. Brookes, R. Stevens and C. A. Boulton*
109 **Using cereal science and technology for the benefit of consumers: proceedings of the 12th International ICC Cereal and Bread Congress, 24–26th May, 2004, Harrogate, UK** *Edited by S. P. Cauvain, L. S. Young and S. Salmon*
110 **Improving the safety of fresh meat** *Edited by J. Sofos*
111 **Understanding pathogen behaviour in food: virulence, stress response and resistance** *Edited by M. Griffiths*
112 **The microwave processing of foods** *Edited by H. Schubert and M. Regier*
113 **Food safety control in the poultry industry** *Edited by G. Mead*
114 **Improving the safety of fresh fruit and vegetables** *Edited by W. Jongen*
115 **Food, diet and obesity** *Edited by D. Mela*
116 **Handbook of hygiene control in the food industry** *Edited by H. L. M. Lelieveld, M. A. Mostert and J. Holah*
117 **Detecting allergens in food** *Edited by S. Koppelman and S. Hefle*
118 **Improving the fat content of foods** *Edited by C. Williams and J. Buttriss*
119 **Improving traceability in food processing and distribution** *Edited by I. Smith and A. Furness*
120 **Flavour in food** *Edited by A. Voilley and P. Etievant*
121 **The Chorleywood bread process** *S. P. Cauvain and L. S. Young*
122 **Food spoilage microorganisms** *Edited by C. de W. Blackburn*
123 **Emerging foodborne pathogens** *Edited by Y. Motarjemi and M. Adams*
124 **Benders' dictionary of nutrition and food technology Eighth edition** *D. A. Bender*
125 **Optimising sweet taste in foods** *Edited by W. J. Spillane*
126 **Brewing: new technologies** *Edited by C. Bamforth*
127 **Handbook of herbs and spices Volume 3** *Edited by K. V. Peter*

154 **Delivery and controlled release of bioactives in foods and nutraceuticals** *Edited by N. Garti*
155 **Fruit and vegetable flavour: recent advances and future prospects** *Edited by B. Brückner and S. G. Wyllie*
156 **Food fortification and supplementation: technological, safety and regulatory aspects** *Edited by P. Berry Ottaway*
157 **Improving the health-promoting properties of fruit and vegetable products** *Edited by F. A. Tomás-Barberán and M. I. Gil*
158 **Improving seafood products for the consumer** *Edited by T. Børresen*
159 **In-pack processed foods: improving quality** *Edited by P. Richardson*
160 **Handbook of water and energy management in food processing** *Edited by J. Klemeš, R. Smith and J-K Kim*
161 **Environmentally compatible food packaging** *Edited by E. Chiellini*
162 **Improving farmed fish quality and safety** *Edited by Ø. Lie*
163 **Carbohydrate-active enzymes** *Edited by K-H Park*
164 **Chilled foods: a comprehensive guide Third edition** *Edited by M. Brown*
165 **Food for the ageing population** *Edited by M. M. Raats, C. P. G. M. de Groot and W. A Van Staveren*
166 **Improving the sensory and nutritional quality of fresh meat** *Edited by J. P. Kerry and D. A. Ledward*
167 **Shellfish safety and quality** *Edited by S. E. Shumway and G. E. Rodrick*
168 **Functional and speciality beverage technology** *Edited by P. Paquin*
169 **Functional foods: principles and technology** *M. Guo*
170 **Endocrine-disrupting chemicals in food** *Edited by I. Shaw*
171 **Meals in science and practice: interdisciplinary research and business applications** *Edited by H. L. Meiselman*
172 **Food constituents and oral health: current status and future prospects** *Edited by M. Wilson*
173 **Handbook of hydrocolloids Second edition** *Edited by G. O. Phillips and P. A. Williams*
174 **Food processing technology: principles and practice Third edition** *P. J. Fellows*
175 **Science and technology of enrobed and filled chocolate, confectionery and bakery products** *Edited by G. Talbot*
176 **Foodborne pathogens: hazards, risk analysis and control Second edition** *Edited by C. de W. Blackburn and P. J. McClure*
177 **Designing functional foods: measuring and controlling food structure breakdown and absorption** *Edited by D. J. McClements and E. A. Decker*

223 **Lifetime nutritional influences on cognition, behaviour and psychiatric illness** *Edited by D. Benton*

224 **Food machinery for the production of cereal foods, snack foods and confectionery** *L-M. Cheng*

Preface

Whilst there are a large number of books available to the manufacturing and retail sectors on food product development in general, there are surprisingly very few covering the development of products for children and adolescents. This is a major oversight, especially in view of the increasing concerns regarding diet and nutrition in children and their potential impact on nutrition-related health issues in later life. For an obviously important and expanding food and drinks sector, this book aims to fill the gap.

There is undoubtedly a broad range of important factors that need to be borne in mind to maximise success in this sector. Many companies have failed in their development of products for children, as they have tended to apply the same principles as for standard product development and, in many cases have used adults to design and test the products. Children can be discerning and opinionated consumers and this means that one can so easily get it wrong. For example, targeting products to the right childhood age group is extremely difficult if the danger of patronising or alienating the target consumer is to be avoided.

This book covers three broad aspects in relation to developing children's food products – nutrition and health, children's food choices, and the design and testing of food and drink products for children.

Part I (*Pre-adult nutrition and health*) covers topical and important children's health issues such as nutritional requirements, fluid intake needs, diet and behaviour, and growing 20th century health problems such as childhood obesity and food allergies.

Part II (*Children's food choices*), covers food promotion and food choice in children and strategies that can be used to improve children's food choices both inside and outside of the home.

Finally, Part III (*Design of food and drink products for children*) covers the design of children's food products, with a focus on working with children and adolescents to design food and drink products and how best to undertake consumer and sensory testing with children. Case studies are given providing an insight into lessons learned from practical sensory and consumer testing experiences.

We have assembled a variety of expert international contributors from academia and industry to provide their excellent contributions. We hope that readers with an interest in the sector will find the book a valuable addition to the literature and are sure that it provides important insights that will assist the product developer to tackle this challenging market.

David Kilcast and Fiona Angus

Part I

Pre-adult nutrition and health

1

Children's dietary needs: nutrients, interactions and their role in health

L. R. Marotz, University of Kansas, USA

Abstract: Children's growth, development and health potentials are dependent on the nutrient quantity and quality of their diet. Insufficient intakes of macro- and micronutrients have deleterious, and in some cases permanent, effects on linear growth, early brain development, cognitive abilities and well-being. In contrast, children's over-consumption of calories, fats, sugars and salt is contributing to alarming increases in obesity, Type 2 diabetes, hypertension and elevated cholesterol, and is raising concerns about the nature of foods being consumed. Given the potential consequences, collaboration among researchers, healthcare professionals, policy makers and the food industry is critical to developing food products that address children's essential dietary and health needs.

Key words: nutrient requirements, dietary deficiencies, eating behaviors, eating characteristics, children's health, diet.

1.1 Introduction

Eating evokes a pleasurable response for most individuals. It provides an opportunity to enjoy favorite foods, experiment with new flavors and combinations, satisfy hunger and engage in social conversation with friends and family. Children's food preferences and eating behaviors are shaped by many of these same factors, but with one exception. Neophobic tendencies limit many children's willingness to try new foods, and cause them to resist items that are either alien or prepared in an unfamiliar manner. This propensity can result in the acceptance of only a few familiar comfort foods.

Consequently, families spend considerable time and effort trying to identify foods that will appeal to children's interests and taste buds. Similarly, manufacturers devote years of research to formulating new food products with unique flavor, color, shape and ingredient combinations in hopes of gaining children's attention and loyalty. Some products, such as functional foods, provide added value; others may offer improved aesthetic and sensory qualities or respond to new market opportunities. Yet, the single most overarching consideration in any of these deliberations should be whether a given food item or meal delivers the nutrients essential to support children's healthy growth and development.

1.2 Children's basic nutrient requirements: an overview of macro- and micronutrients

People often make food decisions without giving much serious thought to their personal nutrient needs or to the nutritive contribution of foods they have chosen. This approach may eventually result in nutrient intakes that are excessive in some areas, and/or deficient in others. It is particularly problematic when it comes to children, who are undergoing dramatic and rapid growth and developmental changes. Careful planning is necessary to ensure that children's diets include macro- and micronutrients in amounts sufficient to meet their nutritional needs, promote good health, and reduce the potential for debilitating diseases.

1.2.1 Macronutrients: protein, carbohydrates and fats

Proteins, carbohydrates and dietary fats are classified as macronutrients because the human body requires them in reasonably large amounts. They are also the only nutrients that supply caloric energy. Each macronutrient group fulfills specific physiological roles and is only able to perform these functions if nutrients are available in adequate amounts.

Daily macronutrient intake guidelines have been established in the United States (US) and the United Kingdom (UK) for food labeling purposes (Table 1.1). Food manufacturers in the US are mandated to provide nutrient information on product labels as a percent of Daily Values (DVs) based on a 2000 calorie intake for persons four years and older. The UK has established a similar system whereby food manufacturers voluntarily report the macronutrient contributions of food items as Guideline Daily Amounts (GDAs) on product packages. Information on calories, sugars, fat, saturates and salt are based on a 1800 daily caloric intake for children (5–10 years). Consumer response to this information has been favorable and has prompted food manufacturers in an increasing number of countries throughout the European Union to adopt the GDA format. Food manufacturers in the US have also begun to offer similar front-of-package nutrient information but guidelines for consistent reporting and use of authorized health claims are undergoing review. These

Table 1.1 Comparison of macronutrient values for food labeling purposes: US Daily Food Values and UK Guideline Daily Amounts

	Daily Values (DV)	Guideline Daily Amounts (GDA)
Calories	2000	1800
Total fat	65 g	70 g
Saturated fat	20 g	20 g
Cholesterol	300 mg	–
Sodium	2400 mg	1400 mg
Total carbohydrate	300 g	220 g
of which sugars	–	85 g
Fiber	25 g	15 g
Protein	50 g	24 g

initiatives have been motivated by increasing obesity rates and efforts to improve consumers' ability to make healthier food choices (CIAA, 2008).

Proteins

Proteins contribute four calories per gram and consist of amino acids, which serve as critical building materials for cellular growth and maintenance and as precursors in the production of biological chemicals such as enzymes, hormones and neurotransmitters. Twelve are considered non-essential because the body recovers and recycles various amino acid components from the proteins in cells that are being broken down. Ten amino acids are considered to be essential because they can only be obtained in sufficient amounts from food sources. Protein deficiencies among adults are relatively uncommon in most industrialized countries unless caloric intake is also inadequate. However, children's rapid growth requires a daily intake of approximately 1 gram of protein per kilogram of body weight daily, and thus places them at higher risk for deficiencies.

Proteins are found abundantly in animal- and many plant-based foods, although there are noteworthy differences in the quality of amino acids derived from each source. Animal products, such as meat, fish, eggs, milk and cheese, yield proteins that include all essential amino acids and are called complete proteins. Plant-based proteins, such as those found in legumes, grains, seeds, nuts and vegetables, typically are deficient in one or more of the essential amino acids, and thus are referred to as incomplete proteins. Each form offers distinct advantages and disadvantages for children. Animal-based foods yield high quality proteins that deliver all required amino acids in a relatively small serving size. However, these food sources also tend to be higher in calories, cholesterol, saturated fats and cost than incomplete proteins. Plant-based proteins are usually readily available, lower in calories and dietary fat, and less expensive to purchase. However, their main limitation in children's diets is that they must be consumed in fairly large quantities in order to obtain all of the essential amino acids.

Carbohydrates

Carbohydrates yield 4 calories per gram, serve as the body's main energy source, and are derived primarily from plant-based foods, such as grains, legumes, dried beans, fruits and vegetables. It is recommended that carbohydrates supply between 50 to 60% of a child's total daily calories or approximately 130 grams. Because foods that yield carbohydrates are relatively plentiful and inexpensive, they satisfy nearly 80% of human energy needs in many countries.

Carbohydrates are present in food as sugars, starches and dietary fiber. Simple sugars, such as glucose and fructose, are single-molecule monosaccharides that are quickly absorbed and their energy is available for immediate use. Two-molecule compounds called disaccharides must undergo digestion and conversion to glucose before their energy stores are in a form that can be utilized. Glucose in excess of a person's immediate energy needs is converted to glycogen and is stored in muscle and liver cells for future use.

Starches are complex, multi-molecule polysaccharides that are reduced to simple glucose during digestion. When glucose enters the blood stream, the pancreas responds by releasing insulin to facilitate its transport to the liver and conversion to glycogen. Complex carbohydrates are found primarily in whole grains, vegetables and fruits. International guidelines recommend that children consume at least 6 ounces of grain, 2½ cups of vegetables and 1½ cups of fruit daily.

Fiber, an indigestible form of carbohydrate, plays an important role in promoting digestive health and waste elimination. Studies have also established a positive relationship between dietary fiber intake and reduced serum cholesterol levels, as well as lowered risk of certain diseases and conditions, including Type 2 diabetes, colon cancer, diverticulitis, heart disease and obesity (Anderson *et al.*, 2009a,b). International guidelines recommend that children older than two years consume between 19–25 grams of fiber daily.

Fats

Fats comprise a third macronutrient group, which includes phospholipids, triglycerides and sterols. Fats supply a rich energy source, and are responsible for transporting fat-soluble vitamins, maintaining body temperature and forming a protective layer around vital organs. Dietary fats also enhance the texture, richness, and satiety of foods, and thus improve their appeal. Each fat gram supplies 9 calories, more than twice the number in proteins or carbohydrates, which can be an important consideration when trying to meet young children's high energy needs. However, US and UK dietary guidelines suggest that no more than 25 to 35% of a child's daily calories should be derived from fats.

Fats are categorized as being either saturated or unsaturated, depending on their chemical composition. Saturated fats are found primarily in animal products, are solid at room temperature and are often associated with increased health risks, including cardiovascular disease and some cancers

(Lucenteforte *et al.*, 2010; Siri-Tarino *et al.*, 2010). Two exceptions are: fish which contain healthy omega 3 unsaturated fatty acids; and plant-based tropical oils (coconut and palm) which have more saturated fat than do most animal products. Unsaturated fats, such as canola, corn and olive, are plant-based oils which are typically liquid at room temperature and have been shown to have positive health effects. Unfortunately, the food industry discovered hydrogenation, a process that transforms liquid vegetable oils into a solid or semi-solid form to create products such as soft and stick margarines. Hydrogenation eliminates the health benefits associated with unsaturated fat consumption by creating trans fats which the human body recognizes and treats as saturated (Micha and Mozaffarian, 2009; Kummerow, 2009). Food manufacturers have begun to show some response to public demands and those of the scientific community calling for the elimination of trans fats in food processing.

1.2.2 Micronutrients: water, vitamins and minerals

Children's growth, development and well-being also depend on adequate dietary intakes of vitamins, minerals and water (Benton, 2008). Micronutrients are responsible for transporting nutrients to cells, regulating essential body functions, and serving as catalysts for energy extraction and utilization (Table 1.2). Some micronutrients can be stored for future use while others must be consumed on a daily basis. Most micronutrients, with the exception of water, are required in quite small amounts.

Water

Water accounts for approximately 65–70% of children's total body weight. It aids in regulating body temperature and serves as a delivery system for transporting nutrients into cells, and removing cell wastes. Children and adolescents need to consume approximately 2 to 3 liters of water daily, due to a high turnover rate which gradually decreases with age (Raman *et al.*, 2004). Fruit, vegetables and beverages easily satisfy the body's basic water needs, although fluid absorption is reduced when beverages contain added sugars.

Vitamins and minerals

Most vitamins and minerals are required only in minute amounts, yet healthy and malnourished children alike are most often at risk for deficiencies (Table 1.3). Unlike macronutrients, vitamins and minerals do not contribute energy but are essential for the daily performance of almost every body function. Their absorption and utilization are improved by the presence of other nutrients in a food item. However, the same benefit is lacking when supplements are taken as substitutes for food sources.

Vitamins are necessary for healthy cell growth, division and maintenance, but they are not a structural component. Although individual vitamins each

Table 1.2 Common micronutrients: functions, deficiencies and food sources

	Function	Signs of deficiency	Food sources
Vitamins			
A	Regulates growth and maintenance of cells, bone, vision, reproductive and immune systems.	Night blindness, loss of visual acuity, skin infections and dryness, stunted growth, hair loss.	Fortified milk and dairy products, eggs, orange and dark green vegetables, orange colored fruits.
B_6	Involved in protein, amino acid, neuro-transmitter and hemoglobin synthesis.	Headache, nausea, stunted growth, tremor, and convulsions.	Fish, poultry, meats, green leafy vegetables, whole grains, nuts, seeds and fortified foods.
B_{12}	Synthesis of RNA, DNA and myelin, promotes blood formation, carbo-hydrate metabolism and healthy nervous system function.	Pernicious and macrocytic anemia, sores on mouth and tongue, nausea and vomiting.	Fish, meats and animal products, eggs, dairy products and milk, fortified foods.
C	Aids in calcium and iron absorption, collagen formation and wound healing. Converts folacin to folic acid.	Scurvy, joint pain, pin-point hemorrhages, bleeding gums, poor wound healing.	Peppers, citrus fruits, strawberries, mangoes, cauliflower, green leafy vegetables, watermelon.
D	Regulates absorption of calcium and phosphorus, promotes bone mineralization.	Rickets, bone deformities.	Oily fish, liver, egg yolk, fortified cereals and dairy products
Minerals			
Calcium	Serves as main com-ponent of teeth and bones, aids nerve transmission, regulates muscle contraction and maintains acid/base balance.	Bone fractures, muscle cramps, numbness and tingling in fingers, poor appetite, heartbeat irregularity.	Milk and dairy products, canned salmon, sardines, soybeans, tofu and leafy greens.
Iron	Involved in energy metabolism, component of neurotransmitters and hemoglobin, carries oxygen, maintenance of myelin.	Microcytic anemia, shortness of breath, pallor.	Red meats, oysters, whole grains, leafy green vegetables, dried fruits.
Zinc	Aids in hemoglobin production, energy metabolism, collagen formation, immune system function, cell growth and reproduction, and vitamin A utilization in the eye.	Stunted growth, skin infections, diarrhea, decreased immune system function, and night blindness due to poor vitamin A utilization.	Eggs, whole grains, legumes, seafood and meats.

Table 1.3 Comparison of US (DRI) and UK (RNI) recommendations for children's intake of select nutrients.

	Daily Reference Intake (DRI)		Reference Nutrient Intake (RNI)	
	4–8 years	9–13 years	4–6 years	7–10 years
Vitamin A	400 μg	600 μg	400 μg	500 μg
Vitamin B_6	0.6 mg	1.0 mg	0.9 mg	1.0 mg
Vitamin B_{12}	1.2 μg	1.8 μg	0.8 μg	1.0 μg
Vitamin C	25 mg	45 mg	30 mg	30 mg
Calcium	800 mg	1300 mg	450 mg	550 mg
Iron	10 mg	8 mg	6.1 mg	8.7 mg

assume a unique role in these processes, they typically work in combinations and seldom alone. Their chemical composition establishes whether they are fat- or water-soluble, which affects the way in which they are absorbed, utilized and excreted. For example, fat-soluble vitamins are found in animal-based foods and vegetable oils, are stored in the liver and fatty tissues, and can be toxic if consumed in large doses. Water-soluble vitamins are prevalent in fruits and vegetables, are absorbed directly into the bloodstream, and any excesses are excreted. They must be consumed daily or at least several times a week to maintain adequate levels because the body is unable to store water-soluble vitamins.

Minerals are inorganic compounds that the body utilizes in their original ingested form. They play a key role in maintaining fluid and electrolyte balance, regulating nerve and muscle fiber responses, and facilitating tooth and bone formation. Several minerals, particularly calcium and iron, are required in larger amounts, and thus are most likely to be deficient in children's diets because food sources rich in these minerals are limited and are not always appealing to children. Additionally, the body is relatively inefficient at absorbing these micronutrients which further increases the risk of deficiency. Other minerals, such as zinc, magnesium, and selenium, are required only in trace amounts and are easily obtained if a child's diet is adequate and varied.

No single food or food group is able to exclusively satisfy the body's basic needs for energy and essential nutrients. For this reason, young children must be introduced to, and have opportunities to taste, a wide variety of foods. Although children may resist initial attempts at dietary variety, their receptiveness will usually improve with repeated exposure and positive adult modeling.

1.3 Determinants of adequate nutrient intake in children

Dietary guidelines based on scientific findings and international recommendations have been established in most countries (Food and Agriculture Organization of the United Nations, 2009). These tools have proven beneficial for government-run nutrition programs and food manufacturers, but their application and functionality for ordinary citizens has sometimes been limited. Cultural and socioeconomic differences, lack of basic nutrition education, environmental challenges and detailed age- and gender-specific values often challenge a family's ability to translate nutrient information into healthy meals. However, government agencies have taken steps to convert basic nutrient information into applied behavioral guidelines that are meaningful for individuals and families: two such initiatives include the UK's '8 Tips for Eating Well' (Food Standards Agency) and the Dietary Guidelines for Americans (US Department of Health & Human Services, 2005). These dietary guidelines reflect what current science knows about the synergistic relationships that exist between food intake and personal health, especially as they relate to supporting children's continued growth, developmental advancement, absence of excessive illness or disease, and sufficient energy for play.

1.3.1 Growth and development

Growth and development occur at an accelerated pace during childhood and depend upon a diet adequate in calories and essential macro- and micronutrients. However, simply having access to food does not guarantee that children's basic nutrient needs will be met. Poor food choices and inactivity may contribute to nutrient deficiencies and weight variations, despite an intake of calories that is sufficient or even excessive. Thus, weight is not considered to be a reliable index of children's nutrient status because intermittent changes in appetite, level of physical activity and/or well-being may lead to temporary fluctuations. However, unexplained weight gains or losses are also not typical in children and should be evaluated by healthcare professionals to prevent interference with typical growth and development.

The long-term adequacy of a child's diet is most effectively measured by continuous gains in linear growth. Factors such as chronic illness, infection and/or malnutrition can disrupt this process and should be examined if a child's growth plateaus for more than a few months.

1.3.2 Absence of illness

A second indicator of adequate nutrient intake is the absence of excessive illness and disease, although caution must be exercised here because young children (under the age of 5–6 years) typically experience a greater incidence of acute and communicable infections than do older children. Immature development of children's immune and respiratory systems leaves them more susceptible to infectious conditions. However, the frequency and duration of communicable illness gradually decreases as children mature and begin developing antibodies to common pathogens. A healthful diet also plays a critical role in improving resilience and boosting immune system function.

1.3.3 Adequate energy

A third indication that children's dietary needs are being adequately met can be determined by their energy levels. By nature, children are curious, physically active and engaged in various forms of play during most of their waking hours. Lethargy is uncharacteristic and may be related to insufficient calories or micronutrients, often iron and B vitamins. Behavioral and cognitive problems, including excessive or undirected activity and inability to focus or concentrate, may also be related to poor diet and should be carefully investigated (Benton, 2008).

1.4 Developmental considerations in children's dietary needs

Many environmental factors, including food availability, family lifestyles, advertising, cultural and religious practices, socio-cultural preferences, eating context and peers, collectively shape children's food preferences and dietary patterns. In addition, children's eating behaviors reflect the skills and abilities typical of their developmental stage. Table 1.4 provides an overview of eating characteristics, but these behaviors are generalizations that may not always be consistent for all children of a given chronological age.

1.4.1 Preschool-age children

Preschoolers (4–5 years) are notorious for their limited interest in food and often finicky eating habits. In part, this behavior reflects a slower growth rate, which translates into a need for fewer calories and smaller food portions. Short attention spans make it difficult for children to sit quietly through a meal. Rudimentary self-feeding skills, which are still being perfected, can quickly become a source of frustration when foods prove difficult to maneuver or manipulate. When children become discouraged or are overly tired, they often resort to picking up food with their fingers. Choking is also quite common because foods tend to be chewed and swallowed quickly. Many preschool-age children display neophobic tendencies or a wariness of unfamiliar foods. However, it is important to continue introducing new foods and variety into children's diets, even if they are initially rejected, because lifelong attitudes regarding nutrition and health are being established (Marotz, 2012; Hill, 2002).

1.4.2 School-age children

School-age children (6–12 years) begin to assume a keen interest in foods, grocery shopping, meal preparation and eating. Preadolescent growth spurts and active play translate into increased hunger at mealtimes and demands

Table 1.4 Children's developmental eating behaviors

4-year-olds	have an unpredictable appetite; hungry then quickly uninterested maintain fairly strong food preferences use eating utensils with fair skill are interested in helping with meal preparation eat slowly and are easily distracted prefer small servings like milk (and soft textured foods).
5-year-olds	are more willing to try 'new foods' preferences are strongly influenced by peers and family members assist with meal preparation; help to make own lunch; spread bread, pour milk need some help pouring liquids and opening packages.
6-year-olds	have healthy appetite, but are not always able to finish larger servings are developing strong food preferences are willing to try some new foods but this behavior is unpredictable prefer finger foods have limited attention span and ability to focus on eating; lose interest if too much effort is required act quickly without thinking: may lead to spills.
7-year-olds	are willing to taste small amounts of unfamiliar foods use utensils well but still have some difficulty cutting with a knife are easily distracted while eating – by conversation, TV, telephone call have a strong desire to serve self and make own food selections.
8-year-olds	take interest in meals have fluctuations in appetite; boys often hungrier than girls open to tasting new foods – often curious and willing to try eat quickly so can resume activities; don't always chew thoroughly, overload their mouths.
9–10-year-olds	experience fluctuations in appetite related to growth and activity prefer to eat when hungry rather than at designated meal times have many favorite foods – pizza, French fries, cookies, but are open to trying others.
11–12-year-olds	always hungry, especially boys; high energy needs due to growth spurts are interested in trying new foods, especially if unfamiliar or what they see others eating make many independent food choices; may prepare own meals/snacks.
14–18-year-olds	are becoming aware of relationships between food, calories and weight gain/loss; concerns about body image may lead to eating disorders have periods of rapid growth which cause voracious appetite, especially among boys may have irregular and impulsive eating patterns due to busy schedules and time commitments know importance of consuming healthful diet but often disregard eat frequently between meals are highly susceptible to media influence.

for between-meal snacks. However, boredom can have the same effect for many children and should be carefully noted and addressed. Fruits, vegetables and combination dishes previously disliked may now become a source of curiosity and something worth trying. Food preferences and eating behaviors are frequently modeled after those of peers and family members. Television commercials and media advertisements also capture children's attention and exert a strong, persuasive influence on their food choices (Dorey, 2009).

1.4.3 Adolescents

Adolescence (14–18 years) is marked by dramatic physical and emotional transformations that alter children's nutrient needs and eating patterns. Rapid growth spurts once again increase the body's demand for calories, protein, vitamins, iron and calcium. Hormonal changes can trigger unpredictable mood swings and heightened concerns about weight, body image and athletic ability. More time is spent with friends and participating in school activities, which result in meals skipped or eaten away from home.

1.5 Children's dietary quality and its impact on well-being

Children's dietary patterns vary significantly throughout the world. While childhood obesity rates in many countries continue to climb at an alarming rate, there are also countless numbers of children who face serious energy and nutrient shortages (UNICEF, 2009: WHO, 2008a). Both realities demand the attention of policy makers, healthcare professionals and the food industry, as indisputable links continue to be established between children's nutrient intakes and their effects on survival, growth, development, health potential, and even injury prevention (Marotz, 2012).

1.5.1 Macronutrient deficiencies

Energy-related deficiencies

Energy balance is achieved when calories taken in are roughly equivalent to those required to sustain basic bodily functions and support physical activity, growth and development. Devastating, lifelong effects can result when food insecurities leave children deprived of sufficient energy and other essential nutrients (Kursmark and Weitzman, 2009). Innumerable childhood deaths are attributed to acute energy malnutrition each year (Christian, 2010). Furthermore, those children who survive are likely to experience brain development and cognitive deficits because of the severe protein shortages that often accompany energy-deficient diets.

Skipped meals, self-imposed calorie restriction, unhealthy choices or excessive participation in physical activity can also lead to energy deficiencies (Storey *et al.*, 2009; Lobera *et al.*, 2008). In some instances, debilitating diseases such as cancer, chronic kidney disease, HIV and unpleasant medication side-effects, may disrupt children's caloric intake (Greenbaum *et al.*, 2009; Houlston *et al.*, 2009). Prolonged energy shortages can lead to delayed menarche, menstrual dysfunction, muscle wasting, lowered resistance to illness and infection, reduced bone density and increased risk of injury (Akuyam, 2007; Heger *et al.*, 2008; Nguyen-Rodriguez *et al.*, 2009). Thus, early comprehensive assessment and individualized dietary interventions are essential to preventing serious complications from interfering with continued development.

Changes in dietary energy and nutrient intakes are also common as children mature and gain greater control over their eating behaviors. More foods are typically eaten away from home, and often include choices high in calories, sodium, sugar and fat, which can create a positive energy balance (Bleich and Pollack, 2010; Di Noia *et al.*, 2008). Over time, energy intake in excess of caloric need can lead to weight gain, obesity and health complications, including hypertension, Type 2 diabetes, cardiovascular changes, sleep apnea, shorter stature, depression and gallbladder disease (Mitchell *et al.*, 2009; Chiarelli and Marcovecchio, 2008; Salvadori *et al.*, 2008).

Global reports show a rising trajectory of childhood obesity in nearly every country (Akinbami and Ogden, 2009; Huang *et al.*, 2009; Ji and Cheng, 2009). Experts continue to search for causative factors and are examining everything from disparities in socio-economic position and environmental design to the lack of parent and nutrition education, abundance of processed and fast foods, genetic predisposition, media advertising and a steady decline in physical activity, in an effort to discover what may be fueling this epidemic (Bradford, 2009; Mitchell, *et al.*, 2009; Wilson *et al.*, 2009). It is becoming increasingly clear that childhood obesity is not the result of a single cause, but rather is a complex social problem that requires a multifaceted approach to treatment and prevention.

Inadequate protein

Optimal growth and development during childhood depend upon a diet that includes high-quality protein. However, feeding protein to children in excess of the Recommended Daily Intakes (RDIs) will not enhance their chances of growing beyond genetic potential. Protein overload can place additional stress on children's kidneys as they work to filter out metabolic by-products (urea and creatinine).

Protein deficiencies are often consistent with poverty and malnutrition, but may also accompany debilitating conditions, such as eating disorders, renal failure, cancer, congenital heart problems and some metabolic disorders in which caloric intake is compromised. Children who experience chronic food shortages are at greatest risk for developing protein-energy diseases, including marasmus and kwashiorkor.

Marasmus is the world's leading cause of childhood death and suffering (UNICEF, 2009). Chronic protein-energy malnutrition (PEM) gradually leads to severe weight loss, muscle wasting, stunted growth and development, anemia, electrolyte and fluid imbalance and decreased resistance to infectious diseases. Some physical impairments can be reversed successfully through the gradual reintroduction of fluids and high-protein foods. However, the negative effects of chronic malnutrition on children's brain development and stature are seldom entirely reversible (Benton, 2008; Kar *et al.*, 2008).

Similarly, Kwashiorkor is a disease caused by severe protein malnutrition that frequently occurs when infants are transitioning from breast milk to solid foods. At this time, their diets may be deficient in replacement protein, or consist of solid foods that have been over-diluted and thus provide insufficient protein. Manifestations of this disease include fluid retention with generalized edema and bloated abdomen, muscle wasting, changes in hair color and texture (brittle), appetite loss, diarrhea, skin lesions, increased susceptibility to infections, stunted growth and delayed development. Treatment involves a gradual reintroduction of fluids, proteins and carbohydrates to correct many of the physical complications associated with Kwashiorkor, but stunted growth is seldom reversible.

Although young children are the most frequent victims of protein-energy malnutrition, these diseases can strike at any age. Homelessness, drug and alcohol use, chronic diseases such as cancer, renal failure, tuberculosis, AIDS, and parasitic infections can also result in severe protein deficiencies (Campanozzi *et al.*, 2009; Wolff, 2008).

Carbohydrate intake

Carbohydrates are often perceived as undesirable dietary components, because they are thought to be fattening and the cause of such health problems as diabetes and childhood hyperactivity (Johnson *et al.*, 2009). However, no direct connections between carbohydrate ingestion and these conditions have been documented to date. Researchers have established that risks for dental caries and obesity are increased among children whose diets consist primarily of highly-refined sugars and grain products (Anderson *et al.*, 2009a; Roberts, 2008). Replacing poor quality foods with whole grains, legumes, fruits and vegetables not only reduces children's sugar intake but also contributes complex carbohydrates, vitamins, minerals, antioxidants and fiber that afford important health benefits.

1.5.2 Micronutrient deficiencies

Throughout the world, vitamin and mineral deficiencies affect millions of children, despite the fact that most micronutrients are required in very small amounts. Food shortages, costs and environmental concerns can impede children's access to micro-nutrient rich fruits, vegetables, legumes and animal products (Powell and Bao, 2009; Campbell *et al.*, 2008). As a result, children's diets may lack micronutrients, including vitamins A, B and C, calcium, iron, zinc and folic acid. Serious health consequences, including early death, disease, growth failure, delayed development and loss of productivity, are commonly associated with dietary intakes that repeatedly fail to meet recommended guidelines. A brief summary of the physiological functions, food sources and deficiencies associate with common at-risk vitamins and minerals is presented in Table 1.2.

Vitamins

Severe vitamin deficiencies are typically more prevalent in developing countries, but the incidence is increasing in some of the world's richest nations because of poverty, homelessness, food insecurity and poor nutritional management (Barrett, 2010; Valendia *et al.*, 2008). Protein shortages impair the body's ability to convert, transport and store vitamin A, and gradually result in a deficit that is the leading cause of childhood blindness in the world. Several groups, including the World Health Organization, have spear-headed initiatives to provide at-risk child populations with vitamin A supplements in an effort to eradicate night blindness and measles infections (WHO, 2009b).

Similar issues of malnutrition and accessibility are responsible for vitamin C and folic acid deficiencies in children. High costs involved in producing, transporting and distributing seasonal fruits and vegetables may prohibit families with limited incomes from purchasing these items (Mosdol *et al.*, 2008). Fruits and vegetables are also not a high priority on many children's lists of favorite foods, which further challenges efforts to meet vitamin C and folic acid recommendations. Similarly, vitamin B_{12} deficiencies in children are often attributed to cost, availability and preference. The lack of adequate refrigeration and prohibitive expense of meat, eggs and dairy products in many countries severely limit children's intake of this essential vitamin. Because B_{12} is found only in animal-based proteins, children who consume a diet that excludes or severely restricts these foods must be given vitamin supplements.

Reduced consumption of fortified dairy products and limited sun exposure are contributing to a resurgence of vitamin D deficiencies among children in many countries (Pearce and Cheetham, 2010; Ginde *et al.*, 2009; Huh and Gordon, 2008). Few unfortified food sources, with the exception of some fish species, provide vitamin D in amounts that adequately meet children's nutrient needs. Although the human body is able to synthesize vitamin D by converting UV rays absorbed through the skin, warnings to limit sun exposure and apply sun screen products have reduced the body's ability to complete this process. Additionally, children's steadily declining intake of dairy products has lowered calcium intake, which is also thought to exacerbate the problem. Consequently, it has been suggested that dairy products be fortified with even more vitamin D and that children, especially those with darker skin, be given daily supplements (Saintonge *et al.*, 2009; Holick and Chen, 2008).

Minerals

Mineral deficiencies are also increasing among children due, in part, to malnutrition and the widespread availability of low nutrient-dense food products. Children's current dietary patterns often fail to meet recommended guidelines for several important minerals, including calcium, iron and zinc, which are essential for healthy growth and development. Calcium intake has shown a steady decline as increasing numbers of soft drinks, energy beverages and fruit juices have been introduced into global markets (CDC, 2007; Storey *et al.*, 2004). Furthermore, Vitamin D deficiencies and sedentary behaviors compound this problem by interfering with calcium absorption, which leaves children at even greater risk of fractures, short stature and adult hypertension (McDevitt and Ahmed, 2010).

International studies have also revealed significant iron and zinc deficiencies among children who live in poverty and experience protein-energy malnutrition (Christian, 2010; WHO, 2008b). Food sources rich in both minerals include meats, dried beans, some nut varieties and fortified grains. However, the form of iron and zinc commonly found in plant-based foods is poorly absorbed by the body, and may leave children who follow a primarily vegetarian diet at higher risk for deficiencies. Some children who are iron deficient also develop iron-deficiency anemia which reduces the amount of oxygen their red blood cells are able to carry. Extreme fatigue, poor appetite and immune dysfunction increase children's vulnerability to HIV/AIDS, malaria, tuberculosis, and parasitic and intestinal infections, and can result in death. The consequences associated with zinc insufficiencies are similar. Strategies designed to improve children's intake of iron and zinc have been aimed at improving access to nutritional foods, fortification, and the administration of preventive supplements.

1.5.3 Childhood hypertension

Negative health effects are commonly associated with nutrient deficiencies, but excessive intakes of some nutrients have also proved to be harmful. For example, although sodium plays an integral role in several body functions, moderate to high intakes have been correlated with increased blood pressure and cardiovascular disease (Mohan and Campbell, 2009; He *et al.*, 2008). Most sodium is consumed in the form of sodium chloride (table salt), which is added to many processed and fast foods including canned vegetables, lunch meats, crackers, cereals and sport drinks. Lifestyle changes have led families to rely more heavily on foods prepared outside of the home, many of which are relatively high in salt and calories (Webster *et al.*, 2010; Ferrara *et al.*, 2008). Not only has this trend contributed to rising obesity rates but it is also being blamed for the increasing incidence and severity of hypertension in children.

1.5.4 Elevated cholesterol

Childhood obesity has quickly become one of the most significant global health concerns in recent decades (WHO, 2009a). Studies have shown that overweight children are often at higher risk for developing elevated blood cholesterol levels (Harel, 2010; Korsten-Reck *et al.*, 2008). Children over the age of two who consume a diet high in saturated and trans fats tend to have higher blood cholesterol levels than those who adhere to the recommended dietary guidelines. Fatty plaque deposits begin to accumulate in arterial walls, reducing blood flow, forcing the heart to pump harder, and placing the child at greater risk of developing atherosclerotic heart disease. The American Academy of Pediatrics (AAP) has issued guidelines recommending early identification and treatment of children with elevated cholesterol levels, especially if they have a family history of cardiovascular heart disease (Daniels *et al.*, 2008). Measures to improve children's dietary and physical activity patterns have demonstrated effective reductions in the potentially life-threatening risk factors associated with high blood cholesterol levels (McGill and McMahon, 2010; Keeton and Kennedy, 2009; WHO, 2009a).

1.6 Implications of children's nutrient requirements for the food industry, healthcare professionals and policy makers

Food insecurity and micronutrient deficiencies affect vast numbers of children and adults worldwide, not just those living in underdeveloped or developing nations. The recent economic downturn, unemployment, and increased homelessness have created a sharp increase in the number of children residing in industrialized countries who are currently suffering from food shortages and malnutrition. The consequences of this reality are disconcerting, given what we know about children's vulnerability to early nutrient deficiencies and their devastating outcomes.

What can we do to improve children's nutrient intake and ultimately their health? Supplementation initiatives have been effective in situations that required the rapid delivery of specific nutrients, such as vitamin A or calcium, but these programs have often proven difficult to sustain. Interventions based on food fortification represent another approach that has been employed by countries and food manufacturers to eliminate specific nutrient-related diseases such as pellagra, goiter, osteoporosis, and iron-deficiency anemia. This technique was initially developed to restore essential vitamins and minerals lost during commercial food processing and it remains an important method for delivering essential micronutrients to at-risk populations. However, fortification has gradually evolved into a method for enriching a product's nutrient quality beyond the value of its original ingredients in order to reduce documented micronutrient deficiencies among the general population. For example, US and Canadian laws passed in the 1990s require manufacturers to enrich grain flours with folic acid which, in turn, has led to significant declines in neural tube birth defects (Wolff *et al.*, 2009).

More recently, the food industry has taken fortification to new enrichment levels through the incorporation of everything from herbal and food supplements to probiotics, prebiotics, stanols, fiber and fish oils into their products. In essence, grocery stores are literally being turned into nutrient pharmacies: foods labels proclaim important health benefits and disease-reducing properties. However, regulation of health claims has lagged behind manufacturers' zealous efforts to attract consumer attention through prominent front-of-package displays (Enserink, 2010; Nestle and Ludwig, 2010). Their marketing success is clearly evidenced by increasing demands for these nutrient-spiked products, commonly known as neutraceuticals or functional foods, as consumers assume a more proactive role in managing their personal well-being and look to food for added health benefits (Grunert, 2010). In turn, manufacturers have responded by expanding their lines of fortified food products – and have improved their profit margins in the process.

The practice of enriching foods with specific vitamins and minerals is based upon years of solid scientific evidence. However, the speed at which foods are currently being fortified with newer additives is outpacing the availability of data necessary to validate manufacturers' claims. Health benefits cited on food products are often based on single-study results or outcomes that have been difficult to replicate. In addition, few definitive studies have specifically examined the effectiveness of herbal and food additives in children, or whether any contraindications are associated with their long-term use (Aggett, 2010). Little is known about the cumulative dose of food additives that may result when children ingest multiple food sources that have been fortified with the same vitamin, mineral or probiotic. To date, safe upper limits of most vitamins and minerals have not been established for children, so the risk of developing toxicities from functional foods is unknown. The increasing number of food additives and their widespread use may also place some children at greater risk for allergic responses – an especially important consideration given the prevalence of food allergies and intolerances among children and the limited disclosure of potential side effects associated with some food additives (Spanjersberg *et al.*, 2010; Branum and Lukacs, 2008).

Functional foods represent an emerging and significant market opportunity for the food industry. Parents today are more health conscious than in previous generations. They are better informed about the diet–health relationship and are interested in providing children with healthy food alternatives (Lazarou *et al.*, 2008). However, rigorous scientific studies involving children are needed to assure the safety of food additives and to protect consumers from false or unsubstantiated health claims.

Additionally, the global nature of crop production, manufacturing and food distribution requires that consistent legal definitions and regulatory policies governing food and drink products replace the highly variable collection of laws and standards that currently exist. Uniform international labeling standards are also needed to aid consumers in making informed decisions about the foods they purchase. The combined implementation of these two measures would also improve efficiency for food manufacturers and enhance consumer access to important nutrient information.

Collaboration among health professionals, scientists, policy makers and members of the food industry is essential if the goal of providing children and families with safe, healthy food is to be achieved. Cooperative efforts are also needed to increase educational initiatives that strengthen families' nutrition knowledge, address diverse food interests and eating patterns, and reinforce an understanding of the critical role that a healthful diet plays in promoting children's health.

1.7 Future trends

Undoubtedly, food manufacturers, distributors, and retailers wish they could discover what the future direction or next 'hot' item will be in children's food products. Changes in lifestyle, economics, diversity, health awareness, and product advertising will continue to have a significant impact on families' food choices and, ultimately, on new food product development, marketing and distribution. Environmental concerns are also likely to elicit major changes in everything from crop production and sustainability to green product packaging. New scientific discoveries may reveal health-promoting nutrients of which we are not yet aware, and possibly determine how foods can be altered to assist in the fight against certain diseases.

It is not certain what effect these factors will have on shaping the future development of new foods and food products. However, several emerging trends are likely to serve as driving forces and realize predictions that consumers will increasingly demand foods and beverages that:

- are unadulterated and incorporate more natural and organic ingredients, such as colorings, flavorings and nutrients that provide health benefits;
- are produced under the highest food safety standards;
- have significantly less sodium and fewer sodium compounds;
- eliminate trans fats, and replace animal fats (saturated) and tropical oils with healthier plant derivatives;
- have reduced sugar content;
- are smaller in portion size to address increasing obesity rates;
- offer nutrient value, not just empty calories;
- are labeled consistently from country to country;
- include health claims on food product labels and in advertising that are backed by reliable scientific evidence;
- offer convenience, can be eaten out-of-hand, and require minimal preparation;

- include additional soluble and insoluble fibers which may improve cholesterol levels and satiety;
- reflect greater cultural, ethnic and religious diversity in product options; and
- deliver quality for the money.

Families expect the food industry to act in a socially responsible fashion by responding to their demands for food items that are healthier, safer and environmentally friendly. In return, the food industry has a pivotal opportunity to improve sales by developing and marketing healthy food products that address children's nutrient requirements and support their well-being.

1.8 Sources of further information and advice

Additional resource information can be found on the following web sites:

American Dietetic Association

www.eatright.org

Includes publications, position papers and international news.

British Nutrition Foundation

www.nutrition.org.uk

Provides resource information on healthy eating, food labeling, nutrient-related diseases, food allergies, health claims and contemporary developments.

European Food Information Council (EUFIC)

www.eufic.org

Disseminates science-based information about nutrition, food safety, food technology, and European Union initiatives.

Food Standards Agency

www.food.gov.uk

Provides information ranging from basic nutrition and healthy eating to food production regulations, labeling guidelines, and research developments, pertinent to the unique interests of consumers and the food industry.

International Food Information Council

www.ific.org

Offers extensive resources on health, nutrition and safety, including links, newsletters and videos.

The Food Institute

www.foodinstitute.com/

Provides international news of interest to food industry personnel, including research, health studies, food regulations and market reports.

United States Department of Agriculture Economic Research Service

www.ers.usda.gov

Includes extensive research and international trade information, an overview of government supported food programs, food policies and regulation, publications and statistical data.

United States Food & Drug Administration
International organizations and Foreign Government Agencies
www.fda.gov/InternationalPrograms/Agreements/ucm131179.htm
Live links to regulatory agencies responsible for overseeing food production and distribution are provided country-by-country.

1.9 References

Aggett, PJ (2010), 'Toxicity due to excess and deficiency', *Journal of Toxicology and Environmental Health*, Part A, Vol. 73, Nos 2 & 3, pp. 175–80.

Akinbami, LJ and Ogden, CL (2009), 'Childhood overweight prevalence in the United States: The impact of parent-reported height and weight', *Obesity*, Vol. 17, No. 8, pp. 1574–80.

Akuyam, SA (2007), 'A review of some metabolic changes in protein-energy malnutrition', *The Nigerian Postgraduate Medical Journal*, Vol. 14, No. 2, pp. 155–62.

Anderson, CA, Curzon, ME, Van Loveren, C, Tatsi, C and Duggal, MS (2009a), 'Sucrose and dental caries: A review of the evidence', *Obesity Reviews*, Vol. 10, No. 1, pp. 41–54.

Anderson, JW, Baird, P, Davis, RH Jr, Ferreri, S, Knudtson, M, Koraym, A, Waters, V and Williams, CL (2009b), 'Health benefits of dietary fiber', *Nutrition Reviews*, Vol. 67, No. 4, pp. 188–205.

Barrett, CB (2010), 'Measuring food insecurity', *Science*, Vol. 327, No. 5967, pp. 825–28.

Benton, D (2008), 'The influence of children's diet on their cognition and behavior', *European Journal of Nutrition*, Vol. 47, No. 3, pp. 25–37.

Bleich, SN and Pollack KM (2010), 'The public's understanding of daily caloric recommendations and their perceptions of calorie posting in chain restaurants', *BMC Public Health*, Vol.10, pp. 121–31.

Bradford, NF (2009), 'Overweight and obesity in children and adolescents', *Primary Care*, Vol. 36, No. 2, pp. 319–39.

Branum, AM and Lukacs, SL (2008), Food allergy among US children: Trends in prevalence and hospitalizations', *NCHS Data Brief,* No. 10, Oct., pp. 1–8.

Campanozzi, A, Russo, M, Catucci, A, Rutigliano, I, Canestrino, G, Giardino, I, Romondia, A and Pettoello-Mantovani, M (2009), 'Hospital-acquired malnutrition in children with mild clinical conditions', *Nutrition*, Vol. 25, No. 5, pp. 540–47.

Campbell, AA, Thorne-Lyman, A, Sun, K, de Pee, S, Kraemer, K, Moench-Pfanner, R, Sari, M, Akhter, N, Bloem, MW and Semba, RD (2008), 'Greater household expenditures on fruits and vegetables but not animal source foods are associated with decreased risk of under-five child mortality among families in rural Indonesia', *Journal of Nutrition*, Vol. 138, No. 11, pp. 2244–49.

Centers for Disease Control and Prevention (CDC) (2007), 'Youth risk behavior surveillance – United States, 2007', *Morbidity and Mortality Weekly Report 2008*, Vol. 57, No. SS-4. pp. 1–31. Accessed on 31 July at http://www.cdc.gov/HealthyYouth/yrbs/pdf/yrbss07_mmwr.pdf.

Chiarelli, F and Marcovecchio, ML (2008), 'Insulin resistance and obesity in childhood', *European Journal of Endocrinology*, Vol. 159, Suppl 1, pp. S67–74.

Christian, P (2010), 'Impact of the economic crisis and increase in food prices on child mortality: Exploring nutritional pathways', *Journal of Nutrition*, Vol. 140, No. 1, pp. 177S–181S.

Confederation of the Food and Drink Industries of the EU (CIAA) (2008), 'GDA nutrition labels gaining ground throughout Europe, survey shows'. Accessed on 11 April, 2010 at http://www.ciaa.be/asp/documents/detailed_doc.asp?doc_id=848.

Daniels, SR, Greer, FR and The Committee on Nutrition (2008), 'Lipid screening and cardiovascular health in childhood', *Pediatrics*, Vol. 122, No. 1, pp. 198–208.

Di Noia, J, Schinke, SP and Contento, IR (2008), 'Dietary fat intake among urban, African American adolescents', *Eating Behavior*, Vol. 9, No. 2, pp. 251–56.

Dorey, E (2009), 'The role of media in influencing children's nutritional perceptions', *Qualitative Health Research*, Vol. 19, No. 5, pp. 645–54.

Enserink, M (2010), 'European food watchdog slashes dubious health claims', *Science*, Vol. 327, No. 5970, pp. 1189.

Ferrara, LA, Pacioni, D, Vitolo, G, Staiano, L, Riccio, E and Gaetano, G (2008), 'Fast food versus slow food and hypertension control', *Current Hypertension Reviews*, Vol. 4, No. 1, pp. 30–5.

Food and Agriculture Organization of the United Nations (2009), 'Food guidelines by country'. Accessed on 5 August (2009) at http://www.fao.org/ag/humannutrition/nutritioneducation/fbdg/en/.

Food Standards Agency, ' *Eat well, be well – 8 tips for eating well'*, accessed on 11 April, 2010 at http://www.eatwell.gov.uk/healthydiet/eighttipssection.

Ginde. AA, Liu. MC and Camargo. CA (2009), 'Demographic differences and trends of vitamin D insufficiency in the US population, 1988–2004', *Archives of Internal Medicine*, Vol. 169, No. 6, pp. 626–32.

Greenbaum, LA, Warady, BA and Furth, SL (2009), 'Current advances in chronic kidney disease in children: Growth, cardiovascular, and neurocognitive risk factors', *Seminars in Nephrology*, Vol. 29, No. 4, pp. 425–34.

Grunert, KG (2010), 'European consumers' acceptance of functional foods', *Annals of the New York Academy of Sciences*, Vol. 1190, pp. 166–73.

Harel, Z (2010), 'Isolated low HDL cholesterol emerges as the most common lipid abnormality among obese adolescents', *Clinical Pediatrics*, Vol. 49, No. 1, pp. 29–34.

He, FJ, Marrero, NM and Macgregor, GA (2008), 'Salt and blood pressure in children and adolescents', *Journal of Human Hypertension*, Vol. 22, pp. 4–11.

Heger, S, Körner, A, Meigen, C, Gausche, R, Keller, A, Keller, E, and Kiess, W (2008), 'Impact of weight status on the onset and parameters of puberty: Analysis of three representative cohorts from central Europe', *Journal of Pediatric Endocrinology and Metabolism,* Vol., 21, No. 9, pp. 865–77.

Hill, A (2002), 'Developmental issues in attitudes to food and diet', *Proceedings of the Nutrition Society'*, Vol. 61, pp. 259–66.

Holick, MF and Chen, TC (2008), 'Vitamin D deficiency: A worldwide problem with health consequences', *American Journal of Clinical Nutrition*, Vol. 87, No. 4, pp. 1080S–86S.

Houlston, A, Buttery, E, and Powell, B (2009), 'Cook to order: Meeting the nutritional needs of children with cancer in hospital', *Paediatric Nursing*, Vol. 21, No. 4, pp. 25–7.

Huang, RC, Stanley, FJ and Beilin, LJ (2009), 'Childhood obesity in Australia remains a widespread health concern that warrants population-wide prevention programs', *The Medical Journal of Australia,* Vol. 191, No. 1, pp. 45–57.

Huh, SY and Gordon, CM (2008), 'Vitamin D deficiency in children and adolescents: Epidemiology, impact and treatment', *Reviews in Endocrine and Metabolic Disorders*, Vol. 9, No. 2, pp. 161–70.

Ji, CY and Cheng, TO (2009), 'Epidemic increase in overweight and obesity in Chinese children from 1985 to 2005', *International Journal of Cardiology*, Vol. 132, No. 1, pp. 1–10.

Johnson, RJ, Perez-Pozo, SE, Sautin, YY, Manitius, J, Sanchez-Lozada, LG, Feig, DL, Shafiu, M, Segal, M, Glassock, RJ, Shimada, M, Roncal, C and Nakagawa, T (2009),

'Hypothesis: Could excessive fructose intake and uric acid cause Type 2 diabetes?', *Endocrine Review*, Vol. 30, No. 1, pp. 96–116.

Kar, BR, Rao, SL and Chandramouli, BA (2008), 'Cognitive development in children with chronic protein energy malnutrition, *Behavior and Brain Functions*, Vol. 24, No. 4, pp. 31–6.

Keeton, VF and Kennedy, C (2009), 'Update on physical activity including special needs populations', *Current Opinions in Pediatrics*, Vol. 21, No. 2, pp. 262–68.

Korsten-Reck, U, Kromeyer-Hauschild, K, Korsten, K, Baumstark, MW, Dickhuth, HH and Berg, A (2008), 'Frequency of secondary dyslipidemia in obese children', *Vascular Health Risk Management*, Vol. 4, No. 5, pp. 1089–94.

Kummerow, FA (2009), 'The negative effects of hydrogenated trans fats and what to do about them', *Atherosclerosis*, Vol. 205, No. 2, pp. 458–65.

Kursmark, M and Weitzman, M (2009), 'Recent findings concerning childhood food insecurity', *Current Opinion in Clinical Nutrition and Metabolic Care*, Vol. 12, No. 3, pp. 310–16.

Lazarou, C, Kalavana, T and Matalas, AL (2008), 'The influence of parents' dietary beliefs and behaviours on children's dietary beliefs and behaviours: The CYKIDS study', *Appetite*, Vol. 51, No. 3, pp. 690–96.

Lobera, IJ, Humanes, SE and Fernández, MJ (2008), 'Physical activity, eating behavior, and pathology', *Archicos Latinoamericanos de Nutriticion,* Vol. 58, No. 3, pp. 280–85.

Lucenteforte, E, Talamini, R, Bosetti, C, Polesel, J, Franceschi, S, Serraino, D, Negri, E and LaVecchia, C (2010), 'Macronutrients, fatty acids, cholesterol and pancreatic cancer', *European Journal of Cancer*, Vol. 46, No. 3, pp. 581–87.

Marotz, L (2012), *Health, Safety and Nutrition for the Young Child*, 8th edn, Wadsworth Cengage Learning, Belmont, CA.

McDevitt, H and Ahmed, SF (2010), 'Establishing good bone health in children', *Paediatrics and Child Health*, Vol. 20, No. 2, pp. 83–7.

McGill, HC and McMahon, CA (2010), 'Starting early to control all risk factors in order to prevent coronary heart disease', *Clinical Lipidology*, Vol. 5, No. 1, pp. 87–93.

Micha, R and Mozaffarian, D (2009), 'Trans fatty acids: Effects on metabolic syndrome, heart disease and diabetes', *Nature Review: Endocrinology*, Vol. 5, No. 6, pp. 335–44.

Mitchell, JA, Mattocks, C, Ness, AR, Leary, SD, Pate, RR, Dowda, M, Blair, SN and Riddoch, C (2009), 'Sedentary behavior and obesity in a large cohort of children', *Obesity*, Vol. 17, No. 8, pp. 1596–602.

Mohan, S and Campbell, NR (2009), 'Salt and high blood pressure', *Clinical Science*, Vol. 117, No. 1, pp. 1–11.

Mosdol, A, Erens, B and Brunner, EJ (2008), 'Estimated prevalence and predictors of vitamin C deficiency within UK's low-income population', *Journal of Public Health*, Vol. 30, No. 4, pp. 456–60.

Nestle, M and Ludwig, D (2010), 'Front-of-package food labels: Public health or propaganda?', *JAMA*, Vol. 303, No. 8, pp. 771–72.

Nguyen-Rodriguez, ST, Unger, JB and Spruijt-Metz, D (2009), 'Psychological determinants of emotional eating in adolescence', *Eating Disorders*, Vol. 17, No. 3, pp. 211–24.

Pearce, S and Cheetham, T (2010), 'Diagnosis and management of vitamin D deficiency', *British Medical Journal*, Vol. 340, pp. 140–47.

Powell, LM and Bao, Y (2009), 'Food prices, access to food outlets and child weight', *Economics and Human Biology*, Vol. 7, No. 1, pp. 64–72.

Raman, A, Schoeller, DA, Subar, AF, Troiano, RP, Schatzkin, A, Harris, T, Bauer, D, Bingham, SA, Everhart, JE, Newman, AB, and Tylavsky, FA (2004), 'Water turnover in 458 American adults 40–79 yr of age', *American Journal of Physiology: Renal Physiology*, Vol. 286, pp. 394–401.

Roberts, MW (2008), 'Dental health of children: Where we are today and remaining challenges', *Journal of Clinical Pediatric Dentistry*, Vol. 32, No. 3, pp. 231–34.

Saintonge, S, Bang, H and Gerber, LM (2009), 'Implications of a new definition of vitamin D deficiency in a multiracial US adolescent population: The National Health and Nutrition Examination Survey III, *Pediatrics*, Vol. 123, No. 3, pp. 797–803.

Salvadori, M, Sontrop, JM, Garg, AX, Truong, J, Suri, RS, Mahmud, FH, Macnab, JJ and Clark, WF (2008), 'Elevated blood pressure in relation to overweight and obesity among children in a rural Canadian community', *Pediatrics*, Vol. 122, No. 4, pp. e821–27.

Siri-Tarino, P, Sun, Q, Hu, F and Krauss, R (2010), 'Saturated fat, carbohydrate, and cardiovascular disease', *American Journal of Clinical Nutrition*, Vol. 91, No. 3, pp. 502–9.

Spanjersberg, MQ, Knulst, AC, Kruizinga, AG, Van Duijn, G, and Houben, GF (2010), 'Concentrations of undeclared allergens in food products can reach levels that are relevant for public health', *Food Additives and Contaminants: Part A*, Vol. 27, No. 2, pp. 169–74.

Storey, KE, Hanning, RM, Lambraki, IA, Driezen, P, Fraser, SN and McCargar, LJ (2009), 'Determinants of diet quality among Canadian adolescents', *Canadian Journal of Dietary Practice and Research,* Vol. 70, No. 2, pp. 58–65.

Storey, ML, Forshee, RA and Anderson, PA (2004), 'Associations of adequate intake of calcium with diet, beverage consumption, and demographic characteristics among children and adolescents', *Journal of the American College of Nutrition,* Vol. 23, No. 1, pp. 18–33.

UNICEF (2009), *The State of the World's Children 2009*. Accessed on 15 July 2009 at http://www.unicef.org/sowc09/report/report.php.

US Department of Health and Human Services (2005), '*Dietary Guidelines for Americans*'. Accessed on 11 April, 2010 at http://www.health.gov/dietaryguidelines.

Valendia, B, Centor, RM, McConnell, V and Shah, M (2008), 'Scurvy is still present in developed countries', *Journal of General Internal Medicine*, Vol. 23, No. 8, pp. 1281–84.

Webster, JL, Dunford, EK and Neal, BC (2010), 'A systematic survey of the sodium contents of processed foods', *American Journal of Clinical Nutrition*, Vol. 91, No. 2, pp. 413–20.

Wilson, TA, Adolph, AL, and Butte, NF (2009), 'Nutrient adequacy and diet quality in non-overweight and overweight Hispanic children of low socioeconomic status: The Viva la Familia Study', *Journal of the American Dietetic Association*, Vol. 109, No. 6, pp. 1012–21.

Wolff, H (2008), 'Homelessness and malnutrition', *International Journal of Public Health*, Vol. 53, No. 1, pp. 7–8.

Wolff, T, Witkop, CT, Miller, T and Syed, SB (2009), 'Folic acid supplementation for the prevention of neural tube defects: An update of the evidence for the US Preventive Services Task Force', *Annals of Internal Medicine*, Vol. 150, No. 9, pp. 632–39.

World Health Organization (WHO) (2009a), *Obesity and Overweight*, accessed on 31 July 2009 at http://www.who.int/dietphysicalactivity/publications/facts/obesity/en/.

World Health Organization (WHO) (2009b), *WHO Global Database on Vitamin A Deficiency*, accessed on 18 July 2009 at http://www.who.int/vmnis/vitamina/en/.

World Health Organization (WHO) (2008a), *The State of Food Insecurity in the World 2008*, accessed on 15 July 2009 at http://www.fao.org/docrep/011/i0291e/i0291e00.htm.

World Health Organization (WHO) (2008b), *Worldwide Prevalence of Anaemia 1993–2005,* accessed on 1 August 2009 at http://www.whqlibdoc.who.int/publications/2008/9789241596657_eng.pdf.

2

Fluids and children's health

R. Muckelbauer, L. Libuda and M. Kersting, University of Bonn, Germany

Abstract: This chapter discusses the influence of beverage consumption on children's health and reveals opportunities to improve drinking habits. It first reviews the effect of total fluid intake and the consumption of the quantitatively and qualitatively most important beverages in the diet of children and adolescents, i.e. water, sugar-containing beverages, and milk, on several health conditions. The chapter then gives the typical beverage intake for children and adolescents in Germany and gives recommendations and implications for the food industry, healthcare professionals and policy makers according to each beverage category.

Key words: beverage consumption, sugar-containing beverages, milk, water, child health.

2.1 Introduction

Beverages are a considerable part of diet with respect to energy (Nielsen and Popkin, 2004; Storey *et al.*, 2006) and nutrient intake (Marshall *et al.*, 2005) and they are a main source to meet water requirements (Table 2.1). Furthermore, beverage consumption influences diet quality in children (Subar *et al.*, 1998) and seems to be associated with various health conditions. For example, milk is the main contributor of calcium intake in children (Subar *et al.*, 1998) and therefore, the observed replacement of milk by sugar-containing beverages is a concern in child nutrition (Marshall *et al.*, 2005; Nielsen and Popkin, 2004). The intake of sugar-containing beverages including soft drinks and juices has increased in children and adolescents (Nielsen and Popkin, 2004) and is linked to weight gain and obesity in children and adolescents (Vartanian *et al.*, 2007).

Table 2.1 Recommendations for water intake in German-speaking countries supplied by beverages, solid foods, and oxidation water. Data from Deutsche Gesellschaft für Ernährung *et al.* (2000)

Age group of children and adolescents	Water supplied by		Oxidation water	Total water intake[2]
	beverages (mL/day)	solid foods[1] (mL/day)	(mL/day)	(mL/day)
1 to under 4 y	820	350	130	1300
4 to under 7 y	940	480	180	1600
7 to under 10 y	970	600	230	1800
10 to under 13 y	1170	710	270	2150
13 to under 15 y	1330	810	310	2450
15 to under 19 y	1530	920	350	2800

[1] Water in solid food about 79 mL/MJ
[2] Including water from oxidation, beverages, and food; equating to 290 mL/MJ in younger children, 250 mL/MJ in older children and adolescents.

2.1.1 Physiological water requirements

Water is quantitatively the most important nutrient in human nutrition (Manz *et al.*, 2002). Water is essential for a number of physiological functions such as nutrient and oxygen transport, the maintenance of a constant body temperature, and urinary excretion of metabolic waste products (Kleiner, 1999). Due to permanent water losses (urine, respiratory and faecal water losses, sweat, and insensible losses), a constant water intake is required to sustain the balance of body water (Sawka *et al.*, 2005). Children's and adults' water needs should be met by water intake from beverages, water from solid foods, and water from the metabolism of macronutrients. Beverages represent the main source of water (Table 2.1).

With the exception of only a few countries, water requirements are often neglected in dietary recommendations (Manz and Wentz, 2005a). The US-American Food and Nutrition Board of the Institute of Medicine (IOM) defined an adequate intake (AI) for total water intake which is derived from the usual intake in apparently healthy people instead of an exact estimated average requirement (EAR) (Food and Nutrition Board, 2004). Recommendations for water intake in German-speaking countries are also based on valuations (Deutsche Gesellschaft für Ernährung *et al.*, 2000). However, fluid requirements vary widely among individuals and populations, and depend on physical activity and climate, which affect water losses due to perspiration. Individual water needs can be multiplied by physical activity and heat through increasing sweat losses (Sawka *et al.*, 2005). Therefore, recommendations of total water intake should be understood as values of orientation.

Children are at particular risk for water imbalances as their body surface per unit body weight is larger, and their percentage of body water and their body water turnover is higher in comparison to adults (Manz, 2007).

Consequences of acute water imbalances range from thirst and headache to impaired physical and cognitive performance and vertigo (Food and Nutrition Board, 2004; Kleiner, 1999). Severe water losses can cause lethal acute kidney failure. However, there is increasing evidence that already a chronic mild dehydration might be associated with a number of morbidities such as urolithiasis, constipation, and exercise asthma (Manz amd Wentz, 2005b).

In infants, the consumption of human milk or formula meets total water needs. In contrast, older infants and children need additional water from beverages. Results from fluid balance studies showed that daily water needs increase from 0.6 L/day to 1.7 L/day in childhood (Sawka *et al.*, 2005). From adolescence onwards, water needs of boys are higher in comparison to girls due to a higher total body water content resulting from a higher lean body mass. Lean body mass consists of 73% water. In contrast, the water content of fat mass is only 10% (Sawka *et al.*, 2005).

Under normal conditions, thirst is an adequate indicator to achieve a constant hydration status (Sawka *et al.*, 2005). Additionally, euhydration can be achieved over a large range of water intake by adaptation of urine osmolality and urinary water losses (Food and Nutrition Board, 2004). However, this ability of adaptation is limited in children, especially in the younger age groups. Results from urine osmolality analyses in healthy German children showed that the usual water intake of school-aged children is about 1 cup (240 mL) too low to reach euhydration (Manz *et al.*, 2002). Therefore, children in Germany, and probably in other populations with similar dietary behaviour and lifestyle, might be at particular risk of suffering from inadequate water intake, with the consequence of acute or chronic mild dehydration. Results from other European countries on children's hydration status are rare. A comparison of the results from these studies showed a slightly lower mean 24 hour urine osmolality in children from France and Switzerland, indicating a marginally better hydration in comparison to German children (Manz and Wentz, 2003). However, these results also showed that the hydration status in children from other European countries, e.g. Poland, might be substantially better (Manz and Wentz, 2003).

2.1.2 Water as a beverage

The main characteristic of water as a beverage is that water is free of energy, which is of particular importance regarding the worldwide rising trend of childhood overweight and obesity (Lobstein *et al.*, 2004). In Germany, tap water is the best and most regularly controlled food available (Grimm, 2002) and, together with mineral water, is the recommended beverage for children to meet their daily fluid needs (Kersting *et al.*, 2005). Also, according to food-based guidelines of other European countries such as Hungary or Portugal, water is the recommended beverage in a healthy diet (Food and Agriculture Organization of the United Nations, 2009). Since the quality of drinking water varies within Europe (European Environment Agency *et al.*, 2002), recommendation of drinking water, mineral water or boiled water depends on the country.

Water and the prevention of overweight

An increased water consumption may support a healthy body weight status primarily by decreasing energy intake if it displaces sugar-containing beverages. Beside this compensating effect on the energy balance, there are other supposed mechanisms of water consumption that may prevent overweight. Although in the general population its widely believed that the plentiful consumption of water can support weight loss in self-management of overweight, the few studies investigating this effect have shown ambiguous results (Negoianu and Goldfarb, 2008). The postulated effect is that water ingestion might suppress hunger and thereby reduce energy intake. In fact, the intake of two glasses of water concurrently with a meal increased subjective satiety during this meal but this effect was not maintained after the meal (Lappalainen *et al.*, 1993). Other studies do not support an influence of water ingestion before or with a meal on the energy intake during the subsequent meal in adults (Flood *et al.*, 2006; Rolls *et al.*, 1990).

Another potential mechanism of water consumption on weight regulation is the thermogenic effect induced by the ingestion of pure water, independently of water temperature. In adults, the ingestion of 500 mL of water increased the energy expenditure by about 60 kJ (Boschmann *et al.*, 2003, 2007). However, this effect could not be found in other studies (Brown *et al.*, 2006) and no such study has been carried out with children. In conclusion, there is surprisingly little data to clarify the potential role of water consumption in the reduction of the overweight epidemic in adults (Negoianu and Goldfarb, 2008) and even less is known about any effects in children.

A large controlled trial found the preventive effect of an intervention that promoted water consumption in school children on the risk of overweight (Muckelbauer *et al.*, 2009b). The intervention resulted in increased water consumption whereas reduction in sugar-containing beverages was not observed in the intervention group. This may indicate a beneficial effect of water consumption independently of the reduction in other caloric beverages.

Water and mineral intake

Water as a beverage is also a dietary source of essential micro-nutrients. The mineral content of water varies qualitatively and quantitatively within wide ranges between the different water types and origins. In Germany, mineral water contains more Na, Ca, and Mg and less Zn and Cu than tap water (Grimm, 2002; Heseker, 2001). Despite these differences, water is generally a minor contributor to the mineral intake, i.e. of Ca and Mg (Heseker, 2001), because the main sources in a children's well balanced diet are solid foods (Kersting *et al.*, 2005). Although certain mineral waters may be useful as partial providers of essential minerals, the World Health Organisation (WHO) is unaware of any convincing evidence to support the beneficial effects of consuming such mineral waters. Therefore, the WHO does not recommend minimum concentrations of micro-nutrients in drinking water (World Health Organisation, 2000).

2.1.3 Sugar-containing beverages

Sugar-containing beverages such as regular soft drinks and fruit juices predominantly consist of water and sugar (Table 2.2). In contrast to regular soft drinks, the term 'low-energy soft drink' includes only sugar-free soft drinks (US Department of Agriculture *et al.*, 1999). While there is a European directive for fruit juices (European Council, 2002), there is no uniform definition of soft drinks as a beverage group, but country-specific regulations (Deutsches Lebensmittelbuch, 2003; Österreichisches Lebensmittelbuch, 2008). In Germany, soft drinks are a heterogeneous group of carbonated and uncarbonated beverages such as fruit drinks, lemonades and soda pop (Deutsches Lebensmittelbuch, 2003). According to the definition from the USDA, only carbonated beverages belong to the group of soft drinks (US Department of Agriculture et al., 1999). These different definitions make a comparison of the results from studies on the health effects of soft drinks difficult.

Body weight

Due to the energy content of sugar-containing beverages (Table 2.2) and their popularity, especially in children, their consumption is a matter of interest. There is increasing evidence, that energy intake from beverage consumption is not fully compensated by a reduction of energy intake from solid foods (Bachman *et al.*, 2006; DiMeglio and Mattes, 2000; Mattes, 1996). This incomplete compensation might rely on a weaker satiation effect of beverages in comparison to solid foods, due to a faster gastrointestinal passage (Mattes, 2006). Accordingly, consumption of sugar-containing beverages might be

Table 2.2 Content of energy and macro-nutrients in categories of milk and sugar-containing beverages per 100 g

	Regular milk (3.5% fat)[1]	Fat reduced milk (1.5% fat)[1]	Chocolate milk[2]	Apple juice[1]	Regular soft drinks[1]
Energy (kJ)	272	201	264	203	185
Water (g)	87	89	85	88	90
Carbohydrates (g)	4.7	4.8	8	11	11
Protein (g)	3.4	3.4	3.6	0.1	0
Fat (g)	3.6	1.6	1.8	0	0

[1] Data from Souci *et al.* (2008)
[2] With 5 g instant cocoa powder per 100 ml fat reduced milk (1.5% fat) according to food-based dietary guidelines for children and adolescents (Forschungsinstitut für Kinderernährung, 2008)

associated with increasing total energy intake and energy imbalances, which might lead to overweight in the long-term.

A number of studies that were predominantly conducted in the USA analysed the association between overweight in children and consumption of sugar-containing beverages and regular soft drinks in particular. Results from these studies are not univocal, but point to a causal link between soft drink consumption and weight gain in total (Malik *et al.*, 2006). However, these results might not be transferable to European children and adolescents due to differences in dietary pattern, lifestyle, and the composition of these beverages. In contrast to European soft drinks, which include sucrose as added sugar (Malik *et al.*, 2006), US-American soft drinks contain High Fructose Corn Syrup (HFCS) (Bray *et al.*, 2004). Due to the supposed high content of free fructose which is metabolised independently from insulin, HFCS-sweetened soft drinks might have a unique impact on body weight.

In fact, consumption of fructose-sweetened drinks was associated with higher weight gain than consumption of sucrose-sweetened drinks in an animal study (Jurgens *et al.*, 2005). However, a recent study in Germany observed an association between consumption of sugar-containing beverages without HFCS and body weight in girls (Libuda *et al.*, 2008b). At this time, it is not clear whether US-American soft drinks act more adipogenically than European soft drinks.

Diet quality

Regular soft drinks usually have a low micronutrient content. There is evidence that regular soft drinks displace nutrient-dense foods such as milk in the diet of children and adolescents (Vartanian *et al.*, 2007). Accordingly, consumption of soft drinks was associated with lower intake of micronutrients such as calcium and folate in German children (Libuda *et al.*, 2009). Such an impaired diet quality is undesirable for the prevention of later, diet-related diseases such as osteoporosis and cardiovascular diseases. Findings from a study in German children and adolescents indicate a stronger diluting effect on diet quality in girls than in boys (Libuda *et al.*, 2009). Since mean diet quality was found to decrease with age in girls, high soft drink consumption might be a cause for concern in adolescent girls in particular.

Bone health

Results from various studies suggest that consumption of soft drinks affects bone parameters such as bone mineral density. Gender specific effects are controversial (Libuda *et al.*, 2008a; McGartland *et al.*, 2003; Whiting *et al.*, 2004). The mechanism of this potential bone catabolic effect of soft drinks is also not fully understood. A commonly suggested pathway is the displacement of milk, which is one of the main sources of calcium in children (Fitzpatrick and Heaney, 2003; Heaney and Rafferty, 2001). However, several studies observed that the association between soft drink consumption and bone parameters remained significant even after consideration of milk consumption (Libuda *et al.*, 2008a; McGartland *et al.*, 2003). Another potential mechanism might rely on the observed negative association between soft drink consumption and protein intake in children and adolescents, since protein showed an anabolic effect on children's bone (Libuda *et al.*, 2008a).

Caffeine-containing beverages

Specific ingredients of caffeinated soft drinks such as caffeine and phosphoric acid might have direct effects on bone. In caffeinated soft drinks, phosphoric acid is used as acidifier. In contrast to citric acid, which is added in uncaffeinated soft drinks and is metabolically oxidized to bicarbonate and water, phosphoric acid in caffeinated soft drinks theoretically increases the dietary acid load (Remer *et al.*, 2003). However, in a recent prospective cohort study, the effect of caffeinated soft drinks on children's bone remained significant even after adjustment for dietary acid load (Libuda *et al.*, 2008a). An experimental study also observed no effect of the acidulant type (phosphoric acid vs. citric acid) on calciuria (Heaney and Rafferty, 2001). Therefore, dietary acid load does not seem to explain the effect of caffeinated soft drinks.

Results from studies that analysed the influence of caffeine on bone are conflicting. An excess calciuria that is known to cause bone losses in long-term was observed after consumption of caffeinated soft drinks, but not after consumption of uncaffeinated soft drinks (Heaney and Rafferty, 2001). Additionally, the consumption of caffeinated soft drinks affected bone parameters in children and adolescents that were not affected by uncaffeinated soft drinks (Libuda *et al.*, 2008a). However, two other studies found no direct effect of self-reported caffeine consumption on bone parameters (Conlisk and Galuska, 2000; Wetmore *et al.*, 2008). Additionally, in a double-blind study, caffeine showed either no or only minor effects on parameters of calcium economy (Barger-Lux *et al.*, 1990). The authors suggested that moderate caffeine intake is not a risk factor for osteoporosis in women with adequate calcium intake. Despite these conflicting results on the effect of caffeinated soft drinks on bone status, their consumption has to be classified as unfavourable for children and adolescents due to their undisputed effect on the central nervous system.

2.1.4 Milk

Milk, and its influence on various health outcomes, is still under discussion, and research is going on. Despite its fat content, the high density in milk of numerous essential nutrients leads to dietary recommendation and guidelines for the daily consumption of milk and milk products by children (Dixey *et al.*, 1999; Kersting *et al.*, 2005).

Milk is known to be an important source of calcium intake as it provides together with dairy products from a third to about a half of children's calcium intake in Germany (Kersting *et al.*, 2005; Kersting and Bergmann, 2008; Mensink *et al.*, 2007a) and other countries (Moynihan *et al.*, 1996; Subar *et al.*, 1998). An adequate intake of calcium in childhood, and especially in adolescence, supports the skeletal growth and is one condition to prevent the later development of osteoporosis (Nicklas, 2003; NIH, 2001).

Furthermore, milk is a main contributor to the protein and phosphorus intake in children (Kersting *et al.*, 2005; Mensink *et al.*, 2007a). Dairy products are also an important source for the dietary iodine intake in adults (Haug *et al.*, 2007; Jahreis *et al.*, 2001) and in children (Als *et al.*, 2003; Jahreis, 2005; Kersting *et al.*, 2005). It is noteworthy that the iodine content in milk can vary substantially as it depends highly on the cow feeds (Als *et al.*, 2003; Haug *et al.*, 2007). Its contribution to the iodine intake in children has increased significantly during the last decade in Germany (Remer *et al.*, 2006) due to raised iodine contents of cow's milk. Formerly, milk was claimed to have a negative impact on the blood lipid profile, weight gain, and coronary heart diseases due to its fat content and composition (Aggett *et al.*, 1994; Berkey *et al.*, 2005). Today, it is evident that milk has no negative effect on health if consumed moderately (Haug *et al.*, 2007). Moreover, milk components as calcium, bioactive peptides of the whey fraction, unsaturated fatty acids, conjugated linoleic acid, and phospholipides are supposed to have beneficial health effects, e.g. by controlling the blood lipid profile, lipid oxidation and lipolysis, blood pressure, and carcinogenesis (Haug *et al.*, 2007; Zemel and Miller, 2004).

Some observational studies in children and adolescents showed an inverse association between dairy products and obesity whereas others did not, and no intervention study has demonstrated an effect on body weight status yet (Huang and McCrory, 2005). Therefore, the potential role of dairy products in the prevention of obesity in children still remains unproven and is controversially discussed (Barba and Russo, 2006; Huang and McCrory, 2005; Nicklas, 2003).

In conclusion, milk is a nutrient-rich food item and can help to achieve the recommended intake of many nutrients. Furthermore, several milk components may have beneficial effects on health. However, milk is not a recommended beverage to cover fluid requirements in children due to its energy content compared to water, and some children have to moderate or modify milk consumption due to intolerance.

2.2 Typical beverage intake in children: data and trends from Germany

The beverage types consumed by children and adolescents depend strongly on the age. In the first four to six months of a child's life, breast milk should be the exclusive diet as it provides the optimal balance between fluid intake and osmolar load that the child can cope with. Modern formula is the alternative for breast milk, but it is not completely equal as it has a higher osmolar load. In the complementary feeding period, starting in month 4 to 6, water requirements are still met by milk and foods. Around the end of the first year of life, infants need additional water, preferably in the form of plain water (Kersting, 2001).

2.2.1 Water as a beverage

Among German children and adolescents, mineral and drinking water have become the predominantly consumed beverages and their proportion has increased in the last two decades in all childhood age groups (Sichert-Hellert *et al.*, 2001). On average, 45% to 51% of the total beverage intake (excluding milk) comes from water, depending on sex and age, in a recent nationwide dietary survey among children and adolescents aged 6 to 17 years (Mensink *et al.*, 2007a). About half of all children and adolescents consume mineral water at least once a day and about one third to a fourth depending on sex and age consume tap water daily (Fig. 2.1).

2.2.2 Sugar-containing beverages

The second most-consumed beverages in children up to the age of 12 years are juices, accounting for 27% of the total beverage intake, followed by soft drinks (19%). In adolescence, the proportion of juice is lower than in childhood, accounting for about 20%. In contrast, soft drinks contribute, at 25%, an increasing part to the total beverage intake in male adolescents but not in female (17%). Generally, boys drink soft drinks more often than girls, with an increasing gap in adolescence as shown in Fig. 2.1 (Mensink *et al.*, 2007b). Time trends observed in a German cohort showed a slight

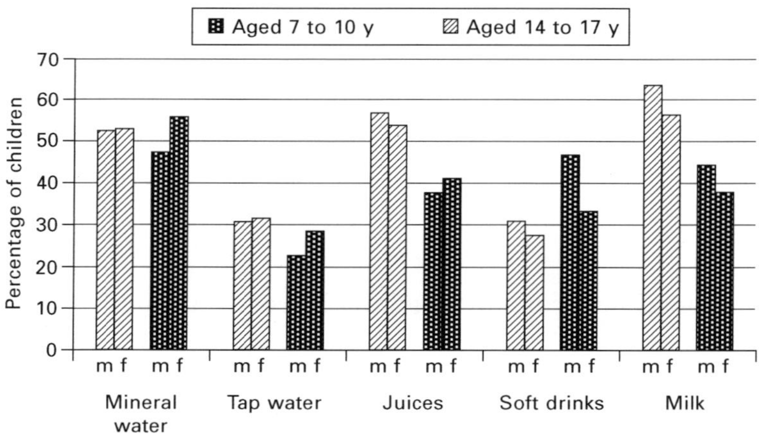

Fig. 2.1 Percentage of male (m) and female (f) children (7 to 10 years) and adolescents (14 to 17 years) with at least daily consumption of different beverage categories (data modified from Mensink *et al.*, 2007b).

decrease in soft drink consumption between 1985 and 1999 and, conversely, an increase in juice consumption (Sichert-Hellert *et al.*, 2001).

2.2.3 Milk

About 60% of children aged 3 to 10 years drink milk daily (Mensink *et al.*, 2007b), but the proportion decreases with age (Mensink *et al.*, 2007b) to about 44% in male and 38% in female adolescents (Fig. 2.1). The median milk consumption per day (including milk with flavoured powder) among male adolescents was 225 mL/day and among females 153 mL/day (Mensink *et al.*, 2007a). Adding dairy products, such as yoghurt, to the milk consumption, the total median consumption was about 250 g in children aged 6 to 11 years. That is much lower than the recommended intake of 400 g for this age group (Forschungsinstitut für Kinderernährung, 2008). In contrast, young children in Belgium had a higher consumption of milk and dairy products (excluding cheese), ranging between 470 and 540 mL/day (Huybrechts *et al.*, 2008), but according to the national food-based dietary guidelines, a proportion of 50 to 70%, depending on age and sex, did not reach the recommended daily amount of 500 mL. With increasing age, the consumption of milk products decreased in Belgian children (Huybrechts *et al.*, 2008). Similarly, total daily intake of milk and milk products in male German adolescents aged 12 to 17 years is about 300 g (240 g in females), whereas the recommended amount is from 420 to 500 g depending on age (420 to 450 g in females). This milk consumption in children and adolescents, lower than the recommendations, may result from a trend of decreased milk consumption observed during recent decades in Germany (Sichert-Hellert *et al.*, 2001) and in the USA (Bachman *et al.*, 2006). Nevertheless, in children older than 4 years, this reduction in milk consumption was compensated for by other milk products, but not in children aged 1 to 3 years (Alexy and Kersting, 2003). A beneficial trend according to dietary recommendations (Aggett *et al.*, 1994; Kersting *et al.*, 2005) is the increased percentage of fat-reduced milk products to nearly 25% of all milk and milk products (Alexy and Kersting, 2003). This time trend of decreased consumption of whole milk and its replacement by low-fat milk was also observed in Spanish children and adolescents (Ribas-Barba *et al.*, 2007).

2.2.4 Other beverages

Tea is a minor contributor to daily total beverage intake in children and adolescents, with a proportion between 5% and 8% (Mensink *et al.*, 2007a). Children younger than 12 years rarely drink coffee and still among adolescents coffee accounts for less than 2% of the total beverage intake. Alcoholic drink contribution to total beverage intake is rising in adolescence, especially from the age of 15 years, reaching an average proportion lower than 5% (Mensink *et al.*, 2007a).

2.3 Implications of typical beverage intake in children for food industry, healthcare professionals and policy makers

2.3.1 Water as a beverage

Although the trend of total fluid intake in children is promising, many children are mildly dehydrated. Therefore, children should drink, additionally, one glass of fluid per day, preferably water, as this is the recommended beverage to meet the fluid needs of children and adolescents from transition from infant diet to family diet around the age of 1 year. Water is a widely-consumed beverage in children but is less attractive to them than sugar-containing beverages. As a compromise, water can be mixed with fruit juice in a proportion water:juice larger than 2:1, to increase the attractiveness for children of drinking more. Nevertheless, children drink also plain water if it is available and it is not unattractive for them. Schools could provide free water access for children and introduce a policy of water as the preferred beverage, for example by environmental and educational interventions that have been proved to be feasible and effective in the school setting (Muckelbauer *et al.*, 2009a, b).

2.3.2 Soft drinks

Due to the effects of soft drinks on body weight and diet quality, their consumption should be restricted in children and adolescents. The recommendation for an upper limit of all sweets, to which soft drinks belong, is 10% of total energy intake in the German food-based dietary guidelines for children and adolescents. This is in line with recommendations from other countries as the upper limit for extrinsic sugars is 11% of total energy in the Dietary Reference Values for the UK. Popkin *et al.* (2006) suggested a drinking pattern for the US population that provides 10% of total energy intake from beverages. To diminish the effect of soft drinks upon weight gain and obesity, a reduction in their energy content might be feasible. Along with the decreasing energy content, the reasonable consumption of these beverages in absolute amounts would increase.

Multiple fortification of high-sugar products with micronutrients should be avoided. The fortification of single critical vitamins might moderate the diluting effect on diet quality but upper intake levels should be considered. Caffeinated soft drinks are not suitable for children and adolescents due to their effect on the central nervous system. Since sensory tests showed that caffeine in common concentrations does not play a major role in the flavour of soft drinks (Griffiths and Vernotica, 2000; Keast and Riddell, 2007), its application in the production of soft drinks is redundant.

2.3.3 Fruit juices

Fruit juices are nutrient-rich beverages. Their consumption in moderate amounts might be a strategy to meet the recommendations for daily fruit consumption in children and adolescents. However, due to the supposed effect on body weight, the consumption of fruit juice should be restricted to one glass per day for displacing one portion of fruit. Because of the high micronutrient and fibre content of the fruit paring, the consumption of fruits as a solid food should be generally preferred. Similar considerations are applicable to the recently introduced beverage category 'smoothies', which contain fruit juices and chunks of fruit.

2.3.4 Milk

The trend towards a decrease in the consumption of milk among children and adolescents is worrying because milk is a food item of a high nutrient density. Today, the recommended intake of milk and dairy products is not reached by a considerable proportion (around 60%) of German children and adolescents, and this gap increases with increasing age (Kersting and Bergmann, 2008). A possibility to enhance the attractiveness of milk consumption can be by flavouring with instant cocoa or other sugared powder. Mixed with milk in a proportion of about 5% powder, as suggested within a recommended diet (Forschungsinstitut für Kinderernährung, 2008), energy and carbohydrate content increases but is still within an acceptable range (Table 2.2). The recommended milk for children and adolescents is fat reduced milk with a fat-content of about 1.5%. Tests with pupils showed that the majority did not taste a difference between fat reduced milk and unskimmed milk (Forschungsinstitut für Kinderernährung, 2008). Skim milk with 0.3% fat is not recommended for children and adolescents due to the low content of fat-soluble vitamin A and D.

A general desire to increase milk consumption among the entire child and adolescent population is not appropriate, but should be addressed to the group of low-consumers of milk. Individual nutritional consulting with simple anamneses can identify concerned children. In the public health context, schools are an ideal setting for programmes, e.g. supported by European Community funds and tailored to age groups.

2.4 Future trends

2.4.1 Declaration of energy, nutrients, and portion sizes

With the background of the epidemic dimension of childhood overweight and obesity, the most important information that should be labelled on beverages is the energy content. As beverages should be consumed abundantly to cover the fluid needs rather than contribute to other nutrient supply, those beverages with the lowest energy content are always to be preferred. Regarding milk, fat-reduced milk with 1.5% fat should be labelled as the recommended milk.

The European regulation (EWG) 90/496 and (EC) 1924/2006 on nutrition and health claims made on foods points to such a direction by regulation the information on food labels. However, there are substantial doubts that large proportions of the population would not use such information, particularly from lower socio-economic backgrounds and education levels, who are also known to have a less favourable diet. Although the composition in fat, carbohydrates and protein may have an influence on health, this can hardly be identified by the customer. Therefore, the emphasis should lay on the energy content, which is easier to interpret and facilitate a comparison between two products. Nevertheless, energy content can only be interpreted correctly in association with a portion size. This portion size should be defined and harmonized by the authorities to exclude a commercial interest. In this context, it is very important that for children and adolescents, portion sizes as well as the food amounts of the dietary guidelines strongly depend on age. Therefore, portion sizes used to indicate energy contents per serving sizes (as already applied on products) should be age-dependent.

2.4.2 Advertisement restrictions

Restrictions on the consumption of sugar-containing beverages in children and adolescents are thought to be one possibility to face the increasing obesity problem. A method to decrease the consumption of sugar-containing beverages might be the promotion of non-caloric beverages such as water, and making non-caloric beverages unrestrictedly available. Such an intervention has been shown to be effective in obesity prevention (Muckelbauer *et al.*, 2009b).

Another approach could be to decrease the access to sugar-sweetened beverages for children and adolescents, for example by removing vending machines from elementary schools as is done in some states in the USA. A further step could be the restriction of the advertisement of energy-dense foods, such as sugar-containing beverages. Currently, there is little evidence for a direct role of advertisement for energy-dense foods in the increasing obesity prevalence in children. However, there is strong evidence that food promotion affects children's food behaviour (Hastings *et al.*, 2003). Therefore, it is reasonable that advertisement of sugar-containing beverages increases the consumption of these beverages. Furthermore, children and adolescents in particular might be influenced by advertisements. Therefore, restraints of advertising might be a useful policy, at least to achieve a decrease in the consumption of sugar-containing beverages in children and adolescents.

2.5 Sources of further information and advice

www.aap.org/ American Academy of Pediatrics

www.espghan.med.up.pt (Committee on Nutrition. European Society of Pediatric Gastroenterology Hepatology, and Nutrition)

www.trinkfit-mach-mit.de. Information on the project: Prevention of overweight in school children through the promotion and provision of drinking water.
www.forum-trinkwasser.de/ Information on health benefits of drinking water.
www.who.org World Health Organisation.
www.fke-do.de Research Institute of Child Nutrition
www.efsa.eu.int European Food Safety Authority (EFSA)
www.usda.gov US Department of Agriculture

2.6 References

Aggett, P. J., Haschke, F., Heine, W., Hernell, O., Koletzko, B., Lafeber, H. *et al.* (1994). Committee report: Childhood diet and prevention of coronary heart disease. ESPGAN Committee on Nutrition. European Society of Pediatric Gastroenterology and Nutrition. *J Pediatr Gastroenterol Nutr, 19*(3), 261–269.

Alexy, U. and Kersting, M. (2003). Time trends in the consumption of dairy foods in German children and adolescents. *Eur J Clin Nutr, 57*(10), 1331–1337.

Als, C., Haldimann, M., Burgi, E., Donati, F., Gerber, H. and Zimmerli, B. (2003). Swiss pilot study of individual seasonal fluctuations of urinary iodine concentration over two years: Is age-dependency linked to the major source of dietary iodine? *Eur J Clin Nutr, 57*(5), 636–646.

Bachman, C. M., Baranowski, T. and Nicklas, T. A. (2006). Is there an association between sweetened beverages and adiposity? *Nutr Rev, 64*(4), 153–174.

Barba, G. and Russo, P. (2006). Dairy foods, dietary calcium and obesity: A short review of the evidence. *Nutr Metab Cardiovasc Dis, 16*(6), 445–451.

Barger-Lux, M. J., Heaney, R. P. and Stegman, M. R. (1990). Effects of moderate caffeine intake on the calcium economy of premenopausal women. *Am J Clin Nutr, 52*(4), 722–725.

Berkey, C. S., Rockett, H. R., Willett, W. C. and Colditz, G. A. (2005). Milk, dairy fat, dietary calcium, and weight gain: A longitudinal study of adolescents. *Arch Pediatr Adolesc Med, 159*(6), 543–550.

Boschmann, M., Steiniger, J., Franke, G., Birkenfeld, A. L., Luft, F. C. and Jordan, J. (2007). Water drinking induces thermogenesis through osmosensitive mechanisms. *J Clin Endocrinol Metab, 92*(8), 3334–3337.

Boschmann, M., Steiniger, J., Hille, U., Tank, J., Adams, F., Sharma, A. M. *et al.* (2003). Water-induced thermogenesis. *J Clin Endocrinol Metab, 88*(12), 6015–6019.

Bray, G. A., Nielsen, S. J. and Popkin, B. M. (2004). Consumption of high-fructose corn syrup in beverages may play a role in the epidemic of obesity. *Am J Clin Nutr, 79*(4), 537–543.

Brown, C. M., Dulloo, A. G. and Montani, J. P. (2006). Water-induced thermogenesis reconsidered: The effects of osmolality and water temperature on energy expenditure after drinking. *J Clin Endocrinol Metab, 91*(9), 3598–3602.

Conlisk, A. J. and Galuska, D. A. (2000). Is caffeine associated with bone mineral density in young adult women? *Prev Med, 31*(5), 562–568.

Deutsche Gesellschaft für Ernährung, Österreichische Gesellschaft für Ernährung, Schweizerische Gesellschaft für Ernährungsforschung, and Schweizerische Vereinigung für Ernährung. (2000). *Referenzwerte für die Nährstoffzufuhr* (Vol. 1. Auflage). Frankfurt am Main: Umschau/Braus.

Deutsches Lebensmittelbuch. (2003). *Leitsätze für Erfrischungsgetränke.*

DiMeglio, D. P. and Mattes, R. D. (2000). Liquid versus solid carbohydrate: Effects on food intake and body weight. *Int J Obes Relat Metab Disord, 24*(6), 794–800.

Dixey, R., Heindl, I., Loureiro, I., Pérez-Rodrigo, C., Snel, J. and Warnking, P. (1999). *Healthy Eating for young people in Europe – A school-based nutrition education guide*: International Planning Committee of the European Network of Health Promoting Schools. ISBN 92 890 1170 X.

European Council (2002). *Richtlinie 2001/112/EG des Rates vom 20. Dezember 2001 über Fruchtsäfte und bestimmte gleichartige Erzeugnisse für die menschliche Ernährung*, Amtsblatt der Europäischen Gemeinschaft.

European Environment Agency and WHO Regional Office for Europe (Eds.) (2002). *Water and Health in Europe: A Joint Report from the European Environment Agency and the WHO Regional Office for Europe* (Vol. 93). Copenhagen: World Health Organization.

Fitzpatrick, L. and Heaney, R. P. (2003). Got soda? *J Bone Miner Res, 18*(9), 1570–1572.

Flood, J. E., Roe, L. S. and Rolls, B. J. (2006). The effect of increased beverage portion size on energy intake at a meal. *J Am Diet Assoc, 106*(12), 1984–1990; discussion 1990–1991.

Food and Agriculture Organization of the United Nations (2009). *Food-based Dietary Guidelines*. Retrieved 27.7.2009, from http://www.fao.org/ag/humannutrition/nutritioneducation/49851/en/

Food and Nutrition Board (2004). *Dietary reference intakes for water, potassium, sodium, chloride, and sulfate*. Retrieved 08.09.2008, from http://www.nap.edu/openbook.php?isbn=0309091691

Forschungsinstitut für Kinderernährung (2008). *Empfehlungen für die Ernährung von Kindern und Jugendlichen – OptimiX*. Dortmund: Forschungsinstitut für Kinderernährung GmbH, Dortmund.

Griffiths, R. R. and Vernotica, E. M. (2000). Is caffeine a flavoring agent in cola soft drinks? *Arch Fam Med, 9*(8), 727–734.

Grimm, P. (2002). Wie gut ist unser Wasser? *Ernährungs-Umschau, 49*(2), 58–59.

Hastings G. *et al.* (2003). *Review of Research on the Effects of Food Promotion to Children*. Prepared for the Food Standards Agency.

Haug, A., Hostmark, A. T. and Harstad, O. M. (2007). Bovine milk in human nutrition – a review. *Lipids Health Dis, 6*, 25.

Heaney, R. P. and Rafferty, K. (2001). Carbonated beverages and urinary calcium excretion. *Am J Clin Nutr, 74*(3), 343–347. Retrieved 07.07.2008, from http://www.forum-trinkwasser.de/downloads/studien07_02.pdf

Heseker, H. (2001). *Untersuchungen zur ernährungsphysiologischen Bedeutung von Trinkwasser in Deutschland*: Forum Trinkwasser.

Huang, T. T. and McCrory, M. A. (2005). Dairy intake, obesity, and metabolic health in children and adolescents: Knowledge and gaps. *Nutr Rev, 63*(3), 71–80.

Huybrechts, I., Matthys, C., Vereecken, C., Maes, L., Temme, E. H., Van Oyen, H. *et al.* (2008). Food intakes by preschool children in Flanders compared with dietary guidelines. *Int J Environ Res Public Health, 5*(4), 243–257.

Jahreis, G. (2005). Milch – wichtige Quelle für Jod. *Phoenix, 3*, 6–7.

Jahreis, G., Hausmann, W., Kiessling, G., Franke, K. and Leiterer, M. (2001). Bioavailability of iodine from normal diets rich in dairy products – results of balance studies in women. *Exp Clin Endocrinol Diabetes, 109*(3), 163–167.

Jurgens, H., Haass, W., Castaneda, T. R., Schurmann, A., Koebnick, C., Dombrowski, F. *et al.* (2005). Consuming fructose-sweetened beverages increases body adiposity in mice. *Obes Res, 13*(7), 1146–1156.

Keast, R. S. and Riddell, L. J. (2007). Caffeine as a flavor additive in soft-drinks. *Appetite, 49*(1), 255–259.

Kersting, M. (2001). Nutrition of the healthy baby. Food and meal related recommendations. *Monatsschr Kinderheilkd, 149*, 4–10.

Kersting, M., Alexy, U. and Clausen, K. (2005). Using the concept of Food Based Dietary Guidelines to Develop an Optimized Mixed Diet (OMD) for German children and adolescents. *J Pediatr Gastroenterol Nutr, 40*(3), 301–308.

Kersting, M. and Bergmann, K. (2008). Calcium and Vitamin D supply to children – Selected results from the DONALD study, focussing on the consumption of milk products. *Ernährungs-Umschau, 55*(9), 523–527.

Kleiner, S. M. (1999). Water: An essential but overlooked nutrient. *J Am Diet Assoc, 99*(2), 200–206.

Lappalainen, R., Mennen, L., van Weert, L. and Mykkanen, H. (1993). Drinking water with a meal: A simple method of coping with feelings of hunger, satiety and desire to eat. *Eur J Clin Nutr, 47*(11), 815–819.

Libuda, L., Alexy, U., Buyken, A. E., Sichert-Hellert, W., Stehle, P. and Kersting, M. (2009). Consumption of sugar-sweetened beverages and its association with nutrient intakes and diet quality in German children and adolescents. *Br J Nutr, 101*, 1549–1557.

Libuda, L., Alexy, U., Remer, T., Stehle, P., Schoenau, E. and Kersting, M. (2008a). Association between long-term consumption of soft drinks and parameters of bone modeling and remodeling in a sample of healthy German children and adolescents. *Am J Clin Nutr, 88*, 1670–1677.

Libuda, L., Alexy, U., Sichert-Hellert, W., Stehle, P. and Kersting, M. (2008b). Pattern of beverage consumption and long-term association with body weight status in German adolescents – Results from the DONALD Study. *Br J Nutr, 99*, 1370–1379.

Lobstein, T., Baur, L. and Uauy, R. (2004). Obesity in children and young people: A crisis in public health. *Obes Rev, 5 Suppl 1*, 4–104.

Malik, V. S., Schulze, M. B. and Hu, F. B. (2006). Intake of sugar-sweetened beverages and weight gain: A systematic review. *Am J Clin Nutr, 84*(2), 274–288.

Manz, F. (2007). Hydration in children. *J Am Coll Nutr, 26*(5 Suppl), 562S–569S.

Manz, F. and Wentz, A. (2003). 24-h hydration status: Parameters, epidemiology and recommendations. *Eur J Clin Nutr, 57 Suppl 2*, S10–18.

Manz, F. and Wentz, A. (2005a). Hydration status in the United States and Germany. *Nutr Rev, 63*(6 Pt 2), S55–62.

Manz, F. and Wentz, A. (2005b). The importance of good hydration for the prevention of chronic diseases. *Nutr Rev, 63*(6 Pt 2), S2–5.

Manz, F., Wentz, A. and Sichert-Hellert, W. (2002). The most essential nutrient: Defining the adequate intake of water. *J Pediatr, 141*(4), 587–592.

Marshall, T. A., Eichenberger Gilmore, J. M., Broffitt, B., Stumbo, P. J. and Levy, S. M. (2005). Diet quality in young children is influenced by beverage consumption. *J Am Coll Nutr, 24*(1), 65–75.

Mattes, R. (2006). Fluid calories and energy balance: The good, the bad, and the uncertain. *Physiol Behav, 89*(1), 66–70.

Mattes, R. D. (1996). Dietary compensation by humans for supplemental energy provided as ethanol or carbohydrate in fluids. *Physiol Behav, 59*(1), 179–187.

McGartland, C., Robson, P. J., Murray, L., Cran, G., Savage, M. J., Watkins, D. *et al.* (2003). Carbonated soft drink consumption and bone mineral density in adolescence: The Northern Ireland Young Hearts project. *J Bone Miner Res, 18*(9), 1563–1569.

Mensink, G. B. M., Heseker, H., Richter A., Stahl, A. and Vohmann, C. (2007a). *Forschungsbericht Ernährungsstudie als KiGGS-Modul (EsKiMo)*: Robert Koch-Institut Berlin, Universität Paderborn.

Mensink, G. B. M., Kleiser, C. and Richter, A. (2007b). Food consumption of children and adolescents in Germany. Results of the German Health Inerview and Examination Survey for Children and Adolescents (KiGGS). *Bundesgesundheitsbl – Gesundheitsforsch – Gesundheitsschutz 50*, 609–623.

Moynihan, P., Adamson, A., Rugg-Gunn, A., Appleton, D. and Butler, T. (1996). Dietary sources of calcium and the contribution of flour fortification to total calcium intake in the diets of Northumbrian adolescents. *Br J Nutr, 75*(3), 495–505.

Muckelbauer, R., Libuda, L., Clausen, K. and Kersting, M. (2009a). Long-term process evaluation of a school-based programme for overweight prevention. *Child Care Health Dev,* 35(6), 851–857.

Muckelbauer, R., Libuda, L., Clausen, K., Reinehr, T., Toschke, A. M. and Kersting, M. (2009b). Promotion and provision of drinking water in schools for overweight prevention: A randomized controlled cluster trial. *Pediatrics, 123(4)*, e661–e667.

Negoianu, D. and Goldfarb, S. (2008). Just Add Water. *J Am Soc Nephrol, 19*(6), 1041–1043.

Nicklas, T. A. (2003). Calcium intake trends and health consequences from childhood through adulthood. *J Am Coll Nutr, 22*(5), 340–356.

Nielsen, S. J. and Popkin, B. M. (2004). Changes in beverage intake between 1977 and 2001. *Am J Prev Med, 27*(3), 205–210.

NIH Consensus Development Panel on Osteoporosis Prevention, Diagnosis, and Therapy (2001). Osteoporosis prevention, diagnosis, and therapy. *JAMA, 285*(6), 785–795.

Österreichisches Lebensmittelbuch. (2008). *Erfrischungsgetränke mit geschmacksgebenden Zusätzen* (Vol. IV. Auflage).

Popkin, B. M., Armstrong, L. E., Bray, G. M., Caballero, B., Frei, B. and Willett, W. C. (2006). A new proposed guidance system for beverage consumption in the United States. *Am J Clin Nutr, 83*(3), 529–542.

Remer, T., Dimitriou, T. and Manz, F. (2003). Dietary potential renal acid load and renal net acid excretion in healthy, free-living children and adolescents. *Am J Clin Nutr, 77*(5), 1255–1260.

Remer, T., Fonteyn, N., Alexy, U. and Berkemeyer, S. (2006). Longitudinal examination of 24-h urinary iodine excretion in schoolchildren as a sensitive, hydration status-independent research tool for studying iodine status. *Am J Clin Nutr, 83*(3), 639–646.

Ribas-Barba, L., Serra-Majem, L., Salvador, G., Castell, C., Cabezas, C., Salleras, L. *et al.* (2007). Trends in dietary habits and food consumption in Catalonia, Spain (1992–2003). *Public Health Nutr, 10*(11A), 1340–1353.

Rolls, B. J., Kim, S. and Fedoroff, I. C. (1990). Effects of drinks sweetened with sucrose or aspartame on hunger, thirst and food intake in men. *Physiol Behav, 48*(1), 19–26.

Sawka, M. N., Cheuvront, S. N. and Carter, R., 3rd. (2005). Human water needs. *Nutr Rev, 63*(6 Pt 2), S30–39.

Sichert-Hellert, W., Kersting, M. and Manz, F. (2001). Fifteen year trends in water intake in German children and adolescents: Results of the DONALD Study (Dortmund Nutritional and Anthropometric Longitudinally Designed Study). *Acta Paediatr, 90*(7), 732–737.

Souci SW, Fachmann W, Kraut H, *Die Zusammensetzung der Lebensmittel Nährwert-Tabellen* [Compositions of Food – Tables of nutrient contents] 7th edn 2008, Stuttgart: Wissenschaftliche Verlagsgesellschaft mbH.

Storey, M. L., Forshee, R. A. and Anderson, P. A. (2006). Beverage consumption in the US population. *J Am Diet Assoc, 106*(12), 1992–2000.

Subar, A. F., Krebs-Smith, S. M., Cook, A. and Kahle, L. L. (1998). Dietary sources of nutrients among US children, 1989-1991. *Pediatrics, 102*(4 Pt 1), 913–923.

US Department of Agriculture and Agricultural Research Service (1999). *Food and Nutrient Intakes by Children 1994-96, 1998*: Food Surveys Research Group.

Vartanian, L. R., Schwartz, M. B. and Brownell, K. D. (2007). Effects of soft drink consumption on nutrition and health: A systematic review and meta-analysis. *Am J Public Health, 97*(4), 667–675.

Wetmore, C. M., Ichikawa, L., Lacroix, A. Z., Ott, S. M. and Scholes, D. (2008). Association between caffeine intake and bone mass among young women: Potential effect modification by depot medroxyprogesterone acetate use. *Osteoporos Int, 19*(4), 519–527.

Whiting, S. J., Vatanparast, H., Baxter-Jones, A., Faulkner, R. A., Mirwald, R. and Bailey,

D. A. (2004). Factors that affect bone mineral accrual in the adolescent growth spurt. *J Nutr, 134*(3), 696S–700S.
World Health Organisation (2000). *Bottled drinking water* – Fact sheet No. 256.
Zemel, M. B. and Miller, S. L. (2004). Dietary calcium and dairy modulation of adiposity and obesity risk. *Nutr Rev, 62*(4), 125–131.

3

Childhood obesity: the contribution of diet

G. Rodríguez,* J. Fernández and L. A. Moreno, University of Zaragoza, Spain

Abstract: Childhood obesity prevalence has increased dramatically due to contemporary environmental factors in almost all developed countries and it needs to be considered as a global health problem nowadays because it could associate many undesirable long-term health effects. This chapter is focused on main environmental determinants of childhood obesity and provides information about the contribution of diet, lifestyle and socioeconomic and cultural factors. Among others, all these aspects have also consequent implications for the food industry, healthcare professionals, policy makers or TV food advertising.

Key words: obesity, diet, lifestyle, food industry, healthcare, policy makers.

3.1 Introduction

In spite of institutional and health services prevention programs, the prevalence of overweight and obesity has increased dramatically during the last few decades both in children and adults from almost all developed countries (Flodmark *et al.*, 2004; Hedley *et al.*, 2004; Wang and Lobstein, 2006). However, it has been reported that, in some areas showing high obesity rates, the prevalence of obesity has started to level off. This is the case for the United States, Sweden and France (Ogden *et al.*, 2008; Sundblom *et al.*, 2008; Péneau *et al.*, 2009). Childhood obesity still needs to be considered as a global health problem because adiposity at the first stages of life will probably persist in later life and is likely to be associated with undesirable

*Also at Instituto Aragonés de Ciencias de la Salud, Spain.

long-term human health effects, including metabolic, physical and psychosocial disorders and a high risk of cardiovascular disease among others (Daniels *et al.*, 2005; Fisberg *et al.*, 2004). Obesity means more than an excessive body fat deposition because of all the associated complications that adversely impacts upon population health status.

Obesity, defined as an excess of body fat, is the result of an imbalance between energy intake and energy expenditure. There is controvery about what factors are really causing the current increase in body fatness. Genetic and environmental factors are the two most important groups of determinants that modify the risk of being obese. Genetic predisposition is always present in each subject, outweighing many of the environmental and physiological factors that influence obesity development during different periods of life (Fig. 3.1) (Moreno and Rodriguez, 2007; Rodriguez and Moreno, 2006). However, despite this individual genetic predisposition, contemporary environmental factors have more influence on the current increase of obesity prevalence because the human genotype has obviously not changed over the last few decades. This chapter is focoused on the main environmental determinants of childhood obesity, in particular, providing information about the contribution of dietary aspects and associated implications for the food industry, healthcare professionals and policy makers.

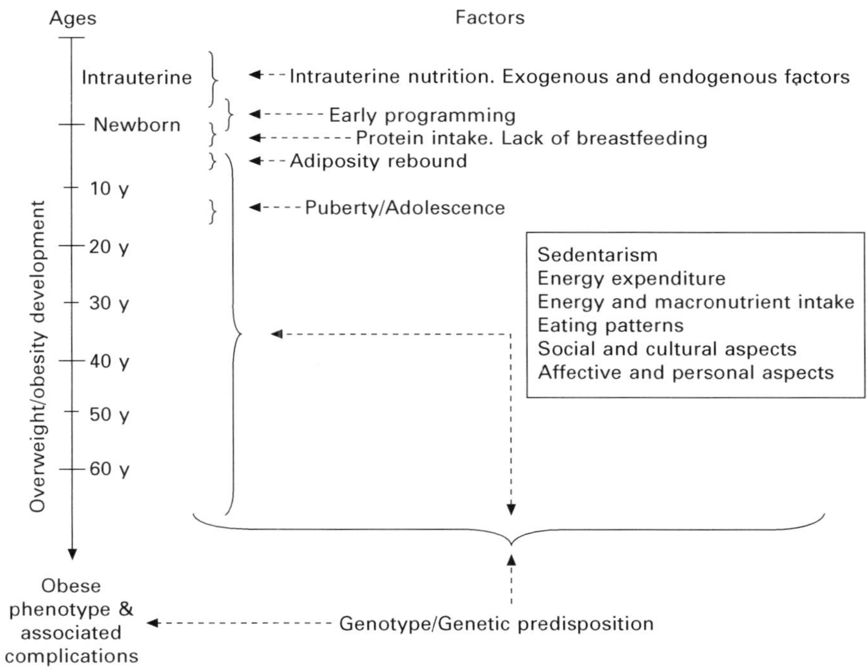

Fig. 3.1 Environmental and genetic factors influencing obesity development along different periods of life. Adapted from Rodriguez and Moreno, 2006.

3.2 Trends in childhood obesity

3.2.1 Current overweight and obesity prevalence

During several decades, overweight and obesity in children and adolescents have dramatically increased all over the world, reaching the grade of a global 'epidemic phenomenon' (Flodmark *et al.*, 2004; Hedley *et al.*, 2004; Wang and Lobstein, 2006). Depending on the demographic origin, population characteristics and criteria definition, epidemiological data show that the prevalence of overweight/obesity in children and adolescents ranges worldwide between 15% and 35%. However, the prevalence remains low in most developing countries from Asia and Africa (overweight <5%, obesity <2%) where under-nutrition is still the major nutrition problem (Wang and Lobstein, 2006). North America and some European countries have the highest prevalence of overweight (approximately 20–30%) and obesity (about 5–15%), as well as the highest rate of increase. In Europe, the combined prevalence of childhood overweight and obesity is higher than 30% in countries such as Spain, Italy or Portugal; and about 20% in many other countries (Lissau, 2004; Moreno *et al.*, 2004).

In overweight and obesity prevalence reports, the body mass index (BMI) is used as the surrogate marker of total body fat, and variations between samples may be partly due to the different BMI cut points and population charts considered. BMI is the parameter most frequently used for the screening of obesity because it is easy to determine and it tends to correlate well with body fat. However, the BMI has limitations at the individual level to identify those children and adolescents with excess body fat (Rodriguez *et al.*, 2004). BMI cutoff values generally accepted for the definition of overweight and obesity in adults are 25 and 30 kg/m^2, respectively. In children and adolescents, as they grow, BMI measures change considerably in both sexes over the years and body mass continuously increases. For this reason, several sex/age-specific cut-off BMI percentiles based on different populations have been used to identify overweight and obesity during childhood and adolescence. A BMI higher than the 95th percentile and a BMI between the 85th and 95th percentile have been generally used for obesity and overweight definitions respectively (Moreno *et al.*, 2000; Must *et al.*, 1991). In 2000, the International Obesity Task Force (IOTF) proposed BMI cut-off points for overweight and obesity screening, for each half-year of age both in males and females, which correspond to BMI values of 25 and 30 kg/m^2 at the age of 18 years (Cole *et al.*, 2000). The IOTF BMI values represent standard unchangeable international references that allow the screening of adiposity in children and adolescents worldwide under the same criterion, without variations depending on geographic, social and secular trends (Cole *et al.*, 2000).

3.2.2 Trends on children and adolescent obesity prevalence

Child and adolescent obesity prevalence has been continuously increasing in developed countries, apart from some areas with high obesity rates that are showing an incipient levelling-off of childhood obesity prevalence (Ogden *et al.*, 2008; Sundblom *et al.*, 2008; Péneau *et al.*, 2009). In these areas, prevention programs, social aspects and institutional actions may have counteracted previous obesity growth rates. For example, in US children and adolescents, the prevalence of high BMI for age showed no significant changes between 2003–2004 and 2005–2006 and no significant trends between 1999 and 2006 (Ogden *et al.*, 2008). A population-based study of 10-year-olds from the Stockholm County (Sweden), showed that rates of obesity, overweight and underweight were stable from 1999 to 2003 (Sundblom *et al.*, 2008). In children aged 6 to 15 years measured at health examination centers in the central/western part of France between 1996 and 2006, overweight prevalence increased between 1996 (11.5%) and 1998 (14.8%), and was stable between 1998 and 2006 (15.2%) (Péneau *et al.*, 2009). The prevalence of overweight in the disadvantaged group increased between 1996 (12.8%) and 2001 (18.9%) and was stable between 2001 and 2006 (18.2%). The stabilization coincides with increasing information on childhood overweight in France, the National Plan on Nutrition and Health being set up in 2001 (Péneau *et al.*, 2009).

High and increasing prevalence of overweight and obesity have, however, been found recently in Spanish children and adolescents when compared with previous rates from one or two decades before (Moreno *et al.*, 2000, 2005a; Serra *et al.*, 2003). In two cross-sectional surveys conducted in Zaragoza (Spain) in 1980 and 1995, with children of ages ranging from 6.0 to 14.9 years, body fat percentage also showed significant increases in all age groups, with percentage increases of 2.46% at 13.5 years and 6.03% at 11.5 years (Moreno *et al.*, 2001a). In the same population samples, we have calculated some indices of fat patterning, derived from skinfold thickness measurements; in males, we observed a significant trend to a central pattern of fat distribution from the ages of 6.5–11.5 y, and in females we also observed a significant trend to a central pattern of fat distribution but only at the ages of 6.5 and 7.5 y (Moreno *et al.*, 2001b). Finally, two studies, undertaken in 1995 and 2000–02, were compared to assess changes in waist circumference in adolescents; between the two time periods, waist circumference increased significantly in males at 13 years and in females at 14 years (Moreno *et al.*, 2005b). All these studies (Moreno *et al.*, 2000, 2001a, b, 2005a, b; Serra *et al.*, 2003) showed a trend towards high BMI and total and regional fat deposition, as has been seen in the great majority of regions all over the world (Wang and Lobstein, 2006).

3.2.3 Main determinants of childhood obesity increasing prevalence

Among other factors, obesity prevalence increases vary, depending on the geographic area where the children and adolescents live, socio-economic and ethnic/racial conditions, and age and sex group considered. The main determinats of current trends are socio-economic, cultural and lifestyle differences between populations exposed to an obesogenic environment (permanent food accessibility and sedentary life). Lifestyle determinants, including all diet and physical activity aspects, are also influenced by socioeconomic and cultural factors. As an example, diets of low nutrient density and high energy density are cheaper (Drewnowski and Specter, 2004) as well as being a risk factor for being obese; socioeconomic factors are also important for diet composition (Guillaume *et al.*, 1998).

Energy imbalance

The established cause of body fat deposition is an energy imbalance during a long period of time when energy intake exceeds energy expenditure. This maintained positive blance could produce significant body composition modifications and then, overweight may appear in a predisposed subject. Regulation of energy balance includes a complex web of processes influencing energy intake, appetite and fat deposition by modifying interactions between genetic (individual predisposition), environmental and behavioral factors. The energy gap is this little positive energy imbalance that causes body fat increase after compensating energy changes have failed in attempting to maintain body weight. Longer-term neuro-endocrine signals depend on the magnitude of energy stores and, when adipose tissue mass has decreased, hunger is activated to restore the loss by stimulating food intake and inhibiting thermogenesis. In contrast, the response to energy excess is relatively weak and food intake is not stopped completely.

In children, an imbalance of around 100–200 kcal/day leads to a significant increase of weight, measured from dual energy X-ray absorptiometry (Butte and Ellis, 2003). In normal-weight children who became overweight, median energy storage was 133 kcal/day and the 90th percentile for energy storage in this group was 171 kcal/day (Butte and Ellis, 2003). Considering an energetic store efficiency of 50%, a deficit of 340–500 kcal/day would be required to prevent further weight gain in most of the overweight children. Data obtained from NHANES III and IV estimate a similar amount of 'Energy Gap' in children (Wang *et al.*, 2006) and, in this group, decreasing energy intake or increasing physical activity energy expenditure around 110–165 kcal/day could be enough to counterbalance the energy gap. In Table 3.1, the daily energy gap implied in excess weight gain is detailed in children and adolescents from NHANES III and IV, depending on their age, gender and family income (Maffeis *et al.*, 1998).

Energy intake

A clear relationship between high energy intake in child populations and subsequent obesity development due to a continuous positive disbalance has not been shown. Results from cross-sectional studies comparing obese children with normo-weight counterparts are controversial and they do not provide sufficient evidence because the obese children already had excess body fat when evaluated. Perhaps obese children (after they become obese)

Table 3.1 Excess weight gain and implied 'energy gap' in children from the NHANES III and IV studies throughout a 10-yr period depending on their age-specific activity level (average activity level or light activity level) (Wang *et al.*, 2006)

		Energy gap	
	Mean 10-y excess weight gain (kg)	Average activity level (Kcal/day)	Light activity level (Kcal/day)
Overall	4.3	131	114
2–4 years	5.1	155	135
5–7 years	3.2	97	85
Boys	4.3	131	114
Girls	4.4	134	116
Lower income *	4.5	137	119
Higher income *	4.2	128	111

(*): Income level on the basis of poverty index ratio (the ratio of annual family income to the USA federal poverty line)

do not eat more than non-obese. Methodology performed to measure energy consumption is not able to find differences; obese children tend to underestimate dietary intake records (consciously or unconsciously) or, probably, obese children are already on a diet for body weight control because of family and health advice.

Longitudinal studies during a controlled period of time are useful to show reliable associations between energy intake and obesity development but, unfortunately, there are not many longitudinal studies in children and adolescents (Berkey *et al.*, 2000; Bogaert *et al.*, 2003; Maffeis *et al.*, 1998; Magarey *et al.*, 2003; Moreno and Rodriguez, 2007; Ong *et al.*, 2006; Rodriguez and Moreno, 2006). In a study with a large group of pre-adolescents and adolescents aged 9–14, the body mass index increase during one year was associated with positive energy intake changes (Berkey *et al.*, 2000). Furthermore, in a birth cohort study of 881 infants, higher total dietary energy intake at 4 months was associated with significantly greater weight gain between birth and 3 years among formula- or mixed-fed infants (not among breastfed infants) and with an increased risk for being overweight at 3 and 5 years (Ong *et al.*, 2006). Except for isolated findings, generally, the rest of the studies have not shown that energy intake is related to significant differences in childhood weight gain (Berkey *et al.*, 2000; Bogaert *et al.*, 2003; Maffeis *et al.*, 1998; Magarey *et al.*, 2003; Moreno and Rodriguez, 2007; Ong *et al.*, 2006; Rodriguez and Moreno, 2006).

Macronutrient intake

The relative proportion of macronutrient intake may able to modify, by itself, the amount of food consumption (by its influence on satiety, hunger or food acceptance), the metabolic efficiency of food and the quantity of energy storage. Over-consumption of energy-dense foods with a high proportion of fat may result in an increase in daily energy intake and energy balance disturbances. However, there are also controversial results obtained from longitudinal studies, carried out in children and adolescents before they become overweight, in relation to macronutrient intake and its association with significant risk for obesity development over time. Diet composition is not easily related to later significant differences in childhood weight gain. As examples of controversial results, Skinner *et al.* (2004) found that mean fat intake recorded in 70 white children aged 2–8 years was a positive predictor of body mass index (BMI) at 8 y; however, conversely, Alexy *et al.* (2004) did not show any fat intake influence on BMI in 228 individuals aged 2–18 years. Proportional macronutrient intake during the first periods of life seems to be related to later body composition differences. A higher protein intake during the early postnatal months has been related to later increases of body size and adiposity, sometimes associated with a short period of breastfeeding that conferred, by itself, a risk of future overweight and obesity (Arenz *et al.*, 2004; Bogen *et al.*, 2004; Gillman *et al.*, 2001; Harder *et al.*, 2005; Heinig *et al.*, 1993; Owen *et al.*, 2005; Scaglioni *et al.*, 2000; Stettler *et al.*, 2002; Veugelers and Fitzgerald, 2005). Mechanisms by which breastfeeding affects the risk of overweight are still unclear.

In prospective studies, there is no current solid evidence that any of the macronutirents is related to obesity development in children but the main positive reported associations can be summarized in the following points: (i) Global dietary energy density and high fat foods have shown positive results in only few studies (McCaffrey *et al.*, 2008; Moreno and Rodriguez, 2007; Rodriguez and Moreno, 2006). (ii) Positive associations have also been reported between protein intake during complementary feeding and transition to adult diet and child obesity (Gunther *et al.*, 2007; Skinner *et al.*, 2004). (iii) Sucrose consumption in children (specially from calorically sweetened beverages) increases the risk for obesity (Gunther *et al.*, 2007; Ludwig *et al.*, 2001; Olsen and Heitmann, 2009) but in a recent meta-analysis, no association between consumption of sugar sweetened beverages and weight gain was found (Forshee *et al.*, 2008).

Dietary habits

Dietary habits are influenced by socio-cultural, personal and family aspects. Favorable economic conditions, constant food availability, fashionable eating habits, poor family supervision, influence of TV advertisements on food selection, low price but non-healthy food industry offers, poor socio-cultural level, among others, are all factors that probably increase the risk of being obese in predisposed subjects in our obesogenic environment. For eating patterns, controversial results have also been reported from longitudinal studies and only little evidence exists of some associations between diet habits and obesity development later in life (Moreno and Rodriguez, 2007; Rodriguez and Moreno, 2006).

Prospective controlled studies in children have found evident associations between obesity development and specific behaviors only rarely. Perhaps methods that are usually performed to search long-term diet and body composition relationships in children are not accurate enough to find associations. The major interesting findings reported can be summarized as follows:

(i) To eat few meals a day (three or fewer) may facilitate weight gain compared with four, five or more daily meals (Toschke *et al.*, 2005).
(ii) Low intake during breakfast or skipping breakfast is associated with weight gain (Niemeier *et al.*, 2006).
(iii) To eat alone without family supervision or while watching TV may be potential risk factors for overweight development (Sen, 2006; Veugelers and Fitzgerald, 2005) but no confirmation data are available from longitudinal studies (Moreno and Rodriguez, 2007; Rodriguez and Moreno, 2006).
(iv) Snacking, fast food and big food portion size consumption have not been consistently related to obesity development in longitudinal studies despite these dietary habits being associated with excessive intake of energy, total fat, saturated fat, carbohydrates, added sugars, and sugar-sweetened beverages (Moreno and Rodriguez, 2007; Rodriguez and Moreno, 2006).
(v) Excessive consumption of sweetened drinks showed, by itself, a predictive influence on overweight prevalence in a few longitudinal studies (Berkey *et al.*, 2004; Ludwig *et al.*, 2001; McCaffrey *et al.*, 2008; Olsen and Heitmann, 2009); however, based on scientific evidence, a recent meta-analysis has found that this association is not fully convincing (Forshee *et al.*, 2008).

3.3 Impact of childhood obesity on children's health and later life

3.3.1 Short- and long-term health problems due to obesity

The main health problem associated with obesity is the cluster of metabolic abnormalities that already appear in obese children and adolescents increasing the risk of cardiovascular diseases. Obesity, also in children, is associated with dyslipidemia, hypertension, insulin resistance/hyperinsulinemia, impaired glucose tolerance/Type 2 diabetes, nonalcoholic fatty liver disease, psychological problems, personal dissatisfaction, orthopedic abnormalities, among others (Csabi *et al.*, 2000; Kang *et al.*, 2006; Schwimmer *et al.*, 2006; Tresaco *et al.*, 2009). Obese children and adolescents with impaired glucose tolerance have peripheral insulin resistance and insulin secretion abnormalities that cause major defects in lipid and carbohydrate metabolism. Early in the natural history of Type 2 diabetes in obese young people, insulin resistance as pre-diabetes status is related to an increased visceral fat and to overall excess body fat (Csabi *et al.*, 2000; Kang *et al.*, 2006; Schwimmer *et al.*, 2006; Tresaco *et al.*, 2009).

Excess body fat and related metabolic disorders begin in childhood and adolescence and remain later into adulthood. Vanhala *et al.* (1999) observed that among children at the age of 7 years with BMIs in the highest quartile, the odds ratio for the metabolic syndrome in adulthood was 4.4 (95% CI 2.1–9.5) compared with the other children in the rest of the quartiles. After adjustment for age, sex and current obesity, the risk of the syndrome still was 2.4 (95% CI 2.1–9.5). Eriksson *et al.* (2003), in a longitudinal study in 8760 children, reported that the cumulative incidence of Type 2 diabetes in adulthood decreased progressively, from 8.6% in persons whose adiposity rebound occurred before the age of 5 years, to 1.8% in those in whom it occurred after 7 years.

Some hemostatic risk factors have also been associated with obesity. Obese children presented significant elevated values for tissue-plasminogen activator (t-PA), plasminogen activator inhibitor-1 (PAI-1), and fibrinogen, compared with their counterparts (Valle *et al.*, 2000). Production of PAI-1 by adipose tissue (Lundgren *et al.*, 1996) can contribute to the elevation of plasma PAI-1 observed in the metabolic syndrome. This increment determines a decrease of the fibrinolytic activity in plasma (Juhan-Vague *et al.*, 1991), which can have an important role in the development of cardiovascular illness in obesity. Obese children also have lower arterial compliance and lower distensibility, as well as higher values for wall stress than their healthy counterparts.

The immunoinflamatory status has also been related with obesity and consequent cardiovascular diseases. Excess body fat may induce a chronic low-grade inflammatory state (Wärnberg *et al.*, 2004). Ford *et al.* (2001) observed that in 5305 children aged 6 to 18 years, after several adjustments, the odds of having an elevated C-Reactive Protein concentration (>2.1 mg/L) were 2.20 (95% CI 1.30, 3.75) for children with a BMI of the 85th–95th percentile and 4.92 (95% CI 3.39, 7.15) for children with a BMI over the 95th percentile, compared with children who had a normal BMI. Adipocytes are a source of cytokines, such as tumor necrosis factor-α and interleukin-6 (Hotamisligil *et al.*, 1993; Mohamed-Ali *et al.*, 1997).

3.3.2 Fat distribution and metabolic risk

Development of metabolic abnormalities associated with adiposity is related to an increased visceral fat more than to excess body fat (Weiss *et al.*, 2003). Waist circumference seems to be the best simple anthropometric predictor for the screening of the metabolic syndrome in children (Moreno *et al.*, 2002a). Waist circumference may be used as an index of abdominal adiposity, which is the sum of visceral and subcutaneous fat at this level. Abdominal fat, measured by nuclear magnetic resonance, showed positive association in obese adolescents with impaired glucose tolerance (Weiss *et al.*, 2003).

So, intra-abdominal fat accumulation is strongly related to insulin resistance and hyperglycaemia in obese children and adolescents.

Other metabolic abnormalities and cardiovascular risk factors have also shown positive relations with central fat distribution in obese children and adolescents, e.g. greater plasma hemostatic factor concentrations (Ferguson *et al.*, 1998); increased intramyocellular lipid content (Weiss *et al.*, 2003); low HDL-cholesterol and high LDL-cholesterol, ApoA1/ApoB and triglycerides plasma levels (Maffeis *et al.*, 2001; Moreno *et al.*, 2002b; Savva *et al.*, 2000; Tresaco *et al.*, 2009); and hypertension (Maffeis *et al.*, 2001; Moreno *et al.*, 2002b; Savva *et al.*, 2000). Metabolic syndrome is characterized in childhood and adolescence by a clustering of several independent cardiovascular risk factors (Moreno *et al.*, 2002b; Chen *et al.*, 1999).

3.4 Implications of childhood obesity for the food industry, healthcare professionals and policy makers

3.4.1 TV food advertising for children

There is evidence suggesting that food advertising causes childhood obesity, although the strength of this effect is unclear (Veerman *et al.*, 2009). The contribution of TV advertising of foods and drinks to the prevalence of childhood obesity differs distinctly by country and is likely to be significant in some countries, depending on the amount of food advertisements and TV use (Goris *et al.*, 2009). Food advertising for children is a very relevant issue: content analyses have shown that food is the most frequently advertised product category on children's TV. The majority of these advertisements target highly-sweetened products, but more recently, the proportion from fast food meal promotions has been growing (Lobstein and Dibb, 2005). Controlled studies on children's choices have consistently shown that children exposed to advertising choose advertised food products at significantly higher rates than do those not exposed (Coon and Tucker, 2002). In addition, greater TV use leads to higher intakes of energy, fat, sweets, salty snacks, carbonated beverages and lower intakes of fruit and vegetables (Coon and Tucker, 2002).

Television watching replaces more vigorous activities, and there is a positive correlation between the time spent watching television and the risk of overweight or obesity on populations of different ages. Obesity prevalence has increased as well as the number of hours that TV networks dedicate to children. The present use of food in movies, shows and cartoons may lead to a misconception of the notion of healthy nutrition and stimulate an excessive intake of poor nutritional food (Caroli *et al.*, 2004).

All these findings justify the need for taking precautionary actions to reduce children's exposure to obesogenic marketing practices. Limiting the exposure of children to marketing of energy-dense foods could be part of a broader effort to make children's diets healthier, in which TV could be a convenient tool to spread correct information on good nutrition and obesity prevention.

3.4.2 Food industry and child obesity

That childhood obesity is an alarming public health problem is clear and is widely appreciated (Sugarman and Sandman, 2007). What is altogether unclear is what our society should do about it. The food industry is a critical factor in any potentially successful long-term strategy to prevent obesity. By producing new, low-energy density products and improving the nutritional quality (and reducing the energy content) of existing products, as well as through advances in responsible marketing and labeling, the food industry can provide foods that enable consumers to achieve lower energy intakes with adequate intake of essential nutrients. Other than the food industry, the consumer is an important player in the solution of obesity because the consumer can make healthy lifestyle choices at an individual level. However, children are usually not fully aware of all the implications their food choices have for health. Therefore, the food industry is committed to providing the consumer with healthy food options and reliable nutrition information (Verduin *et al.*, 2005).

The food industry is not the sole factor and other factors, such as government policies regarding agriculture, prices and subsidies are equally essential. Intensive collaboration between all these players will only be attained if obesity prevention is given the priority it deserves in future public health planning (Seidell, 1999).

3.4.3 Fun food, fast-food restaurants, snacks, sodas and sweet beverages

The major causes of obesity and overweight are lifestyle related, in particular excessive diet intake together with increasingly sedentarism (Grüters *et al.*, 2002). Fast-food has become a prominent feature in the diet of children throughout the world. However, few studies have examined the effects of fast-food consumption on any nutrition or health-related outcome. Anyway, the current evidence shows that consumption of fast food among children in the United States seems to have an adverse effect on dietary quality and this fact could increase the risk of obesity (Bowman *et al.*, 2004).

There is an inconsistent association between obesity and consumption of soft drinks. Even without scientific evidence, the replacement of soft drinks and other sugar-containing beverages such as fruit juices by noncaloric alternatives seems to be a logical approach for the prevention of overweight in childhood and adolescence (James and Kerr, 2005). In the United Kingdom, a school-based initiative focusing on reducing the consumption of these drinks has also been effective in preventing a further increase in obesity (Libuda and Kersting, 2009). However, since the cause of overweight and obesity is multifactorial, the limitation of soft drink, snack and fast food consumption needs to be incorporated into a broader complex strategy for obesity prevention.

3.4.4 Healthcare programs against childhood obesity: diet and physical activity

Institutional policy strategies

Both physical activity and food intake contribute to the energy balance, but research increasingly points to physical inactivity as the primary culprit in weight gain. Singling out and restricting specific foods and beverages is unlikely to be fully effective in reducing the prevalence of overweight children. In general, preventing and treating pediatric obesity are fairly similar: adhering to a healthy lifestyle which emphasizes healthy food choices and habits, regular physical activity, and limiting screen time and other sedentary behaviors (Dubnov-Raz *et al.*, 2009). Treating and preventing obesity is an extremely difficult task, but prevention remains the best option. There are several barriers for obesity prevention and treatment that impair the final outcome: unmotivated parents, unmotivated children, overweight parents, families that often eat fast food, excessive watching of TV, not practicing enough exercise, etc.

Nutrition educators need to emphasize overall lifestyles in childhood overweight intervention efforts, including physical activity and dietary aspects, with particular focus on the motivation of the family as a whole. Long-lasting solutions to the obesity epidemic must be comprehensive and must include all of the key stakeholders: children, parents, schools, health professionals, businesses, and community leaders and organizations (Marr, 2004). The focus of the obesity prevention programs should not be only on nutrition and physical activity, but also account for the complete sociocultural environment of the child. Community participation can be successfully used in the development and implementation of childhood obesity prevention programs.

Public health experts consider a host of overarching and powerful influences beyond any one person's control to be the pivotal causes of childhood obesity (Friedman and Schwartz, 2008). Consequently, it is more useful from a prevention and policy standpoint to examine the increasingly 'toxic environments' in which we live, consider a comprehensive strategy, and introduce, implement and enforce public health policy to change those environments, instead of focusing only on the specific individual determinants of obesity. Current studies show that geographical distribution of childhood obesity varies, with a high prevalence in deprived areas (Edwards *et al.*, 2009). These findings suggest how policy can be tailored to the specific needs of each micro-area in order to achieve better prevention results, taking into account local factors such as area socioeconomic status, shopping facilities, traffic barriers, green areas, sport facilities, etc.

Childhood obesity and overweight is not a problem regarding only the individual, but is a social concern. As a community, we all have responsibility to build healthier environments. Public policy and community partnerships that include all health professionals, the food industry, national and local goverments and stakeholders who have a responsibility in the prevention of childhood obesity should be established.

3.5 Future trends

Childhood obesity prevalence continues to increase in developed, and in many undeveloped, countries, in spite of institutional concerns. The hope is that, as is already occurring in some areas, increasing prevalence will start to level-off according to well-planned prevention programs. We have a difficult future challenge aiming to reverse current rates. Whether we achieve this goal, all obesity-related problems during childhood and adulthood will decrease, considerably improving our population health and, especially, the risk of cardiovascular diseases. In the future, it will be necessary to perform new epidemiological studies about trends on obesity prevalence, monitoring population-rate changes according to environmental and institutional preventive actions.

To measure diet intake, physical activity level and longitudinal body composition changes due to diet and activity habits is problematic, especially in growing populations of any age. Without any doubt, there is a clear need to develop and improve all instruments and methods for these aims. Prospective longitudinal designs provide stronger evidence for causal associations than cross-sectional ones, but unfortunately there are not many longitudinal studies. With a suitable methodology, it will be possible to identify certain 'obesogenic' factors and their real influence on the increasing prevalence of overweight. The evidence regarding obesogenic macronutrients is weak and controversial. Potentially, a cluster of these and other dietary and activity patterns could be involved in the development of obesity in children.

Food industry future responsibilities fall into two main areas. The first is to propose and to advertise new products adapted to current consumer demands: low energy-dense foods, fun products, and nutritive and functional foods. The second is to protect consumers by avoiding food advertisements with misleading information about nutritional and health properties. Manipulated information encourages people to consume certain foods more frequently, thinking that they are better or healthier but, sometimes, they do not provide the required nutrients or they may even lead to an excessive energy intake. TV sources might contribute by taking precautionary actions to reduce children's exposure to obesogenic marketing practices (it could even be a convenient tool to spread correct information on good nutrition and obesity prevention), and parents must limit the exposure of children to advertisements of energy-dense foods.

Government policies and intensive collaboration between institutions must be a priority to improve population health by preventing overweight development. Public health efforts should be emphasized in order to decrease the current trend. Regular family meals could serve as role models for healthy eating behaviors. Educational intervention among parents and the community, aimed at the modification of the whole diet and activity patterns from a healthy perspective, seems to be the most adequate tool to deal with the worldwide obesity epidemic. The focus of the obesity prevention programs should consider the complete sociocultural environment of the child.

3.6 References

Alexy U, Sichert-Hellert W, Kersting M and Schultze-Pawlitschko V (2004), Pattern of long-term fat intake and BMI during childhood and adolescence – results of the DONALD Study, *Int J Obes Relat Metab Disord*, 28, 1203–1209.

Arenz S, Ruckerl R, Koletzko B and von Kries R (2004), Breast-feeding and childhood obesity – a systematic review, *Int J Obes Relat Metab Disord*, 28, 1247–1256.

Berkey CS, Rockett HR, Field AE, Gillman MW, Frazier AL, Camargo CA Jr and Colditz GA (2000), Activity, dietary intake, and weight changes in a longitudinal study of preadolescent and adolescent boys and girls, *Pediatrics*, 105, E56.

Berkey CS, Rockett HR, Field AE, Gillman MW and Colditz GA (2004), Sugar-added beverages and adolescent weight change, *Obes Res*, 12, 778–788.

Bogaert N, Steinbeck KS, Baur LA, Brock K and Bermingham MA (2003), Food, activity and family – environmental vs biochemical predictors of weight gain in children, *Eur J Clin Nutr*, 57, 1242–1249.

Bogen DL, Hanusa BH and Whitaker RC (2004), The effect of breast-feeding with and without formula use on the risk of obesity at 4 years of age, *Obes Res*, 12, 1527–1535.

Bowman SA, Gortmaker SL, Ebbeling CB, Pereira MA and Ludwig DS (2004), Effects of fast-food consumption on energy intake and diet quality among children in a national household survey, *Pediatrics*, 113, 112–118.

Butte NF and Ellis KJ (2003), Comment on 'Obesity and the environment: Where do we go from here?', *Science*, 301, 598.

Caroli M, Argentieri L, Cardone M and Masi A (2004), Role of television in childhood obesity prevention, *Int J Obes Relat Metab Disord*, 28 (Suppl 3), S104–108.

Chen W, Srinivasan SR, Elkasabany A and Berenson GS (1999), Cardiovascular risk factors. Clustering features of insulin resistance syndrome (Syndrome S) in a biracial (Black–White) population of children, adolescents, and young adults: The Bogalusa Heart Study, *Am J Epidemiol*, 150, 667–674.

Cole TJ, Bellizzi MC, Flegal M and Dietz WH (2000), Establishing a standard definition for child overweight and obesity worldwide: International survey, *British Medical Journal*, 320, 1240–1243.

Coon KA and Tucker KL (2002), Television and children's consumption patterns. A review of the literature, *Minerva Pediatr* 54, 423–436.

Csabi G, Torok K, Jeges S and Molnar D (2000), Presence of metabolic cardiovascular syndrome in obese children, *Eur J Pediatr*, 159, 91–94.

Daniels SR, Arnett DK, Eckel RH, Gidding SS, Hayman LL, Kumanyika S, Robinson TN, Scott BJ, St Jeor S and Williams CL (2005), Overweight in children and adolescents: Pathophysiology, consequences, prevention, and treatment, *Circulation*, 111, 1999–2012.

Drewnowski A and Specter SE (2004), Poverty and obesity: The role of energy density and energy costs, *Am J Clin Nutr*, 79, 6–16.

Dubnov-Raz G, Berry EM and Constantini NW (2009), Childhood obesity – assessment, prevention and treatment, *Harefuah*, 148, 831–836.

Edwards KL, Clarke GP, Ransley JK and Cade J (2010), The neighbourhood matters: Studying exposures relevant to childhood obesity and the policy implications in Leeds, UK, *J Epidemiol Community Health*, Mar, 64(3), 194–201.

Eriksson JG, Forsen T, Tuomilehto J, Osmond C and Barker DJ (2003), Early adiposity rebound in childhood and risk of Type 2 diabetes in adult life, *Diabetología*, 46, 190–4.

Ferguson MA, Gutin B, Owens S, Litaker M, Tracy RP and Allison J (1998), Fat distribution and hemostatic measures in obese children, *Am J Clin Nutr*, 67, 1136–1140.

Fisberg M, Baur L, Chen W, Hoppin A, Koletzko B, Lau D, Moreno L, Nelson T, Strauss R, Uauy R and Latin American Society for Pediatric Gastroenterology, Hepatology, and Nutrition (2004), Obesity in Children and Adolescents: Working Group Report of the Second World Congress of Pediatric Gastroenterology, Hepatology, and Nutrition, *J Pediatr Gastroenterol Nutr*, 39, S678–S687.

Flodmark CE, Lissau I, Moreno LA, Pietrobelli A and Widhalm K (2004), New insights into the field of children's and adolescents' obesity: The European perspective, *Int J Obes*, 28,1189–1196.

Ford ES, Galuska DA, Gillespie C, Will JC, Giles WH and Dietz WH (2001), C-reactive protein and body mass index in children: Findings from the Third National Health and Nutrition Examination Survey, 1988-1994, *J Pediatr*, 138, 486–492.

Forshee RA, Anderson PA and Storey ML (2008), Sugar-sweetened beverages and body mass index in children and adolescents: A meta-analysis, *Am J Clin Nutr*, 87, 1662–1671.

Friedman RR and Schwartz MB (2008), Public policy to prevent childhood obesity, and the role of pediatric endocrinologists, *J Pediatr Endocrinol Metab*, 21, 717–725.

Gillman MW, Rifas-Shiman SL, Camargo CA Jr, Berkey CS, Frazier AL, Rockett HR, Field AE and Colditz GA (2001), Risk of overweight among adolescents who were breastfed as infants, *JAMA*, 285, 2461–2467.

Goris JM, Petersen S, Stamatakis E and Veerman JL (2009), Television food advertising and the prevalence of childhood overweight and obesity: A multicountry comparison, *Public Health Nutr*, 17, 1–10.

Grüters A, Wiegand S and Krude H (2002), Gene, fast food and no motion. Causes of childhood obesity, *MMW Fortschr Med*, 144, 34–36.

Guillaume M, Lapidus L and Lambert A (1998), Obesity and nutrition in children. The Belgian Luxembourg child study IV, *Eur J Clin Nutr*, 52, 323–328.

Gunther A L, Buyken A E and Kroke A (2007), Protein intake during the period of complementary feeding and early childhood and the association with body mass index and percentage body fat at 7 year of age, *Am J Clin Nutr*, 85, 1626–1633.

Harder T, Bergmann R, Kallischnigg G and Plagemann A (2005), Duration of breastfeeding and risk of overweight: A meta-analysis, *Am J Epidemiol*, 162, 397–403.

Hedley AA, Ogden CL, Johnson CL, Carroll MD, Curtin LR and Flegal KM (2004), Prevalence of overweight and obesity among US children, adolescents, and adults, 1999-2002, *JAMA*, 291, 2847–2850.

Heinig MJ, Nommsen LA, Peerson JM, Lonnerdal B and Dewey KG (1993), Energy and protein intakes of breast-fed and formula-fed infants during the first year of life and their association with growth velocity: The DARLING Study, *Am J Clin Nutr*, 58, 152–161.

Hotamisligil GS, Shargill NS and Spiegelman BM (1993), Adipose expression of tumor necrosis factor-alpha: Direct role in obesity-linked insulin resistance, *Science*, 259, 87–91.

James J and Kerr D (2005), Prevention of childhood obesity by reducing soft drinks, *Int J Obes (Lond)*, 29 (Suppl 2), S54–57.

Juhan-Vague I, Alessi MC and Vague P (1991), Increased plasma plasminogen activator inhibitor 1 levels: A possible link between insulin resistance and atherothrombosis, *Diabetologia*, 34, 457–462.

Kang H, Greenson JK, Omo JT, Chao C, Peterman D, Anderson L, Foess-Wood L, Sherbondy MA and Conjeevaram HS (2006), Metabolic syndrome is associated with greater histologic severity, higher carbohydrate, and lower fat diet in patients with NAFLD, *Am J Gastroenterol*, 101, 2247–2253.

Libuda L and Kersting M (2009), Soft drinks and body weight development in childhood: Is there a relationship?, *Curr Opin Clin Nutr Metab Care*, 12, 596–600.

Lissau I (2004), Overweight and obesity epidemic among children: Answer from European countries, *Int J Obes*, 28 (Suppl), S10–S15.

Lobstein T and Dibb S (2005), Evidence of a possible link between obesogenic food advertising and child overweight, *Obes Rev*, 6, 203–208.

Ludwig DS, Peterson KE and Gortmaker SL (2001), Relation between consumption of sugar-sweetened drinks and childhood obesity: A prospective, observational analysis, *Lancet*, 357, 505–508.

Lundgren CH, Brown SL, Nordt TK, Sobel BE and Fujii S (1996), Elaboration of type-1 plasminogen activator inhibitor from adipocytes. A potential pathogenetic link between obesity and cardiovascular disease, *Circulation*, 93, 106–110.

Maffeis C, Talamini G and Tato L (1998), Influence of diet, physical activity and parents' obesity on children's adiposity: A four-year longitudinal study, *In J Obes*, 22, 758–764.

Maffeis C, Pietrobelli A, Grezzani A, Provera S and Tatò L (2001), Waist circumference and cardiovascular risk factors in prepubertal children, *Obes Res*, 9, 179–187.

Magarey AM, Daniels LA, Boulton TJ and Cockington RA (2003), Does fat intake predict adiposity in healthy children and adolescents aged 2–15 y? A longitudinal analysis, *Eur J Clin Nutr*, 55, 471–481.

Marr L (2004), Soft drinks, childhood overweight, and the role of nutrition educators: Let's base our solutions on reality and sound science, *J Nutr Educ Behav*, 36, 258–265.

McCaffrey TA, Rennie KL, Kerr MA, Wallace JM, Hannon-Fletcher MP, Coward WA, Jebb SA and Livingstone MB (2008), Energy density of the diet and change in body fatness from childhood to adolescence; Is there a relation?, *Am J Clin Nutr*, 87, 1230–1237.

Mohamed-Ali V, Goodrick S, Rawesh A, Katz DR, Miles JM, Yudkin JS, Klein S and Coppack SW (1997), Subcutaneous adipose tissue releases interleukin-6, but not tumor necrosis factor-alpha, *in vivo*, *J Clin Endocrinol Metab*, 82, 4196–4200.

Moreno LA, Sarría A, Fleta J, Rodríguez G and Bueno M (2000), Trends in body mass index and overweight prevalence among children and adolescents in the region of Aragón (Spain) from 1985 to 1995, *International Journal of Obesity*, 24, 925–931.

Moreno LA, Fleta J, Sarría A, Rodríguez G and Bueno M (2001a), Secular increases in body fat percentage in male children of Zaragoza, Spain, 1980–1995, *Prev Med*, 33, 357–363.

Moreno LA, Fleta J, Sarría A, Rodríguez G, Gil C and Bueno M (2001b), Secular changes in body fat patterning in children and adolescents of Zaragoza (Spain), 1980–1995, *Int J Obes*, 25, 1656–1660.

Moreno LA, Pineda I, Rodríguez G, Fleta J, Sarría A and Bueno M (2002a), Waist circumference for the screening of the metabolic syndrome in children, *Acta Paediatr*, 91, 1307–1312.

Moreno LA, Pineda I, Rodríguez G, Fleta J, Giner A, Juste MG, Sarría A and Bueno M (2002b), Leptin and the metabolic syndrome in obese and non-obese children, *Horm Metab Res*, 34, 394–399.

Moreno LA, Tomás C, González-Gross M, Bueno G, Pérez-González JM and Bueno M (2004), Micro-environmental and socio-demographic determinants of childhood obesity, *Int J Obes Relat Metab Disord*, 28 (Suppl 3), S16–S20.

Moreno LA, Mesana MI, Fleta J, Ruiz JR, González-Gross MM, Sarría A, Marcos A, Bueno M and the AVENA Study Group (2005a), Overweight, obesity and body fat composition in Spanish adolescents. The AVENA Study, *Ann Nutr Metab*, 49, 71–76.

Moreno LA, Sarría A, Fleta J, Marcos A and Bueno M (2005b), Secular trends in waist circumference in Spanish adolescents, 1995 to 2000–02, *Arch Dis Child*, 90: 818–819.

Moreno LA and Rodriguez G (2007), Dietary risk factors for development of childhood obesity, *Curr Opin Clin Nutr Metab Care*, 10, 336–341.

Must A, Dallal GE and Dietz WH (1991), Reference data for obesity: 85th and 95th percentiles of body mass index (wt/ht^2) and triceps skinfold thickness, *American Journal of Clinical Nutrition*, 53, 839–846.

Niemeier HM, Raynor HA, Lloyd-Richardson EE, Rogers ML and Wing RR (2006), Fast food consumption and breakfast skipping: Predictors of weight gain from adolescence to adulthood in a nationally representative sample, *J Adolesc Health*, 39, 842–849.

Ogden CL, Carroll MD and Flegal KM (2008), High body mass index for age among US children and adolescents, 2003–2006, *JAMA*, 299, 2401–2405.

Olsen NJ and Heitmann BL (2009), Intake of calorically sweetened beverages and obesity, *Obes Rev*, 10: 68–75.

Ong KK, Emmett PM, Noble S, Ness A, Dunger DB and ALSPAC Study Team (2006), Dietary energy intake at the age of 4 months predicts postnatal weight gain and childhood body mass index, *Pediatrics*, 117, e503–508.

Owen CG, Martin RM, Whincup PH, Smith GD and Cook DG (2005), Effect of infant feeding on the risk of obesity across the life course: a quantitative review of published evidence, *Pediatrics*, 115, 1367–1377.

Péneau S, Salanave B, Maillard-Teyssier L, Rolland-Cachera MF, Vergnaud AC, Méjean C, Czernichow S, Vol S, Tichet J, Castetbon K, *et al.* (2009), Prevalence of overweight in 6- to 15-year-old children in central/western France from 1996 to 2006: Trends toward stabilization. *Int J Obes (Lond)*, 33, 401–407.

Rodriguez G, Moreno LA, Blay MG, Blay VA, Garagorri JM, Sarria A and Bueno M (2004), Body composition in adolescents: Measurements and metabolic aspects, *Int J Obes*, 28 (Suppl 3), S54–8.

Rodriguez G and Moreno LA (2006), Is dietary intake able to explain differences in body fatness in children and adolescents? *Nutr Metab Cardiovasc Dis*, 16, 294–301.

Savva SC, Tornaritis M, Savva ME, Kourides Y, Panagi A, Silikiotou N, Georgiotou C and Kafatos A (2000), Waist circumference and waist-to-height ratio are better predictors of cardiovascular disease risk factors in children than body mass index, *Int J Obes*, 24, 1453–1458.

Scaglioni S, Agostoni C, Notaris RD, Radaelli G, Radice N, Valenti M, Giovannini M and Riva E (2000), Early macronutrient intake and overweight at five years of age *Int J Obes*, 24, 777–781.

Schwimmer JB, Deutsch R, Kahen T, Lavine JE, Stanley C and Behling C (2006), Prevalence of fatty liver in children and adolescents, *Pediatrics*, 118, 1388–1393.

Seidell JC (1999), Prevention of obesity: The role of the food industry, *Nutr Metab Cardiovasc Dis*, 9, 45–50.

Sen B (2006), Frequency of family dinner and adolescent body weight status: Evidence from the national longitudinal survey of youth, 1997, *Obesity*, 14, 2266–2276.

Serra L, Ribas L, Aranceta J, Pérez C, Saavedra P and Peña L (2003), Childhood and adolescent obesity in Spain. Results of the enKid study (1998–2000), *Med Clin (Barc)*, 121, 725–732.

Skinner JD, Bounds W, Carruth BR, Morris M and Ziegler P (2004), Predictors of children's body mass index: A longitudinal study of diet and growth in children aged 2–8 y, *Int J Obes Relat Metab Disord*, 28, 476–482.

Stettler N, Zemel BS, Kumanyika S and Stallings VA (2002), Infant weight gain and childhood overweight in a multicenter, cohort study, *Pediatrics*, 109, 194–199.

Sugarman SD and Sandman N (2007), Fighting childhood obesity through performance-based regulation of the food industry, *Duke Law J* 56, 1403–1490.

Sundblom E, Petzold M, Rasmussen F, Callmer E and Lissner L (2008), Childhood overweight and obesity prevalences levelling off in Stockholm but socioeconomic differences persist, *Int J Obes (Lond)*, 32, 1525–1530.

Toschke AM, Kuchenhoff H, Koletzko B and von Kries R (2005), Meal frequency and childhood obesity, *Obes Res*, 13, 1932–1938.

Tresaco B, Moreno LA, Ruiz JR, Ortega FB, Bueno G, González-Gross M, Wärnberg J, Gutiérrez A, García-Fuentes M, Marcos A, Castillo MJ, Bueno M and AVENA Study Group (2009), Truncal and abdominal fat as determinants of high triglycerides and low HDL-cholesterol in adolescents, *Obesity (Silver Spring)*, 17, 1086–91.

Valle M, Gascón F, Martos R, Ruiz FJ, Bermudo F, Ríos R and Cañete R (2000), Infantile obesity: A situation of atherothrombotic risk? *Metabolism*, 49, 672–675.

Vanhala MJ, Vanhala PT, Keinanen-Kiukaanniemi SM, Kumpusalo EA and Takala JK (1999), Relative weight gain and obesity as a child predict metabolic syndrome as an adult, *Int J Obes*, 23, 656–659.

Veerman JL, Van Beeck EF, Barendregt JJ and Mackenbach JP (2009), By how much would limiting TV food advertising reduce childhood obesity? *Eur J Public Health*, 19, 365–369.

Verduin P, Agarwal S and Waltman S (2005), Solutions to obesity: Perspectives from the food industry, *Am J Clin Nutr*, 82 (1 Suppl), 259S–261S.

Veugelers PJ and Fitzgerald AL (2005), Prevalence of and risk factors for childhood overweight and obesity, *CMAJ*, 173, 607–613.

Wang Y and Lobstein T (2006), Worldwide Trends in Childhood Obesity, *Int J Pediatr Obes* 1, 11–25.

Wang YC, Gortmaker SL, Sobol AM and Kuntz KM (2006), Estimating the energy gap among US children: A counterfactual approach, *Pediatrics*, 118, e1721–33.

Wärnberg J, Moreno LA, Mesana MI, Marcos A and the AVENA group (2004), Inflamatory mediators in overweight and obese Spanish adolescents. The AVENA Study, *Int J Obes Relat Metab Disord*, 28, S59–63.

Weiss S, Dufour S, Taksali SE, Tamborlane WV, Petersen KF, Bonadona RC, Boseli L, Barbetta G, Allen K, Rife F, Savoye M, Dziura J, Sherwin R, Shulman GI and Caprio S (2003), Prediabetes in obese youth: A syndrome of impaired glucose tolerance, severe insulin resistance, and altered myocellular and abdominal fat partitioning, *Lancet*, 362, 951–957.

4

Diet, behaviour and cognition in children

D. Benton, University of Swansea, UK

Abstract: Both the structural components of the brain and the energy it uses to function come from the diet. The possibility that a child's behaviour and cognition may be influenced by what is eaten while the brain is initially developing has therefore attracted attention: nutritional deficiencies, for example an early shortage of iodine, zinc or iron, permanently decrease cognitive ability. In addition, by serving as coenzymes or as a constituent of important molecules, micronutrients influence general metabolism. A series of trials have found that micronutrient supplementation improved both behaviour and cognition, although the details are not as yet clear. Finally, there are reports that the macronutrient composition of meals influences the cognition of children, possibly reflecting the rate at which glucose is released into the blood-stream.

Key words: cognition, behaviour, essential fatty acids, micronutients, glycaemic load.

4.1 Introduction

The human brain develops rapidly towards the end of pregnancy and during the following two years. At birth, the brain represents about 10% of body weight, although in the adult it is only 2%. By the age of two, the brain is about 80% of its final weight (Dekaban and Sadowsky, 1978). A question that arises during this period of rapid growth is whether the demands placed on the diet can be too great, with adverse consequences for brain development. If nutrition is inadequate during brain growth, is there permanent damage with implications for cognitive functioning throughout life? Although without any doubt the period before and after birth is important, the brain's development continues beyond this stage, although the impact of dietary status has been little explored. After reviewing the evidence, Epstein (1986) concluded that there are periods of rapid brain growth around seven, eleven and fifteen years of age.

That even in industrialized countries the nature of diet during early life is important is illustrated by a unique study that related early dietary status to cognition in later life. Lucas *et al.* (1990) took advantage of the fact that premature infants are fed initially by a nasogastric tube. Randomly, children consumed a traditional cows-milk based formula or one enriched with protein, vitamins and minerals. The enriched formula was associated at eighteen months with greater social and psycho-motor development. By eight years, the enriched formula led to higher verbal intelligence scores in boys but not the girls (Lucas *et al.*, 1998). At fifteen years of age, the boys who had received the enriched formula had a larger caudate nucleus as measured using MRI, and still displayed higher verbal intelligence (Isaacs *et al.*, 2008). This study produced strong evidence that even in industrialized countries, relatively small differences in early nutrition can have long-term consequences. The boys fed the enriched standard formula for a median duration of four weeks had a 12.2 point advantage in intelligence at eight years (Lucas *et al.*, 1998). This study does little more than prove, in principle, that small differences in diet for short periods of time can have long-term consequences. The enriched diet was, however, no more than a best guess and we have no way of knowing the active ingredients and the optimal dose. With full-term infants whose brains will be more developed, the impact of diet may be different.

In addition to influencing periods of brain growth, dietary factors influence all aspects of bodily functioning. A major function of the vitamins is to serve as cofactors for enzymatic reactions and, in this way, metabolism in general is affected. Thus, vitamins are required for the formation of hormones, blood cells and most of the chemicals in the body. Micro-nutrients are also constituents of particular molecules; for example, iron is necessary to form haemoglobin and iodine to create thyroid hormones. Therefore potentially short-term micronutrient deficiencies in later life can have reversible consequences for the functioning of the brain as well as for the rest of the body.

The brain is the most metabolically active organ in the body, yet it has very limited stores of energy and it cannot reduce its needs if energy supplies are low. The brain is unusual in that, unless you have starved, or have eaten a diet devoid of carbohydrate for several days, it does not metabolize ketones and normally almost exclusively uses glucose as its source of energy. As without replacement the glucose in the brain would last about ten minutes, it needs a continuous supply (Benton, 2005). Although studied to only a limited degree, there are suggestions that the patterning of meals and the rate at which glucose is released into the blood stream may influence the cognition of children (Benton *et al.*, 2007).

It is clear that the above agenda lists many ways in which diet can potentially influence the cognition and behaviour of children. To fully consider this range of topics would demand several books, so a single chapter can offer no more than a brief overview. The approach taken is to outline the findings in a series of areas, quoting both in the text, and in the sources of further information section, review articles that will allow the reader to go further.

4.2 Essential fatty acids in children's diets

The dry weight of the brain is about 60% lipid: a figure that is higher in nerve cells where it represents 80%. More specifically, the n-3 (omega-3) fatty acid docosahexaenoic acid (DHA) accounts for about 20% of the brain's mass. DHA, along with the n-6 (omega-6) fatty acid arachidonic acid (AA), is the major long chain poly-unsaturated fatty acids (LCPUFA) in the nervous system. n-3 and n-6 fatty acids are described as essential fatty acids because the body is not able to make them: that is why they should be part of the diet.

Fatty acids fulfil various functions, including playing an important structural role in cell membranes where the presence of unsaturated rather than saturated fatty acids is associated with a more fluid membrane, so that communication both from and to the cell is facilitated (Bourre, 2006). The phospholipids that play a structural role in cell membranes consist of two fatty acids linked to a phosphate group. Prostaglandins are messengers derived from fatty acids that act at many sites. However, although they have potent effects, these influences are local as they have a short half-life. Amongst other effects, prostaglandins can sensitize spinal neurones to pain; influence the inflammatory process; regulate the movement of calcium; and control the growth of cells. Similarly, leukotrienes are metabolized from AA and one role is to help to sustain inflammatory reactions; another is to increase vascular permeability, in this way increasing the passage of small molecules in and out of blood vessels.

4.2.1 Long chain poly-unsaturated fatty acids and cognitive development

The human brain develops faster than other organs, particularly in the last third of pregnancy and the first two years of life. Clearly, such rapid growth places great demands on the diet to supply the nutrients required for brain growth. During the final third of pregnancy, the mother is transferring to the child the fatty acids required for brain development, the nature of which will depend on her diet. Given this context, it is natural that the possibility of a limited supply of fatty acids having long-term implications for brain development has attracted attention. The importance of LCPUFA in the nutrition of the young child has resulted in them being added to infant formula, but is there evidence of lasting benefits, even though, unlike a traditional cow's milk based formula, human milk contains LCPUFA? The level of DHA in human milk is 0.32% of total fatty acids, with 0.47% being the comparable figure for AA. Traditionally, formula-fed infants had to rely on the conversion of the dietary essential fatty α-linolenic acid to DHA, and the conversion of the essential fatty acid linoleic acid to AA. Consequently, post-mortem examination of the cortex of the brain has found less DHA in formula-fed rather than breast-fed infants (Hoffman *et al.*, 2009).

The many reports that the offspring of mothers who breast feed perform better on intelligence tests has led to speculation that the LCPUFA in the milk may be responsible. Such studies are, however, difficult to interpret as the decision to breast feed is associated with more affluent and better educated mothers, so socio-cultural differences may be influential. Der *et al.* (2006) considered the impact of a range of potential confounding variables on the effect of breast feeding on cognitive ability. The intelligence of the mother was the factor most predictive of the decision to breast feed. Although having been breast fed was associated with a four IQ points advantage, when the intelligence of the mother was taken into account, the form of infant feeding had 'little or no effect on intelligence'. The situation may, however, be complex as Caspi *et al.* (2007) reported that the effect of breastfeeding on intellectual development was moderated by a gene involved in the control of fatty acid metabolism.

Given the large effect of psycho-social correlates of the decision to breast feed, randomized trials are helpful as confounding factors should be, on average, similar, irrespective of the type of feeding. In Belarussia, 13 889 healthy breastfeeding infants were followed up at six and a half years of age (Kramer *et al.*, 2008). The offspring of mothers who were randomly chosen to take part in a breast feeding initiative had full scale intelligence scores 5.9 points greater than those who had been bottle fed. The teacher's assessments of both reading and writing skills were also significantly higher. A problem with this study is that some assessments were not carried out blind. It is also not possible to distinguish the role played by LCPUFA in the human milk as opposed to other factors, such the transfer or hormones and anti-bodies from the mother and the social and psychological consequences of breast feeding.

A more certain way of establishing a role for LCPUFA is to randomly allocate infants to formula feeds to which they have and have not been added. In such studies, it is reasonable to suggest that the impact of LCPUFA will be greater in pre-term infants as the brain will be at an earlier developmental stage. Therefore, the Cochrane review of the influence of adding LCPUFA to the formula feeds of preterm infants is instructive (Simmer *et al.*, 2008). As there are high levels of DHA in the retina, attention has been directed to the development of visual acuity. The review concluded that most studies had found that supplementation did not significantly influence vision. Similarly, the meta-analysis of the Bayley Scales of Infant Development, when used at either twelve or twenty-four months, found no significant effect on the rate of development. These authors concluded that, although the studies had tended to use relatively mature and healthy preterm infants, there was no evidence of long-term benefits when a formula feed was supplemented with LCPUFA. Smithers *et al.* (2008) similarly concluded that, to date, the studies of LCPUFA supplementation of premature infants had not found an increased performance on the Bayley Scales of Infant Development, although they recommended further research on the topic.

The stage of brain development may, however, be significant. It is interesting that Eilander *et al.* (2007) suggested that there was a beneficial effect of giving n-3 LCPUFA supplements to mothers during pregnancy and lactation, in so much that cognitive development had been found to benefit, although vision was not influenced. It may be that whether LCPUFAs are supplied as a constituent of human rather than cow's milk is important. More recently, Helland *et al.* (2008) gave mothers cod liver oil or corn oil from the eighteenth week of pregnancy until twelve weeks after birth, but did not find differences in cognitive development when the children were seven years old. However, the concentrations of alpha-linolenic acid (18:3n-3) and DHA during pregnancy correlated with the child's ability to perform sequential processing when seven years old. The authors concluded that the maternal concentration of n-3 LCPUFA during pregnancy might be of importance for some aspects of later cognitive functioning, although they observed no significant effect of n-3 fatty acid intervention on global measures of intelligence.

Hadders-Algra *et al.* (2007) concluded that when term infants were supplemented with LCPUFA, in particular if the DHA represented at least 0.30 % of total milk fat, there was a beneficial effect on neuro-developmental outcomes until four months of age. However, beyond that age, a consistent influence has not been demonstrated. Hoffman *et al.* (2009) specifically reviewed the influence of dietary supplementation of term infants with LCPUFA and found a number of studies had reported a positive correlation between the levels of blood DHA and cognitive or visual functioning. However, randomized trials had reported mixed findings, although they suggested that 'formulas providing close to the worldwide human milk mean of 0.32% DHA were more likely to yield functional benefits'. This review also pointed to evidence suggesting that a ratio of AA to DHA that is greater than one to one resulted in cognitive improvement.

It may well be that future research should systematically consider both the absolute and relative amount of n-3 and n-6 fatty acids in the diet. In fact Fleith and Clandinin (2005) concluded that the blood levels of fatty acids were more similar to breast-fed babies if formula-fed infants were supplemented with both n-3 and n-6 LCPUFA. They found, however, that less than half of studies had reported a significant effect of LCPUFA supplementation on measures of cognitive development. The view of Eilander *et al.* (2007) was that the evidence that n-3 LCPUFA supplementation helped the cognitive development of children of more than two years was too limited to allow a conclusion.

In summary, those reviewing the area have tended to conclude that the consumption of LCPUFA is important for infant development although the evidence that supplementation is beneficial is equivocal (Fleith *et al.*, 2005). Eilander *et al.* (2007) concluded that 'the evidence for potential benefits of LCPUFA supplementation is promising but yet inconclusive'. Hadders-Algra *et al.* (2007) concluded that the effects of supplementation were subtle and depended both on the dose and the gestational stage when it was supplied.

4.3 Vitamins and minerals in children's diets

4.3.1 Iodine

Thyroid hormones are essential for the metabolism of all cells and play an important role in the growth of most organs; more specifically the development of the brain. From a nutrition perspective, the trace element iodine is needed for synthesis of thyroid hormones. A lack of iodine during the end of the first third and the beginning of the second third of pregnancy can result in Iodine Deficiency Disorder (congenital hypothyroidism; cretinism), with a long-term marked reduction in intellectual ability. However, many of those affected will have few symptoms, particularly if thyroid hormone production is only mildly reduced. There is, however, even in those who appear normal, reduced cognitive ability. In China, a 10 to 15 IQ point deficit has been reported in areas of severe iodine deficiency, even in those who appear normal (Tai, 1997). In Europe, Zimmermann and Delange (2004) found that although 'most women in Europe are iodine deficient during pregnancy, less than 50% receive supplementation with iodine', but the implications of a mild deficiency are unclear as the topic has not been studied (Zimmermann, 2007).

The evidence of the influence of an iodine deficiency in later life is even more limited, although the supplementation of iodine-deficient children in Albania was reported to improve various measures of cognition and motor skill (Zimmermann *et al.*, 2006).

4.3.2 Iron

Throughout the world, an inadequate intake of iron occurs commonly, potentially resulting in iron-deficit anaemia that is associated with a poor mood, tiredness and problems of memory and attention. The World Health Organization (2008) concluded that anaemia is a public health problem for pregnant women and preschool-age children in all member states. They estimated that, in the majority of their member states, there was a moderate-to-severe public problem. That a problem can exist in industrialized countries was demonstrated by the findings of Aukett *et al.* (1986), who found in the United Kingdom that eighteen month old children who received iron supplements, in a double-blind trial, had a greater than expected psychomotor development.

There is general agreement that in terms of child development, the age at which iron deficiency occurs is critical. If iron deficiency occurs in the first years of life, problems of cognition will persist into later life, even when the subsequent iron consumption is adequate. In contrast, although a deficiency at a later stage causes problems in the short-term, they will be overcome if the diet improves (Beard and Connor, 2003; Lozoff, 2007). Animal studies find that an iron deficiency during the critical early stage of brain development has a lasting influence on the myelination of neurones and dopamine metabolism (Lozoff, 2007).

4.3.3 Zinc

Similarly to iron, it has been estimated that 20% of the world's population have a deficient zinc intake (Maret and Sandstead, 2008). Also like iron, the influence of zinc on development depends on the age of the child. Animal studies find that a deficiency in late pregnancy impairs neuronal replication and synaptogenesis, and that learning and memory are poorer in later life (Tahmasebi Boroujeni *et al.*, 2008).

Preterm human infants, in particular, benefit from supplementation. In a Canadian study, the consumption by low birth-weight babies of a baby formula with added zinc resulted in faster growth and better motor development (Friel *et al.*, 1993). At older ages, there is less evidence that supplementation benefits cognition. Again in Canada, zinc supplementation at five to seven years of age did not influence attention although it was suggested that those with poor zinc status grew more quickly (Gibson *et al.*, 1989). The first report that supplementation improved cognition studied Chinese children aged six to nine years (Penland *et al.*, 1997). A combination of zinc and other micronutrients had the greatest impact on cognition; zinc alone was the least influential and the micronutrients alone had an intermediate effect.

4.3.4 Folic acid and vitamin B_{12}

Folate and vitamin B_{12} metabolism are closely associated. Women who are intending to become pregnant are encouraged to consume folic acid to prevent neural tube defects (Pitkin, 2007). Folate status is important for brain development as it influences nucleotide synthesis, DNA integrity and transcription (Reynolds, 2006).

A vegan diet can potentially cause developmental problems as only animal products offer significant amounts of vitamin B_{12}, although milk, cheese and eggs offer a source for the vegetarian. Major functions of this nutrient include a role in red blood cell formation, the synthesis of DNA, and the maintenance of a healthy nervous system. Vitamin B_{12} deficiency results in pernicious anaemia, with associated fatigue. As the vitamin has a role in fatty acid metabolism, its absence is associated with damage to the myelin sheath and thus a deficiency may result in irreversible brain damage. A review of the effects of vitamin B_{12} deficiency in infancy found a pattern of irritability, anorexia and developmental delay (Graham *et al.*, 1992). Louwman *et al.* (2000) considered the cognitive functioning of adolescents who had consumed a vegan diet up to six years of age, but subsequently consumed a vegetarian or omnivorous diet. An early deficiency of vitamin B_{12} deficiency was associated with poorer fluid intelligence when adolescence was reached.

4.3.5 Multi-vitamins and minerals

As a poor diet is likely to offer an inadequate intake of many nutrients, it is arguable that, rather than concentrating on a single nutrient, a multi-vitamin/mineral supplement is more likely to beneficial. There are two topics where double-blind placebo controlled trials in industrialized countries have reported a positive response: the study of intelligence and the examination of violent behaviour.

Benton and Roberts (1988), in a randomized double-blind trial, gave 12- and 13-year-old children a multi-vitamin/mineral supplement or a placebo. After eight months, whereas verbal intelligence was not affected, non-verbal intelligence scores had increased significantly. When the subsequent studies (that this finding stimulated) were reviewed, 10 out of 13 reported a positive response in at least a sub-group of children (Benton, 2001). That the response was always with non-verbal and never with verbal measures of intelligence suggested a genuine phenomenon. Non-verbal measures are thought to assess biological potential. Logically, micronutrient supplementation can influence only biology and, at least in the short-term, will not increase the information required to enhance the performance of verbally-based tests.

In Australia and Indonesia, Osendarp *et al.* (2007) gave a multi-vitamin/mineral supplement, with or without omega-3 fatty acids, for a year. In Indonesian girls, and Australian boys and girls the supplement improved verbal learning, although intelligence was not affected. In contrast, the fatty acid supplement was without effect. The study concluded that 'in well-nourished school-aged children, fortification with multiple micronutrients can result in improvements in verbal learning and memory.'

Benton (2001) concluded that this topic was at an early stage and there was a need for large-scale trials that considered the composition of the supplement and the dietary styles of the children. There was no suggestion that all children responded; rather it was suggested that only those who were poorly nourished respond to supplementation.

The study of anti-social behaviour is a second characteristic that has been suggested to respond to micronutrient supplementation. In a well-designed study of young offenders, Gesch *et al.* (2002) found that the disciplinary record benefited from micronutrient supplementation: in particular, the instances of more serious violent offences decreased. Although it is unclear whether the response in this study was to vitamins, minerals or fatty acids, there are reports of similar effects when only vitamin and mineral supplements were administered (Schoenthaler *et al.*, 1997). A role for fatty acids cannot, however, be excluded, as Benton (2007), in a meta-analysis of eight studies, found that DHA decreased aggressive behaviour. Benton (2007) discussed three well-designed studies that had all reported that micronutrient supplementation resulted in a decline in anti-social behaviour. In addition, the Dutch Government replicated the Gesch *et al.* (2002) findings by giving young prisoners micronutrient supplements for three months. Taking the supplements decreased violence 34% whereas the rate in those who received the placebo increased by 13% (Zaalberg *et al.*, 2010).

This series of similar findings, obtained in three countries by three different research groups, suggests a robust phenomenon although we have not begun to establish the active ingredients or the underlying mechanism.

4.4 Behavioural problems in children resulting from diet

A number of studies have considered the influence of food intolerance on Attention Deficit Hyperactivity Disorder (ADHD). An example is Egger *et al.* (1985), who introduced children with the hyperkinetic syndrome to an oligoantigenic diet (a few foods chosen because they were unlikely to produce an adverse response). Additional foods were then reintroduced and retained if they caused no reaction. Critically, if there was an adverse reaction, these foods were tested using a double-blind procedure by creating two similar meals, only one of which contained the problematic item. Nearly fifty foods were found to which at least one child responded, although the most common problems were associated with cow's milk (64% of children), chocolate (59%), grapes (49%), wheat (49%) and oranges (45%). Benton (2007) considered the findings of five such double-blind studies and integrated the results using meta-analysis. When the placebo rather than the test meal was consumed, there were significantly fewer symptoms of hyperactivity. It should be remembered that these findings were obtained with children with ADHD-related symptoms whose parents prior to the study suspected an adverse reaction to diet. As such, the findings are unlikely to generalize either to all children with ADHD or to children without a history of behavioural problems.

4.4.1 Sucrose

There is a common misconception that high sugar consumption is associated with hyperactivity and other behavioural problems of childhood. There are, however, few topics that have been subject to more systematic study in double-blind randomized trials. For example, children have been challenged by asking them to consume drinks that either do or do not contain sugar. A meta-analysis of such trials concluded that sugar consumption does not adversely influence the behaviour of children (Benton, 2008a), irrespective of whether they had been diagnosed with ADHD. However, although there is clearly no general reaction to sucrose, it is logically impossible to exclude the chance that there is a small subset that reacts adversely. In fact the examination of food intolerance supports such a view. Egger *et al.* (1985) found that 16% of a sample of hyperkinetic children, whose parents believed that they react to food, in fact responded to sugar. However, it should be remembered that there were nearly 50 foods to which at least one child responded and there were 13 other foods that were more commonly a problem than sucrose. In addition, there were few children who responded to only one food item.

Benton (2008a) discussed various mechanisms by which sucrose might conceivably influence behaviour. Although he found that a tendency to develop low blood glucose levels was associated with irritability and violence (not low enough that they can be described clinically as hypoglycaemic), sucrose is not the predominant cause of swings in blood glucose levels. Similarly, although there are several reports that micronutrient supplementation decreases anti-social behaviour, there was little evidence that sucrose intake resulted in a low micronutrient status. It was argued that sugar consumption is not a major cause of food intolerance, hypoglycaemia or micronutrient deficiency.

4.4.2 Additives

The Egger *et al.* (1985) study of food intolerance found that the artificial colourant tartrazine and the preservative sodium benzoate more commonly induced an adverse response than any particular food. Recent reviewers of the topic have concluded that additives can adversely affect children. Schab and Trinh (2004) considered fifteen trials in a meta-analysis and concluded that the administration of additives in well-designed trials caused behavioural problems. They concluded, however, that those trials that had examined children whose parents believed that they responded to additives demonstrated the greatest response. It is therefore important to distinguish the reaction of the general population, from a reaction in a self-selected group of children whose parents had reason previously to believe that they responded to additives.

In this context, Bateman *et al.* (2004) distinguished groups of children who displayed high and low symptoms of hyperactivity and a high and low tendency to develop allergic reactions. A reaction to a cocktail of additives, as judged by parental ratings, was found in all groups of children, irrespective of whether they initially displayed hyperactive symptoms or whether there was a pre-existing allergic tendency. The reaction was to a cocktail including the artificial colours sunset yellow, tartrazine, carmoisine, ponceau, and the preservative sodium benzoate. It is unclear whether the reaction was to one, a few, or all of these substances, and to what extent there might have been synergistic interactions such that several might need to be consumed together to induce a reaction. Importantly, the finding was subsequently replicated. McCann *et al.* (2007) found an adverse reaction in three and eight/nine year old children, the first study to consider a non-clinical community-based sample. The colours studied were tartrazine, quinoline yellow, sunset yellow, carmoisine, ponceau 4R and allura red. As a result of this study, the United Kingdom Government proposed the voluntary removal of these substances by food manufacturers by the end of 2009. However, when the European Food Standards Agency reviewed the topic, they found the findings to be inconclusive.

There are several thousand additives that are added to diet for one reason or another, and only a small minority have been considered as potentially inducing adverse behavioural reactions. Some have contrasted artificial from 'natural' substances, with the implication that the latter are safe. As some of the most poisonous substances known are of 'natural' origin, and laboratory-produced substances can be beneficial, there is no alternative to considering each substance individually. Additives cannot be treated as a homogeneous group. Schab and Trinh (2004) concluded that strong clinical recommendations cannot be made before the means of identifying responders is established. Additives need to be kept in context, because a meta-analysis of studies of additives and food intolerance together (Benton, 2007) resulted in an effect size four times greater than when only food colourings were considered (Schab and Trinh, 2004). It is also important to remember that Egger *et al.* (1985) never found a child who responded to only one food and no child in their study responded only to additives. One could not single out an additive, or a particular food, as a unique or universal cause of problems. Given the idiosyncratic nature of children's reaction to their diet, to a large extent advice will need to be given on an individual basis. As those who react to additives tend also to react to other food items, any advice will need to be more than the recommendation to remove an item of food or a single additive.

4.5 The nature of meals and their impact on diet, behaviour and cognition in children

Although traditionally it has been believed that, with a normal dietary regime, homeostatic mechanisms maintain blood glucose levels in the range that is needed for the brain to function (Benton, 2005), there are reports that the nutritional composition of meals can influence cognitive functioning. One suggestion is that the speed at which glucose is released into the blood stream after eating influences brain functioning.

The brain is the most metabolically active organ in the body, yet it has very limited stores of energy and it cannot reduce its needs if energy supplies are low. The brain is unusual in that unless you have starved, or have eaten a diet devoid of carbohydrate for several days, the brain does not metabolize ketones and normally almost exclusively uses glucose as its source of energy. As without replacement the glucose in the brain would last about ten minutes, it needs a continuous supply (Benton, 2005). The hormonal mechanisms that maintain blood glucose values within a prescribed range may reflect evolutionary pressures to maintain a relatively constant supply of glucose to the brain. As such, the existence of these homeostatic mechanisms might suggest that the food consumed should not normally influence brain functioning and hence cognition. It is therefore of interest that there are reports that the composition of meals influence cognition, although the underlying mechanism is not necessarily the provision of glucose.

It is possible that children, rather than adults, may be more susceptible to the provision of glucose: in relation to their bodies, the brain is larger and a given weight of brain tissue from a child uses more glucose (Kalhan and Kilic, 1999). The use of glucose by brain tissue increases up to four years of age and a high rate of glucose utilization continues until about ten years of age, after which it then falls to reach adult values in the late teenage years (Chugani, 1998). Such data suggest that we should consider whether children benefit from eating regularly. Reports that a glucose-containing drink influences the cognition of children are consistent with this view. For example, after consuming a glucose-containing drink, children aged nine to eleven years were found to have better memories and spent more time on task when working in class, although the ability to sustain attention was not influenced (Benton and Stevens, 2008).

In young adults, when the nature of the carbohydrate in breakfasts was varied to influence the speed with which blood glucose levels changed, the meals that released glucose more slowly were associated with better memory in the late morning (Benton *et al.*, 2003). When children ate iso-caloric meals on different days, memory, attention and the time on task in the classroom were better if the breakfast released glucose more slowly (Benton *et al.*, 2007). Ingwersen *et al.* (2007) compared the eating of breakfast cereals that differed in their glycaemic response. The attention of children was better two hours after eating a low rather than high glycaemic load meal.

A working hypothesis is that the gradual release of energy from meals benefits the cognitive functioning of children. Benton and Jarvis (2007) reported data consistent with this view. They related the size of breakfast, and whether a snack was subsequently eaten, to cognitive functioning in the late morning. In nine year old children, a small breakfast, on average

61 kcal, resulted in spending less time performing school work. However, eating a mid-morning snack overcame this adverse effect.

4.6 The impact of hydration on diet, behaviour and cognition in children

Water makes up between half and three-quarters of body weight and is critical to nearly every major function of the body, including maintaining body temperature, carrying nutrients and oxygen to cells, and the removal of waste. It has been suggested that children in particular are at risk of dehydration, as they are often dependent upon others for the provision of fluid and they have the potential to lose more water as they have a greater surface-to-mass ratio than adults. However, when D'Anci *et al.* (2006) reviewed the association between the hydration of children and cognition, they were unable to report a single intervention study that had examined the phenomenon. In fact, at the time there had been only one study of the topic. Bar-David *et al.* (2005) studied children aged ten to twelve years and measured dehydration by examining urine osmolarity. In the morning, the scores on five cognitive tests did not differ in those who were and were not dehydrated. However, in the afternoon, the scores on one out of the five tests favoured the hydrated group. The interpretation of this finding is not straightforward. Stahl *et al.* (2007), in German children aged four to eleven years, used 24-hour urine samples to determine the hydration status and three-day weighed food records to describe the diet. The more hydrated children drank more water, ate more water-supplying foods and consumed less energy from fat. They concluded that overall well hydrated children had a better diet. As such it is difficult to attribute any correlation between hydration status and cognition to a lack of water, since dehydration may be no more than a marker for generally poorer nutrition. More easily interpreted data come from intervention studies that relate drinking or not drinking water to cognition.

In Sicily, Fadda *et al.* (2008) estimated the hydration status of school children and found that those who were more dehydrated tended to have poorer memories. However, when additional water was supplied there was no improvement in memory, perhaps because already there was a free availability of water. Subsequently, more positive findings were reported. In the afternoon, Benton and Burgess (2009) assessed eight year old children twice: once after drinking 300 mL of water and on another occasion when no water was provided. Memory was significantly better when water had been consumed, although the ability to sustain attention was not affected. In a similar study, Edmonds and Burford (2009) compared two groups of seven to nine year olds, half of whom drank on average 211 mL of water. Those who had drunk were better when performing tests of memory and visual attention.

4.7 Implications of trends in children's diet for the food industry, heathcare professionals and policy makers

There is ample evidence in developing countries that nutritional deficiencies during critical periods of brain development have a lasting impact on intellectual functioning: examples include the adverse consequences of a shortage of iodine, zinc or iron. The scale of the problem is immense, with consequences for the individual but also the prosperity of entire nations. In fact, in developing countries, the World Health Organization (2002) lists iron, zinc and vitamin A deficiency in the top ten causes of death. If death is not a consequence, then the impact of nutritional deficiencies on physical and cognitive development will still have serious implications. Fortification of food items is one solution and in this context the World Bank (1993) commented that no other 'technology available today offers as large an opportunity to improve lives and accelerate development at such low cost and in such a short time'. In an ideal world, the goal would be to provide whole foods and thus adequate nutrition, but realistically, fortification has a role to play in many parts of the world. The widespread adding of iodine to salt occurs in many developing countries. As a more specific example, South Africa has a programme of adding of calcium, iron, zinc, vitamins A, B_1, B_2, B_3, B_6 and folate to wheat, maize flour and sugar.

In industrialized countries, the body of evidence is not such that we can make many recommendations: simply, the topic has not received enough attention. Perhaps the strongest evidence is associated with iron deficiency. There are consistent reports that anaemia is a widespread problem and there is agreement that a deficiency in the early years has life-long implications (Beard and Connor, 2003; Sachdev *et al.*, 2005; Iannotti *et al.*, 2006; Lozoff, 2007). In California, Schneider *et al.* (2005) found anaemia in 11% of those between one and two years who attended a Special Supplemental Nutrition Program. The widespread screening of infants for iron status is to be recommended. In the United Kingdom, 3% of boys and 8% of girls aged four to six years had blood haemoglobin levels below 11.0 g/dL, the level that defines anaemia (Gregory and Lowe, 2000).

There are other indications that aspects of diet might influence the cognition and behaviour of children, although they need further examination. We need to establish the optimal diet in the peri-natal stage. There are suggestions that both the incidence of anti-social behaviour (Benton, 2007) and intellectual functioning (Benton, 2001) may be influenced by diet; however, we cannot begin to suggest the active ingredients or the optimal dose.

Assuming that nutritional mechanisms are established, policy makers will have to keep their significance in context. In much of the general population there is a ready tendency to see diet as both causing and offering a simple means of solving complex problems. Diet can only modify our potential by influencing our basic biology. Whether that potential is realized will depend on an interaction with a supportive and stimulating environment. That reaction will be modified by a life-time of experience, sub-cultural norms and the current situation. In many instances, a change in diet will be only one of several interventions that are required. The desired outcome will reflect optimal nutrition acting in an appropriate psychological and social context. Changing the diet is not by itself going to overcome poor teaching or the attitudes that have resulted from a life-time of failure in school. Dietary changes may, however, help to encourage a positive reaction.

4.8 Future trends

The study of the influence of diet on the cognition and behaviour of children is an area where there is relatively little that can as yet be concluded with the confidence needed to make public health recommendations, or to offer clinical advice to the individual. In fact, beyond conditions of gross malnutrition there is little that can be concluded. There are, however, a growing number of well-designed randomized trials that have been carried out in industrialized countries and have demonstrated an impact of dietary manipulation on a child's behaviour or cognitive functioning. We have reached the stage where the principle that certain aspects of the diet have the potential to influence development has been established: we lack, however, the body of data that would justify specific advice. The usual conclusion of scientists that we need more research is unavoidable.

The evidence to date suggests that only rarely will the conclusions be simple. For example, it will be necessary to take into account the developmental stage of the child such that only at particular critical stages of brain development will some aspects of nutritional status have long-term consequences. This is an area where nutrition will interact with individual differences in genetics and physiology, so on occasions we will need to look at interactions between the diet and individual differences in basic biology. One likely development involves nutriomics where the polymorphisms of genes associated with nutrition and energy metabolism are studied. Similarly nutrigenomics examines the ability of nutrition to influence a genetic response. In the future, we may be able to screen for those who are likely to respond adversely to aspects of their diet.

We will need to be able to distinguish those individuals who are nutritionally at risk and to establish the nutrients that are most likely to be deficient and their optimal intake. The time-scale over which nutrition is influential is also likely to increase. To date, the time-scale has been relatively short, so for example the effect of peri-natal diet has been followed up for a few years at the most. It is, however, conceivable that early metabolism programming and early brain development might have consequences for cognitive decline and the development of dementia after many decades. These are topics that we have barely begun to consider.

4.9 Sources of further information and advice

General: Black (2003b); Georgieff (2007); Benton (2008b,c)
Fatty acids: McCann and Ames (2005); Eilander *et al.* (2007); Carlson (2009a,b);
Innis (2009)
Iodine: Zimmermann (2007); de Escobar *et al.* (2007); Rivas and Naranjo (2007)
Iron: Sachdev *et al.* (2005) Iannotti *et al.* (2006); Lozoff (2007)
Folate/vitamin B_{12}: Reynolds (2006); Black (2008); Gordon (2009)
Zinc: Black (1998, 2003a); Sandstead (2003)
Behavioural problems: Liu and Raine (2006); Benton (2007)
Sucrose: Wolraich *et al.* (1995); Benton (2008a)
Additives: Egger *et al.* (1985); Schab and Trinh (2004); McCann *et al.* (2007)
Meals: Benton *et al.* (2003, 2007)
Hydration: D'Anci *et al.* (2006); Lieberman (2007).

4.10 References

Aukett MA, Parks YA, Scott PH, Wharton BA (1986), 'Treatment with iron increases weight gain and psychomotor development', *Arch Dis Child*, 61, 849–857.

Bar-David Y, Urkin J and Kozminsky E. (2005), 'The effect of voluntary dehydration on cognitive functions of elementary school children', *Acta Paediatrica*, 94, 1667–1673.

Bateman B, Warner JO, Hutchinson E, Dean T, Rowlandson P, Gant C, Grundy J, Fitzgerald C and Stevenson J (2004), 'The effects of a double blind, placebo controlled, artificial food colourings and benzoate preservative challenge on hyperactivity in a general population sample of preschool children', *Arch Dis Child*, 89, 506–511.

Beard JL and Connor JR (2003), 'Iron status and neural functioning', *Ann Rev Nutr*, 23, 31–58.

Benton D (2001), 'Micro-nutrient supplementation and the intelligence of children', *Neurosci Biobehav Rev*, 25, 297–309.

Benton D (2005), 'Diet, cerebral energy metabolism and psychological functioning', in Lieberman H. and Kanarek R, Prasad C, *Nutrition, Brain & Behavior, Volume 3, Nutritional Neuroscience: Overview of an Emerging Field*, 57–71, Taylor & Francis, Boca Raton, USA.

Benton D (2007), 'The impact of diet on anti-social behaviour', *Neurosci Biobehav Rev*, 31, 752–774.

Benton D. (2008a), 'Sucrose and behavioural problems', *Crit Rev Food Sci Nutr*, 48, 385–401.

Benton D (2008b), 'Micronutrient status, cognition and behavioural problems in childhood', *Eur J Nutr*, 47(suppl 3), 38–50.

Benton D (2008c), 'The influence of children's diet on their cognition and behaviour', *Eur J Nutr*, 47 (suppl 3), 25–37.

Benton D, Burgess N (2009), 'The effect of the consumption of water on the memory and attention of children', *Appetite*, 53, 143–146.

Benton D, Jarvis M (2007), 'The role of breakfast and a mid-morning snack on the ability of children to concentrate at school', *Physiol Behav*, 90, 382–385.

Benton D, Maconie A and Williams C (2007), 'The influence of the glycaemic load of breakfast on the behaviour of children in school', *Physiol Behav*, 92, 717–724.

Benton D and Roberts G (1988), 'Vitamin and mineral supplementation improves the intelligence of a sample of school children', *Lancet*, 140–143.

Benton D, Ruffin M-P, Lassel T, Nabb S, Messaoud N, Vinoy S, Desor D and Lang V (2003), 'The delivery rate of dietary carbohydrates affects cognitive performances in both rats and humans', *Psychopharmacol*, 166, 86–90.

Benton D and Stevens M (2008), 'The influence of a glucose containing drink on the behavior of children in school', *Biol Psychol*, 78, 242–245.

Black MM (1998), 'Zinc deficiency and child development', *Am J Clin Nutr*, 68 (suppl), 464S–469S.

Black MM (2003a), 'The evidence linking zinc deficiency with children's cognitive and motor functioning', *J Nutr*, 133(5 Suppl 1), 1473S–6S.

Black MM (2003b), 'Micronutrient deficiencies and cognitive functioning', *J Nutr*, 133(11 Suppl 2), 3927S–3931S.

Black MM (2008), 'Effects of vitamin B12 and folate deficiency on brain development in children', *Food Nutr Bull*, 29(2 Suppl), S126–31.

Bourre JM (2006), 'Effects of nutrients (in food) on the structure and function of the nervous system: update on dietary requirements for brain. Part 2: Macronutrients'; *J Nutr Health Aging*, 10, 386–99.

Carlson SE (2009a), 'Early determinants of development: A lipid perspective', *Am J Clin Nutr*; 89, 1523S–1529S.

Carlson SE (2009b), 'Docosahexaenoic acid supplementation in pregnancy and lactation', *Am J Clin Nutr*, 89, 678S–84S.

Caspi A, Williams B, Kim-Cohen J, Craig IW, Milne BJ, Poulton R, Schalkwyk LC, Taylor A, Werts H and Moffitt TE (2007), 'Moderation of breastfeeding effects on the IQ by genetic variation in fatty acid metabolism', *Proc Natl Acad Sci USA*, 2104(47), 18860–5.

Chugani HT (1998), 'A critical period of brain development: Studies of cerebral glucose utilization with PET', *Prev Med*, 27, 184–188.

D'Anci KE, Constant F and Rosenberg IH (2006), 'Hydration and cognitive function in children', *Nutr Rev*, 64, 457–464.

de Escobar GM, Obregón MJ and del Rey FE (2007), 'Iodine deficiency and brain development in the first half of pregnancy', *Pub Health Nutr*, 10(12A), 1554–70.

Dekaban AS and Sadowsky D (1978), 'Changes in brain weights during the span of human life: Relation of brain weights to body heights and body weights', *Ann Neurol*, 4, 345–356.

Der G, Batty GD and Deary IJ (2006), 'Effect of breast feeding on intelligence in children: Prospective study, sibling pairs analysis, and meta-analysis', *Brit Med J*, 333(7575), 945.

Edmonds CJ and Burford D (2009), 'Should children drink more water? The effects of drinking water on cognition in children', *Appetite*, 52, 776–779.

Egger J, Carter CM, Graham PJ, Gumley D and Soothill JF (1985), 'Controlled trial of oligoantigenic treatment in the hyperkinetic syndrome', *Lancet*, 1, 540–545.

Eilander A, Hundscheid DC, Osendarp SJ, Transler C and Zock PL (2007), 'Effects of n-3 long chain polyunsaturated fatty acid supplementation on visual and cognitive development throughout childhood: A review of human studies', *Prostaglandins Leuko Essent Fatty Acids*, 76, 189–203.

Epstein HT (1986), 'Stages in human brain development', *Brain Res*, 395, 114–119.

Fadda R, Rapinett G, Grathwohl D, Parisi M, Fanari R and Schmitt J (2008),' The benefits of drinking supplementary water at school on cognitive performance in children', Washington DC, *Abstracts*: International Society for Developmental Psychobiology.

Fleith M and Clandinin MT (2005), 'Dietary PUFA for preterm and term infants: Review of clinical studies', *Crit Rev Food Sci Nutr*, 45, 205–29.

Friel JK, Andrews WL, Matthew JD, Long DR, Cornel AM, Cox AM, McKim E and Zerbe GO (1993), 'Zinc supplementation in very low birth weight infants', *J Pediatr Gastroenterol Nutr*, 17, 97–104.

Georgieff MK (2007), 'Nutrition and the developing brain: Nutrient priorities and measurement', *Am J Clin Nutr*, 85, 614S–620S.

Gesch CB, Hammond SM, Hampson SE, Eves A and Crowder MJ (2002), 'Influence of supplementary vitamins, minerals and essential fatty acids on the antisocial behaviour of young prisoners. Randomised, placebo-controlled trial', *Brit J Psychiat*, 181, 22–28.

Gibson RS, Vanderkooy PD, MacDonald AC, Goldman A, Ryan BA and Berry M (1989), 'A growth-limiting, mild zinc-deficiency syndrome in some southern Ontario boys with low height percentiles', *Am J Clin Nutr*, 49, 1266–1273.

Gordon N (2009), 'Cerebral folate deficiency', *Dev Med Child Neurol*, 51, 180–2.

Graham SM, Arvela OM and Wise GA (1992), 'Long-term neurologic consequences of nutritional vitamin B_{12} deficiency in infants', *J Pediatr*, 121, 710–714.

Gregory J, Lowe S (2000) *National diet and nutrition survey: Young people aged 4 to 18 years*, London, The Stationery Office.

Hadders-Algra M, Bouwstra H, van Goor SA, Dijck-Brouwer DA and Muskiet FA. (2007), 'Prenatal and early postnatal fatty acid status and neurodevelopmental outcome', *J Perinat Med*, 35 Suppl 1, S28–34.

Helland IB, Smith L, Blomén B, Saarem K, Saugstad OD and Drevon CA (2008), 'Effects of supplementing pregnant and lactating mothers with n-3 very-long-chain fatty acids on children's IQ and body mass index at 7 years of age', *Pediatrics*, 122(2), e472–9.

Hoffman DR, Boettcher JA and Diersen-Schade DA (2009), 'Toward optimizing vision and cognition in term infants by dietary docosahexaenoic and arachidonic acid supplementation: A review of randomized controlled trials', *Prostaglandins, Leuko Essential Fatty Acids*, 81, 151–8.

Iannotti LL, Tielsch JM, Black MM, Black RE (2006), 'Iron supplementation in early childhood: Health benefits and risks', *Am J Clin Nutr*, 84, 1261–1276.

Ingwersen J, Defeyter MA, Kennedy DO, Wesnes KA and Scholey AB (2007), 'A low glycaemic index breakfast cereal preferentially prevents children's cognitive performance from declining throughout the morning', *Appetite*, 49, 240–244.

Innis SM (2009), 'Omega-3 fatty acids and neural development to 2 years of age: Do we know enough for dietary recommendations?' *J Pediatr Gastroenterol Nutr,* 48 Suppl 1, S16–24.

Isaacs EB, Gadian DG, Sabatini S, Quinn BT, Fischl BR and Lucas A (2008), 'The effect of early human diet on caudate volumes and IQ', *Pediat Res*, 63, 308–14.

Kalhan SC and Kilic I (1999), 'Carbohydrate as nutrient in the infant and child: Range of acceptable intake', *Eur J Clin Nutr*, 53 (Suppl. 1), S94–S100.

Kramer MS, Aboud F, Mironova E, Vanilovich I, Platt RW, Matush L, Igumnov S, Fombonne E, Bogdanovich N, Ducruet T, Collet JP, Chalmers B, Hodnett E, Davidovsky S, Skugarevsky O, Trofimovich O, Kozlova L and Shapiro S (2008), 'Breastfeeding and child cognitive development: New evidence from a large randomized trial', *Arch Gen Psychiat*, 65, 578–84.

Lieberman HR (2007), Hydration and cognition: A critical review and recommendations. *J Am Coll Nutr*, 26(5 Suppl), 555S–561S.

Liu J, Raine A (2006), The effect of childhood malnutrition on externalizing behavior. *Curr Opin Pediatr*, 18, 565–70.

Louwman MW, van Dusseldorp M, van de Vijver FJ, Thomas CM, Schneede J, Ueland PM, Refsum H, van Staveren WA (2000), Signs of impaired cognitive function in adolescents with marginal cobalamin status. *Am J Clin Nutr*, 72, 762–769.

Lozoff B (2007), 'Iron deficiency and child development', *Food Nutr Bull,* 28(4 Suppl), S560–71.

Lucas A, Morley R and Cole TJ (1998), 'Randomised trial of early diet in preterm babies and later intelligence quotient', *Brit Med J*, 317, 1481–1487.

Lucas A, Morley R, Cole TJ, Gore SM, Lucas PJ, Crowle P, Pearse R, Boon AJ and Powell R (1990), 'Early diet in preterm babies and developmental status at 18 months', *Lancet*, 335, 1477–1481.

Maret W and Sandstead HH (2008), 'Possible roles of zinc nutriture in the fetal origins of disease', *Exp Gerontol*, 43, 378–81.

McCann D, Barrett A, Cooper A, Crumpler D, Dalen L, Grimshaw K, Kitchin E, Lok K, Porteous L, Prince E, Sonuga-Barke E, Warner JO and Stevenson J (2007), 'Food additives and hyperactive behaviour in 3-year-old and 8/9-year-old children in the community: A randomised, double-blinded, placebo-controlled trial', *Lancet*, 370, 1560–1567.

McCann JC and Ames BN (2005), 'Is docosahexaenoic acid, an n-3 long-chain polyunsaturated fatty acid, required for development of normal brain function? An overview of evidence from cognitive and behavioral tests in humans and animals', *Am J Clin Nutr*, 82, 281–295.

Osendarp SJ, Baghurst KI, Bryan J, Calvaresi E, Hughes D, Hussaini M, Karyadi SJ, van Klinken BJ, van der Knaap HC, Lukito W, Mikarsa W, Transler C and Wilson C (2007), 'Effect of a 12-mo micronutrient intervention on learning and memory in well-nourished and marginally nourished school-aged children: Two parallel, randomized, placebo-controlled studies in Australia and Indonesia', *Am J Clin Nutr*, 86, 1082–1093.

Penland JG, Sandstead HH, Alcok NW, Dayal HH, Chen XC, Li JS, Zhao F and Yang JJ (1997), 'A preliminary report: Effects of zinc and micro-nutrient repletion on growth and neuro-psychological function of urban Chinese children', *J Am Coll Nutr*, 16, 268–272.

Pitkin RM (2007), 'Folate and neural tube defects', *Am J Clin Nutr*, 85, 285S–288S.

Reynolds E (2006), 'Vitamin B12, folic acid, and the nervous system', *Lancet*, 5, 949–960.

Rivas M and Naranjo JR (2007). 'Thyroid hormones, learning and memory', *Genes Brain Behav*, 6 Suppl 1, 40–44.

Sachdev H, Gera T and Nestel P (2005), 'Effect of iron supplementation on mental and motor development in children: Systematic review of randomised controlled trials', *Public Health Nutr*, 8, 117–132.

Sandstead HH (2003), 'Zinc is essential for brain development and function', *J Trace Elements Exp Med*, 16, 165–173.

Schab DW and Trinh NH (2004), 'Do artificial food colors promote hyperactivity in children with hyperactive syndromes? A meta-analysis of double-blind placebo-controlled trials'. *J Dev Behav Pediatr*, 25, 423–434.

Schneider JM, Fujii M, Lamp CL, Lonnerdal B, Dewey KG and Zidenberg-Cherr S (2005), 'Anemia, iron deficiency, and iron deficiency anemia in 12–36 mo old children from low-income families', *Am J Clin Nutr*, 82, 1269–1275.

Schoenthaler SJ, Amos S, Doraz W, Kelly MA, Muedeking G and Wakefield J (1997), 'The effect of randomized vitamin-mineral supplementation on violent and non-violent anti-social behavior among incarcerated juveniles', *J Nutr Environ. Med*, 7, 343–352.

Simmer K, Schulzke SM and Patole S (2008), 'Long chain polyunsaturated fatty acid supplementation in preterm infants', *Cochrane Database Syst Rev*, 23(1), CD000375.

Smithers LG, Gibson RA, McPhee A and Makrides M (2008), 'Effect of long-chain polyunsaturated fatty acid supplementation of preterm infants on disease risk and neurodevelopment: A systematic review of randomized controlled trials', *Am J Clin Nutr*, 87, 912–20.

Stahl A, Kroke A, Bolzenius K and Manz F (2007), 'Relation between hydration status in children and their dietary profile – results from the DONALD study', *Eur J Clin Nutr*, 61, 1386–1392.

Tahmasebi Boroujeni S, Naghdi N, Shahbazi M, Farrokhi A, Bagherzadeh F, Kazemnejad A and Javadian M (2008), 'The effect of severe zinc deficiency and zinc supplement on spatial learning and memory' *Biol Trace Elem Res*, 130, 48–61.

Tai M (1997), 'The devastating consequences of iodine deficiency', *Southeast Asian J Trop Med Public Health,* 28 Suppl 2, 75–77.

Wolraich ML, Wilson DB and White JW (1995), 'The effect of sugar on behavior or cognition in children. A meta-analysis', *J Am Med Assoc*, 274, 1617–1621.

World Bank (1993), *Enriching Lives*, Washington DC, World Bank.

World Health Organization (2002), *The World Health Report*, Geneva, WHO.

World Health Organization (2008), 'Worldwide prevalence of anaemia 1993–2005'. In de Benoist B, McLean E, Egli I and Cogswell M, *Global Database on Anaemia*, Geneva, WHO.

Zaalberg A, Nijman H, Bulten E, Stroosma L and van der Staak C (2010), 'Effects of nutritional supplements on aggression, rule-breaking and psychopathology among young adult prisoners', *Aggress Behav*, 36, 117–26.

Zimmermann MB (2007), 'The adverse effects of mild-to-moderate iodine deficiency during pregnancy and childhood: A review', *Thyroid*, 17, 829–835.

Zimmermann MB, Connolly K, Bozo M, Bridson J, Rohner F and Grimci L (2006), 'Iodine supplementation improves cognition in iodine-deficient schoolchildren in Albania: A randomized, controlled, double-blind study', *Am J Clin Nutr*, 83, 108–114.

Zimmermann M and Delange F (2004), 'Iodine supplementation of pregnant women in Europe: A review and recommendations', *Eur J Clin Nutr*, 58, 979–984.

5

Food allergies and food intolerances in children

H. Mackenzie and T. Dean, University of Portsmouth, UK

Abstract: The needs of food-allergic and intolerant consumers are an increasingly important consideration for food manufacturers. This chapter first examines the definition of food allergy and food intolerance in children and adolescents, the prevalence of these conditions, and their impact on health and quality of life. The role of food in the development and management of food allergies and intolerances is also discussed. The chapter also considers the implications of food allergies and intolerances in children for the food industry, healthcare professionals and policy makers, including future trends in the prevalence and nature of food allergies and intolerances.

Key words: food allergy, food intolerance, 'may contain' labelling, allergen labelling, novel food allergens.

5.1 Introduction

Food allergies and intolerances affect a sizeable minority of consumers and, given the possible severity of the consequences of allergen ingestion, the needs of this group of consumers are an increasingly important consideration for food manufacturers. Food allergic and food intolerant children, teenagers and their caregivers also have particular needs which should be considered by the food industry.

5.2 What are food allergies and intolerances?

Adverse reactions to food can occur by a variety of different mechanisms and cause different symptoms, and although the terms 'food allergy' and 'food intolerance' are often used interchangeably, they actually refer to quite different illnesses. Non-toxic reactions to food are termed 'food hypersensitivity' and are divided into those that are immune mediated and those that are non-immune mediated (Fig. 5.1).

Immune mediated reactions are termed 'food allergies'. Such reactions are either mediated by the antibody IgE (IgE mediated food allergies), or occur via other immune mechanisms (Non-IgE-mediated food allergies) (Johansson *et al.*, 2001). Non-IgE-mediated food allergies present as a range of diseases including coeliac disease, food-protein-induced enterocolitis, Heiner syndrome and contact dermatitis (Ortolani and Pastorello, 2006; Venter and Meyer, 2010). Those reactions that are not mediated by the immune system are termed non-allergic food hypersensitivities, commonly termed food intolerances, and these can occur via a variety of mechanisms, e.g. by enzyme deficiencies and by pharmacological effects on certain individuals (Ortolani and Pastorello, 2006).

The symptoms experienced differ according to the mechanism, and range from mild to severe, affecting one or more organs, typically: the *skin* (causing hives, angioedema (swelling), atopic dermatitis), the *gastrointestinal tract* (causing mild pruritis (itching), angioedema of the *lip* or *tongue*, tingling in the *throat*; reflux, dysphagia (difficulty swallowing), and *abdominal* pain; nausea, *abdominal* cramps, vomiting and diarrhoea) or the *respiratory system* (causing periocular pruritis (itchy *eyes*), conjunctivitis (runny, itchy *eyes*) and rhinitis (runny, itchy or congested *nose*) and asthma) (Ortolani and Pastorello, 2006). Coeliac disease is an auto-immune disease, with a range of mild to severe symptoms, including serious long-term illnesses, when gluten is ingested (McGough, 2009).

In severe cases of IgE-mediated food allergy, a reaction may be systemic, resulting in potentially fatal anaphylactic shock (Holgate *et al.*, 2001). Between 1992 and 2006, there were 87 deaths in the UK as a result of food-related anaphylactic shock (Pumphrey, 2000; Pumphrey and Gowland, 2007). Foods responsible for the majority of deaths were peanuts, tree nuts, milk and seafood although in many cases the food responsible was uncertain, and fatalities

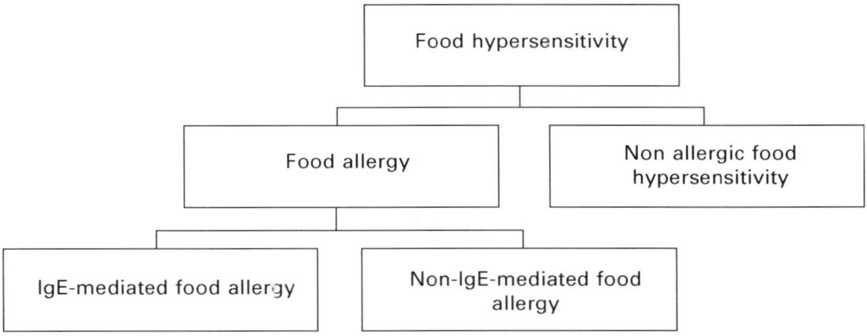

Fig. 5.1 Classifications of adverse reactions to food (Johansson *et al.*, 2001).

did occur with other foods, including chickpea, sesame, banana and egg. In younger children, fatalities are mostly due to milk, whereas in older children and teenagers, peanuts and tree nuts are largely responsible (Pumphrey, 2004). Although not broken down by age, the majority of reactions occurred as a result of eating food prepared outside of the home, including at restaurants, parties, school, and canteens, at camp and at nursery, or packaged/labelled food (Pumphrey, 2000; Pumphrey and Gowland, 2007).

5.3 Prevalence of food allergies and intolerances in children

Studies conducted to determine the prevalence of food allergy and intolerance in children in the UK indicate that 1.6–2.5% of children aged 6 years (Venter *et al.*, 2006), 1.4–2.3% of children aged 11 years and 2.1–2.3% of children aged 15 years (Pereira *et al.*, 2005) in the UK, have food allergy or intolerance. Coeliac disease affects 1% of children in the UK (Bingley *et al.*, 2004). The discrepancy between self-reported and confirmed food hypersensitivity in adults (Young *et al.*, 1994) is also present in childhood; food allergy is not confirmed in a large number of children whose parents report food allergy or intolerance (Pereira *et al.*, 2005; Venter *et al.*, 2006), although the reasons for this are not well understood.

The foods children are commonly allergic/intolerant to vary according to age (Table 5.1) and most children will outgrow their milk or egg allergy during childhood, although it is much rarer for children to outgrow their peanut allergy. There is less evidence for the natural history of other food allergies, but available research suggests that soy and wheat allergies are likely to be outgrown and that those to tree nuts, seeds, fish and shellfish are likely to persist (Wood, 2003).

5.4 Impact of food allergies and intolerances on children's health and quality of life

Given that food avoidance for food allergies and intolerances necessarily persists for a long period of time, it can have a large impact on health,

Table 5.1 Common food allergens by age

3 years and under (Venter *et al.*, 2008):	6 years (Venter *et al.*, 2006):	11 and 15 years (Pereira, *et al.*, 2005):
• Milk	• Milk	• Peanut
• Egg	• Peanut	• Tree nuts
• Peanut	• Wheat	• Shellfish

particularly where a number of foods must be excluded from the diet, where the foods being excluded are common ingredients or are high in important nutrients, and where they form an important part of the diet (Venter and Meyer, 2010). Particularly in toddlers and babies, there are cases where food avoidance (typically milk avoidance or multiple food avoidance) has affected the nutritional adequacy of the diet, including inadequate energy consumption (Arvola and Holmberg-Marttila, 1999) and deficiencies in essential fatty acids (Aldamiz-Echevarria *et al.*, 2008) and nutrients (Henriksen *et al.*, 2000) which may result in impaired growth (Arvola and Holmberg-Marttila, 1999; Isolauri *et al.*, 1998), rickets (Fox *et al.*, 2004; Yu *et al.*, 2006) and Kwashiorkor (Liu *et al.*, 2001). Although there is less research in this area, issues are also evident beyond toddling age, where nutrient intake and growth may still be affected by food allergy (Christie *et al.*, 2002). Further, those with oral allergy syndrome to many fruits may be at risk of scurvy (Des Roches *et al.*, 2006).

Quality of life is also an important aspect of health, particularly for chronic conditions such as food hypersensitivity (Higginson and Carr, 2003). Research suggests that the quality of life of children and teenagers is affected by food allergy. Children themselves worry about having a reaction and eating away from home, especially without their parents (Avery *et al.*, 2003). Children and teenagers report having more limitations in their social activities and having less vitality because of their food allergy (Flokstra-de Blok *et al.*, 2010). Teenagers in particular have higher anxiety because of their food allergy (Lyons and Forde, 2004), and may be more frequently absent from school, and feel less confident in starting relationships (Calsbeek *et al.*, 2002). They may worry about their food allergy, feel that they are different from their peers, and that they are missing out (Mackenzie *et al.*, 2009). However, research suggests that food manufacturers and the catering industry have the potential to significantly improve the lives of teenagers with food allergy (Mackenzie *et al.*, 2009; Mandell *et al.*, 2005; Marklund *et al.*, 2007).

Parents of children and teenagers with food allergy highlight problems with separation anxiety (LeBovidge *et al.*, 2009) and limits on the social activities of their child (Bollinger *et al.*, 2006), as well as poorer physical functioning and general health (Marklund *et al.*, 2006; Ostblom *et al.*, 2008; Sicherer *et al.*, 2001).

From the perspective of the parent and the family, food allergy affects meal preparation, family social activities and parental stress levels (Bollinger *et al.*, 2006; Primeau *et al.*, 2000). Parents of teenagers worry about handing over responsibility for managing food allergy to their son or daughter as they become more independent, and about the possibility of their teenage son or daughter having an anaphylactic reaction (Akeson *et al.*, 2007).

5.5 Role of foods in the development and management of allergies and intolerances

5.5.1 Development of allergies

The onset of allergic disease is affected by genetics and by environmental factors, including diet, and it is likely that early childhood has an important influence on the development of childhood and adult allergic disease (Greer *et al.*, 2008). Research has explored the effect of maternal food intake during pregnancy and lactation, breast feeding and hydrolysed milk formulas, and of weaning, into the role of foods in the development and management of allergies and intolerances; although more research is required.

A clinical report suggests that there is, at present, insufficient evidence to determine the potential role of diet in pregnant and lactating women on the development of atopic disease in children (Greer *et al.*, 2008). For infants at risk of developing atopic disease, there is evidence that, compared with cows' milk-based formulas, exclusive breastfeeding and breastfeeding supplemented by hydrolysed formula for at least four months decreases the risk of atopic dermatitis but not of eczema or asthma. The effect of breastfeeding on the development of food allergies is not yet clear. Whether hydrolysed formulas have a protective effect on atopic disease has not been agreed upon (Greer *et al.*, 2008; Host *et al.*, 1995; Muraro *et al.*, 2004; National Institute for Health and Clinical Excellence, 2008). As yet, there is no convincing evidence that maternal avoidance of food allergens, with the exception of peanut, has a protective effect for atopic disease (Greer *et al.*, 2008; Muraro *et al.*, 2004). Research into the timing of the introduction of complementary foods into the diet has also given mixed results, and until further research has been conducted it is not clear how this might affect development of allergic disease (Greer *et al.*, 2008).

On the basis of existing research evidence, current guidance in the UK recommends that, even where there is a familial history of atopy or atopic disease, it is not necessary to avoid consuming peanuts or peanut products during pregnancy, lactation or infancy. However, it is recommended that infants at risk of developing atopic disease be breastfed until four–six months old (Committee on Toxicity of Chemicals in Food, 2008).

5.5.2 Dietary management of food allergies and intolerances

At present there is no cure or treatment for food allergy or food intolerance, and elimination of the food allergen from the diet is the key to avoiding an adverse reaction. The level of avoidance required depends on a number of factors and varies on an individual basis (Venter and Meyer, 2010). IgE-mediated food allergies (nut allergies in particular), some non-IgE-mediated food allergies and coeliac disease require strict avoidance, since even the smallest amount of the offending food can trigger a severe reaction, whereas food intolerances (non-allergic food hypersensitivities) need larger amounts to provoke symptoms and require less strict avoidance (Venter and Meyer, 2010). In some cases, individuals with IgE-mediated egg or milk allergy may tolerate small amounts of the allergen when it has been thoroughly cooked, but not when it is raw (Lemon-Mule *et al.*, 2008; Nowak-Wegrzyn *et al.*, 2008).

In younger children, parents take on the main responsibility for managing an elimination diet. However, teenagers are often away from their parents and need to learn to manage their allergy or intolerance for themselves. In either case, managing such a diet requires careful checking of all food labels, avoiding high-risk restaurants (such as Indian or Thai restaurants for those with nut allergy and buffets for those with any food allergy) and loose food products (such as delicatessens or bakeries), and asking restaurant staff the ingredients of meals on the menu. Schools and other clubs must be informed about the child's allergy or intolerance and appropriate measures to ensure their safety, as should any other people looking after the child (e.g. friend's parents, extended family) (Munoz-Furlong, 2003; Sampson, 1999; Venter and Meyer, 2010).

5.6 Implications of food allergies and intolerances in children for the food industry, healthcare professionals and policy makers

Food-allergic and intolerant consumers and their caregivers, health professionals, public regulators (regulators and compliance authorities), food retailers, food manufacturers, caterers, and the general public are the key stakeholders who need to be aware of and understand adverse reactions to food (Miles *et al.*, 2004). Since the management of food allergy and intolerance involves avoidance of the problem food, issues around food production, food labelling and novel foods are of extreme importance. This is especially salient given that some fatalities from food allergy have occurred even in individuals who were taking extreme care to avoid food allergens (Pumphrey and Gowland, 2007).

The labelling of food products is of extreme importance to food allergic and intolerant consumers to enable them to make informed decisions about the safety of the food they eat. As will be discussed, food allergen labelling must be accurate, clear and unequivocal. Manufacturers should bear in mind that they are not only conveying such information for adults. If caregivers make mistakes and find labels problematic, this will only be exacerbated for children and teenagers, who may be reading labels unsupervised, for example, when buying sweets at the local shop, or, at an older age, perhaps shopping and preparing meals for themselves.

5.6.1 Food production

Where food production is concerned, potential cross-contamination is a highly salient issue for food hypersensitive consumers (particularly those who require strict avoidance). Cross-contamination could occur at any point in production and in a number of ways; for example, through inappropriate storage and transport of food allergens, rework practices and use of shared equipment. Reactions, and even fatalities, have occurred as a result of cross-contamination by an unlisted allergen (Altschul *et al.*, 2001; Pumphrey, 2000) as even minute amounts of a food allergen can produce a severe reaction in sensitive individuals (Hourihane *et al.*, 1997). Furthermore, establishing the thresholds at which a food might produce a reaction is 'enormously problematic' (Warner, 2005; p. 2.). Hence, it is essential that a realistic appraisal of risk is communicated to consumers.

Although no legislation exists for the labelling of allergen risk with regard to cross-contamination, food manufacturers are bound by the Food Safety Act (as amended; HMSO, 1990) to ensure the safety of the food they produce, be aware of potential risks and have plans in place to control for these. The Food Standards Agency has produced voluntary guidelines on the assessment and monitoring of the risk of cross-contamination with food allergens (Food Standards Agency, 2006a). However, it is important to note that these guidelines were written before the most recent amendment to the EU directive on allergen labelling (see below) in 2007, and hence the list of allergens included is out-of-date. They have also produced an online training package for food manufacturers and their staff on dealing with food allergens (http://allergytraining.food.gov.uk/english/default.aspx).

5.6.2 Labelling

Labelling of food allergens as intended ingredients

There have been several EU directives concerning the labelling of food allergens (European Commission, 2003, 2005, 2006, 2007), under which 14 food allergens (and all products thereof) *must* be listed on labels for all pre-packed food and alcoholic drinks. These directives removed the '25% rule' so if any of these food allergens are present in a final product (either as an ingredient, carry-over additive, additive used as a processing aid, or as a solvent or media for additives or flavourings, and regardless of the proportion of the food in the total product), this must be indicated on the label (Table 5.2). Should a product contain a food allergen as an ingredient, it must be named on the packaging so that it is clear that the ingredient is, or is derived from, a listed food allergen. The 2006 directive states that the list 'will be systematically re-examined and, where necessary, updated on the basis of the most recent scientific knowledge' (European Commission, 2006). Hence, although Table 5.2 lists the food allergens which must be listed on packaging at the time of publication, this may be updated and the

Table 5.2 Food allergens which must be labelled on pre-packed food and alcoholic drinks (adapted from FSA guidance)

Food allergen	Except...
Cereals containing gluten (i.e. wheat, rye, barley, oats, spelt, kamut or their hybridised strains)	• wheat-based glucose syrups including dextrose[1]; • wheat-based maltodextrins[1]; • glucose syrups based on barley; • cereals used for making distillates or ethyl alcohol of agricultural origin for spirit drinks and other alcoholic beverages.
Crustaceans	
Eggs[2]	
Fish	• fish gelatine used as a carrier for vitamin or carotenoid preparations; • fish gelatine or isinglass used as a fining agent in beer and wine.
Peanuts	
Soybeans	• fully refined soybean oil and fat[1] • natural mixed tocopherols (E306), natural D-alpha tocopherol, natural D-alpha tocopherol acetate, natural D-alpha tocopherol succinate from soybean sources; • vegetable oils derived from phytosterols and phytosterol esters from soybean sources; • plant stanol ester produced from vegetable oil sterols from soybean sources.
Milk (including lactose)[3]	• whey used for making distillates or ethyl alcohol of agricultural origin for spirit drinks and other alcoholic beverages; • lactitol.
Nuts i.e. almonds (*Amygdalus communis L.*), hazelnuts (*Corylus avellana*), walnuts (*Juglans regia*), cashews (*Anacardium occidentale*), pecan nuts (*Carya illinoiesis (Wangenh.) K.Koch*), Brazil nuts (*Bertholletia excelsa*), pistachio nuts (*Pistacia vera*), macadamia nuts and Queensland nuts (*Macadamia ternifolia*)	• nuts used for making distillates or ethyl alcohol of agricultural origin for spirit drinks and other alcoholic beverages.
Celery	
Mustard	
Sesame seeds	
Sulphur dioxide and sulphites at concentrations of more than 10 mg/kg or 10 mg/litre expressed as SO_2	

Table 5.2 Continued

Food allergen	Except...
Lupin	
Molluscs.	

[1] The exception applies only to products derived from these products insofar as the process they have undergone is not likely to increase the level of allergenicity assessed by the European Food Safety Authority for the relevant product from which they originated.
[2] There is a temporary exemption from labelling for egg albumin used as a fining agent for wine and lysozyme (produced from egg) used in wine until December 2010.
[3] There is a temporary exemption from labelling for milk (casein) used as a fining agent for wine until December 2010.

most recent directives must be followed. These directives can be found on the Food Standards Agency website (www.fsa.gov.uk).

The current legislation does not apply to foods sold loose, e.g. pick and mix, bakery items or delicatessens do not have to comply with this legislation. From the consumer's perspective this is very restrictive. The Food Standards Agency does, however, provide best practice guidelines on food allergen labelling for manufacturers or retailers of loose foods (Food Standards Agency, 2004). A further point is that the legislation applies only to foods produced within the EU; those produced outside of the EU do not have to comply. Hence, retailers importing packaged foods need to be aware that there may not be sufficient information provided to food-allergic consumers, and may wish to consider the labelling of such products to aid this group.

Labelling errors

Food manufacturers may discover that the labelling of their product is misleading to food-allergic consumers; for example, that a food allergen has been included in the product as an ingredient, but is not listed on the label, or that a food allergen has contaminated a food product. Food-allergic consumers and their caregivers have reported many issues with the labelling of food allergens, including: discovering visible ingredients that were not listed on the label, the outer label differing from the inner label on multipacks, the contents differing from those intended, and ambiguous terminology (Altschul *et al.*, 2001).

Given the gravity of the potential consequences, labelling errors are a serious issue for food-allergic consumers. Should a mistake occur, under the Food Safety Act (as amended; 1990), the manufacturer must alert the Food Standards Agency and their Local Authority. In the UK, the Food Standards Agency and The Anaphylaxis Campaign both offer services to disseminate this information promptly to food-allergic consumers (the details of these organisations can be found at the end of this chapter).

Advisory or 'may contain' labelling

Advisory (or 'may contain') labelling is often used by food manufacturers to indicate that a product may, through cross-contamination, contain a food allergen that is not listed as an ingredient in the product. It is important that consumers are aware of a genuine risk to their health, however: excessive use of advisory labelling serves to restrict consumer choice and may lead some consumers to distrust, and ignore, such labels (Boden *et al.*, 2005). Indeed, some parents of food-allergic children are uncertain as to whether their children should avoid food that has an advisory label (Joshi *et al.*, 2002). Teenagers may not pay sufficient attention to 'may contain' labels, and their overuse may have encouraged a belief that their aim is not to convey a genuine risk, but rather to prevent legal action against the manufacturer (Akeson *et al.*, 2007; Mackenzie *et al.*, 2009). For these reasons, the FSA recommend that 'advisory labelling should only be used when, following a thorough risk assessment, there is a real risk of allergen cross-contamination' (Food Standards Agency, 2006b; p. 5), and that it should not be used as a long-term measure since 'it should be normal practice for foods to be free from common allergens which are not ingredients' (Food Standards Agency, 2002; p. 54). They also provide best practice guidelines for food manufacturers and retailers on issues not currently covered by the legislation; for example, on advisory labelling (Food Standards Agency, 2006a).

Clarity of labelling

Food manufacturers use food labels to communicate ingredients and risk to food-allergic and intolerant consumers. However, this is not always successfully achieved. A US study found that parents of food-allergic children made a large number of mistakes when reading labels for allergy information; most errors resulted when terms such as 'trace peanuts' were not located in or close to the main ingredient list (Joshi *et al.*, 2002). Another study (Simons *et al.*, 2005) found that 16% of food allergic consumers or caregivers had attributed a reaction to a misunderstanding of a label term and 86% had contacted a manufacturer for further information about the ingredients of a product. What is promising for food manufacturers and retailers is that most consumers (86%) said that the brands they bought were 'very much influenced by' the labelling; hence, clear labelling will often be rewarded by more loyalty from food-allergic consumers.

Consumers make assumptions about food labelling which may not match the legal responsibilities of food manufacturers. For example, consumers may expect food manufacturers to declare a change in ingredients if the product contains an allergen it did not previously, even though this is not a legal requirement, and may inadvertently ingest a food allergen as a result (Altschul *et al.*, 2001). Problems may also occur when an English language label has been placed over a foreign language one (Altschul *et al.*, 2001). All are things that food manufacturers may wish to address when considering food-allergic consumers. The Food Standards Agency have considered such issues and provide clear guidance for the food industry on labelling in general, and also on allergen labelling; for example, that the allergen alert box be placed as close to the ingredients as possible and that they highlight the allergen name, e.g. milk, rather than the ingredient name, e.g. casein (Food Standards Agency, 2008).

5.6.3 Novel foods

All foods have the potential to be allergenic; hence, the introduction of new and exotic foods into the European diet may result in the emergence of novel food allergies and intolerances, while existing or genetically-modified crops may produce novel proteins, which could produce an allergic response (Meredith, 2005; Miles *et al.*, 2004). It is not, at present, possible to predict future food allergens (Meredith, 2005); therefore, under the Novel Foods Regulation, all novel foods (foods that do not have a significant history of consumption within the European Union (EU) before 15 May 1997) must be subjected to a pre-market safety assessment (in the UK by the Advisory Committee on Novel Foods and Processes (ACNFP)), including the assessment of their allergenic properties, to decide whether they will be authorised for sale within the EU (European Commission, 1997).

5.6.4 Food colouring and preservatives

Research has suggested that certain food colourings and preservatives (sodium benzoate) can increase hyperactivity in children (Bateman *et al.*, 2004; McCann *et al.*, 2007). Those food colourings studied were E102 Tartrazine, E104 Quinoline Yellow, E110 Sunset Yellow, E122 Carmoisine, E124 Ponceau 4R, E129 Allura Red. As a result, the European Parliament and Council have issued a regulation stating that food products containing these food colourings must include the following warning on the packaging '*name or E number of the colour(s)*: may have an adverse effect on activity and attention in children,' unless the colouring has been used to mark meat products or on decorative eggshells (European Parliament and Council, 2008). This regulation is enforced in England by The Food Additives (England) Regulations (HMSO, 2009). Further guidance can be found on the website of the Food Standards Agency (Food Standards Agency, 2010).

5.7 Future trends

5.7.1 Changes in prevalence rates

The prevalence of food allergy and intolerance does not appear to have changed a large amount over time. A US study conducted in 1987 (Bock, 1987) found a prevalence of 7.4% in the first three years of life, compared with 5–6% in the same age group in a UK study conducted in children born in 2001/2002 (Venter *et al.*, 2008). Research does suggest that there was an increase in peanut allergy in the UK when comparing 3–4 year olds born in 1989 (0.5%) with those born between 1994 and 1996 (1.4%). However, more recently this appears to have stabilised: although there was a decrease evident in those 3–4 year olds born in 2001 and 2002 (1.2%), this was not statistically significant (Venter *et al.*, 2010). It is not clear how the prevalence rates will change in the future.

5.7.2 Novel food allergies/intolerances

Case reports suggest that two particular emerging food allergens are green and gold kiwi (*Actinidia deliciosa* and *Actinidia chiensis* respectively) (Lewis *et al.*, 2004; Lucas *et al.*, 2003). However, changes to the UK diet may result in further novel food allergens. An important source of information about novel food allergens is the InformAll EU Project (2005), which is compiling information about allergenic foods, food proteins and epitopes, which are being continually added to a publicly accessible database (see Section 5.8 for more details).

5.8 Sources of further information and advice

The Food Standards Agency (www.fsa.gov.uk) has thorough guidance on the appropriate food allergen labelling legislation and provides other information for food manufacturers on food allergies, including an online training package. There are several organisations that provide further information about food allergy and food intolerance. Consumer organisations include:

- The Anaphylaxis Campaign (UK) – www.anaphylaxis.org.uk
- Allergy Action (UK) – www.allergyaction.co.uk
- Allergy UK (UK) – www.allergyuk.org
- The Food Allergy and Anaphylaxis Network (US) – www.foodallergy.org
- Coeliac UK – www.coeliac.org.uk

Relevant professional bodies include:

- British Society for Allergy and Clinical Immunology – www.bsaci.org
- European Academy of Allergy and Clinical Immunology – www.eaaci.net
- American Academy of Asthma, Allergy and Immunology – www.aaaai.org

Information on food allergens can be found at http://foodallergens.ifr.ac.uk/

5.9 References

Akeson, N., Worth, A., and Sheikh, A. (2007). The psychosocial impact of anaphylaxis on young people and their parents. *Clinical and Experimental Allergy, 37*(8), 1213–1220.

Aldamiz-Echevarria, L., Bilbao, A., Andrade, F., Elorz, J., Prieto, J. A., and Rodríguez-Soriano, J. (2008). Fatty acid deficiency profile in children with food allergy managed with elimination diets. *Acta Paediatrica, 97*(11), 1572–1576.

Altschul, A. S., Scherrer, D. L., Munoz-Furlong, A., and Sicherer, S. H. (2001). Manufacturing and labeling issues for commercial products: Relevance to food allergy [Letter to editor]. *Journal of Allergy and Clinical Immunology, 108*(3), 468.

Arvola, T., and Holmberg-Marttila, D. (1999). Benefits and risks of elimination diets. *Annals of Medicine, 31*, 293–298.

Avery, N. J., King, R. M., Knight, S., and Hourihane, J. O. B. (2003). Assessment of quality of life in children with peanut allergy. *Pediatric Allergy and Immunology, 14*(5), 378–382.

Bateman, B., J. O. Warner *et al.* (2004). The effects of a double blind, placebo controlled, artificial food colourings and benzoate preservative challenge on hyperactivity in a general population sample of preschool children. *Archives of Disease in Childhood, 89*, 506–511.

Bingley, P., Williams, A. J. K., Norcross, A. J., Unsworth, J., Lock, R. J., Ness, A. R. *et al.* (2004). Undiagnosed coeliac disease at age seven: Population based prospective birth cohort study. *BMJ, 328*, 322–323.

Bock, S. A. (1987). Prospective appraisal of complaints of adverse reactions to foods in children during the first 3 years of life. *Pediatrics, 79*, 683–688.

Boden, M., Dadswell, R., and Hattersley, S. (2005). Review of statutory and voluntary labelling of food allergens. *Proceedings of the Nutrition Society, 64*, 475–480.

Bollinger, M. E., Dahlquist, L. M., Mudd, K., Sonntag, C., Dillinger, S., and McKenna, K. (2006). The impact of food allergy on the daily activities of children and their families. *Annals of Allergy, Asthma and Immunology, 96*(3), 415–421.

Calsbeek, H., Rijken, M., Bekkers, M., Kerssens, J. J., Dekker, J., and van Berge Henegouwan, G. P. (2002). Social position of adolescents with chronic digestive disorders. *European Journal of Gastroenterology and Hepatology, 14*(5), 543–549.

Christie, L., Hine, R. J., Parker, J. G., and Burks, W. (2002). Food allergies in children affect nutrient intake and growth. *Journal of the American Dietetic Association, 102*(11), 1648–1651.

Committee on Toxicity of Chemicals in Food, Consumer Products and the Environment (2008). *Statement on the review of the 1998 COT recommendations on peanut avoidance*. London: Department of Health.

Des Roches, A., Paradis, L., Paradis, J., and Singer, S. (2006). Food allergy as a new risk factor for scurvy. *Allergy, 61*(12), 1487–1488.

European Commission. (1997). REGULATION (EC) No 258/97 OF THE EUROPEAN PARLIAMENT AND OF THE COUNCIL of 27 January 1997 concerning novel foods and novel food ingredients THE EUROPEAN PARLIAMENT AND THE COUNCIL OF THE EUROPEAN UNION. *Official Journal of the European Union, L 43/1.*

European Commission. (2003). DIRECTIVE 2003/89/EC OF THE EUROPEAN PARLIAMENT AND OF THE COUNCIL of 10 November 2003 amending Directive 2000/13/EC as regards indication of the ingredients present in foodstuffs. *Official Journal of the European Union, L 308/15.*

European Commission. (2005). COMMISSION DIRECTIVE 2005/26/EC of 21 March 2005 establishing a list of food ingredients or substances provisionally excluded from Annex IIIa of Directive 2000/13/EC of the European Parliament and of the Council. *Official Journal of the European Union, L 75/33.*

European Commission. (2006). COMMISSION DIRECTIVE 2006/142/EC of 22 December 2006 amending Annex IIIa of Directive 2000/13/EC of the European Parliament and of the Council listing the ingredients which must under all circumstances appear on the labelling of foodstuffs. *Official Journal of the European Union, L 368/110.*

European Commission. (2007). COMMISSION DIRECTIVE 2007/68/EC of 27 November 2007 amending Annex IIIa to Directive 2000/13/EC of the European Parliament and of the Council as regards certain food ingredients. *Official Journal of the European Union, L 310/11.*

European Parliament and Council (2008). Regulation (EC) No 1333/2008 of the European Parliament and Council of 16th December 2008 on food additives. *Official Journal of the European Union,* L354/16.

Flokstra-de Blok, B. M. J., Dubois, A. E. J., Vlieg-Boerstra, B. J., Oude Elberink, J. N. G., Raat, H., DunnGalvin, A. *et al.* (2010). Health-related quality of life of food allergic patients: Comparison with the general population and other diseases. *Allergy, 65*, 238–244.

Food Standards Agency. (2002). *'May Contain' Labelling – The Consumer's Perspective* (No. FSA/0582/0502). London: Food Standards Agency.

Food Standards Agency. (2004). *Advice for caterers on allergy and intolerance*. From http://www.food.gov.uk/safereating/allergyintol/guide/caterers/

Food Standards Agency. (2006a). *Guidance on Allergen Management and Consumer Information* (No. FSA/1064/0606). London: Food Standards Agency.

Food Standards Agency. (2006b). *What to consider when labelling food* (No. FSA/1105/1206). London: Food Standards Agency.

Food Standards Agency. (2008). *Clear food labelling guidance*. London: Food Standards Agency.

Food Standards Agency (2010). *Guidance on the labelling of certain food colours as set out in Regulation* 1333/2008. London, Food Standards Agency.

Fox, A. T., Du, T. G., Lang, A., and Lack, G. (2004). Food allergy as a risk factor for nutritional rickets. *Pediatric Allergy and Immunology, 15*(6), 566–569.

Greer, F. R., Sicherer, S. H., Burks, A. W., and and the Committee on Nutrition and Section on Allergy and Immunology. (2008). Effects of Early Nutritional Interventions on the Development of Atopic Disease in Infants and Children: The Role of Maternal Dietary Restriction, Breastfeeding, Timing of Introduction of Complementary Foods, and Hydrolyzed Formulas. *Pediatrics, 121*(1), 183–191.

Henriksen, C., Eggesbø, M., Halvorsen, R., and Botten, G. (2000). Nutrient intake among two-year-old children on cows' milk-restricted diets. *Acta Paediatrica, 89*, 272–278.

Higginson, I. J., and Carr, A. J. (2003). 'The clinical utility of quality of life measures.' In A. J. Carr (Ed.), *Quality of Life* (pp. 63–78). London: Sage.

HMSO. (1990). *Food Safety Act c. 16 (as amended).*

HMSO (2009). The Food Additives (England) Regulations 2009. *Statutory Instruments* (No. 3238).

Holgate, S. T., Church, M. K., and Lichtenstein, L. M. (2001). *Allergy* (2nd ed.). London: Mosby.

Host, A., Jacobsen, H. P., Halken, S., and Holmenlund, D. (1995). The natural history of cow's milk protein allergy/intolerance. *European Journal of Clinical Nutrition, 49*(S1), S13–S18.

Hourihane, J. O. B., Kilburn, S. A., Nordlee, J. A., Hefle, S. L., Taylor, S. L., and Warner, J. O. (1997). An evaluation of the sensitivity of subjects with peanut allergy to very low doses of peanut protein: A randomized, double-blind, placebo-controlled food challenge study. *Journal of Allergy and Clinical Immunology, 100*(5), 596–600.

InformAll EU Project. (2005). InformAll database on allergenic foods. From http://foodallergens.ifr.ac.uk/

Isolauri, E., Sutas, Y., Salo, M. K., Isosomppi, R., and Minna, K. (1998). Elimination

diet in cow's milk allergy: Risk for impaired growth in young children. *Journal of Pediatrics, 132*, 1004–1009.
Johansson, S. G. O., Hourihane, J. O. B., Bousquet, J., Bruijnzeel-Koomen, C., Dreborg, S., Haahtela, T. *et al.* (2001). A revised nomenclature for allergy: An EAACI position statement from the EAACI nomenclature task force. *Allergy, 56*(9), 813–824.
Joshi, P., Mofidi, S., and Sicherer, S. H. (2002). Interpretation of commercial food ingredient labels by parents of food-allergic children. *Journal of Allergy and Clinical Immunology, 109*(6), 1019–1021.
LeBovidge, J. S., Strauch, H., Kalish, L. A., and Schneider, L. C. (2009). Assessment of psychological distress among children and adolescents with food allergy. *Journal of Allergy and Clinical Immunology, 124*, 1282–1288.
Lemon-Mule, H., Sampson, H. A., Sicherer, S. H., Shreffler, W. G., Noone, S., and Wegrzyn, A. (2008). Immunologic changes in children with egg allergy ingesting extensively heated egg. *Journal of Allergy and Clinical Immunology, 122*(5), 977–983.
Lewis, S. A., Warner, J. O., Hourihane, J. O. B., and Lucas, J. S. A. (2004). Gold Kiwi Fruit – A New Allergen. *Journal of Allergy and Clinical Immunology, 113*(2), S153.
Liu, T., Howard, R. M., Mancini, A. J., Weston, W. L., Paller, A. S., Drolet, B. A. *et al.* (2001). Kwashiorkor in the United States: Fad diets, perceived and true milk allergy and nutritional ignorance. *Archives of Dermatology, 137*(5), 630–636.
Lucas, J. S. A., Lewis, S. A., and Hourihane, J. O. B. (2003). Kiwi fruit allergy: A review. *Pediatric Allergy and Immunology, 14*, 420–428.
Lyons, A. C., and Forde, E. M. E. (2004). Food allergy in young adults: Perceptions and psychological effects. *Journal of Health Psychology, 9*(4), 497–504.
Mackenzie, H., Roberts, G., Van Laar, D., and Dean, T. (2009). Teenagers' experiences of living with food hypersensivity: A qualitative study. *Pediatric Allergy and Immunology*, 21(4 Part 1), 595–602.
Mandell, D., Curtis, R., Gold, M., and Hardie, S. (2005). Anaphylaxis: How Do You Live with It? *Health and Social Work, 30*(4), 325–335.
Marklund, B., Ahlstedt, S., and Nordström, G. (2006). Health-related quality of life in food hypersensitive schoolchildren and their families: Parents' perceptions, *Health and Quality of Life Outcomes, 4*(48).
Marklund, B., Wilde-Larsson, B., Ahlstedt, S., and Nordström, G. (2007). Adolescents' experiences of being food-hypersensitive: A qualitative study. *BMC Nursing, 6*(8).
McCann, D., A. Barrett *et al.* (2007). Food additives and hyperactive behaviour in 3-year-old and 8/9-year-old children in the community: A randomised, double-blinded, placebo-controlled trial. *Lancet, 37,* 1560–1567.
McCough, N. (2009). 'The Role of Allergy and Intolerance in Coeliac Disease'. In I. Skypala and C. Venter (Eds.), *Food Hypersensitvity: Diagnosing and Managing Food Allergies and Intolerance* (pp. 85–95). Oxford: Blackwell Ltd.
Meredith, C. (2005). Allergenic potential of novel foods. *Proceedings of the Nutrition Society, 64*, 487–490.
Miles, S., Crevel, R., Chryssochoidis, G., Frewer, L., Grimshaw, K., Guidnoet Riera, A. *et al.* (2004). 'Communication needs and food allergy: An analysis of stakeholder views'. In L. J. W. J. Gilissen, H. J. Wichers, H. Savelkoul and R. J. Bogers (Eds.), *Allergy Matters: New Approaches to Prevention and Management* (pp. 171–192). New York: Springer.
Munoz-Furlong, A. (2003). Daily Coping Strategies for Patients and Their Families. *Pediatrics, 111*(6), 1654–1661.
Muraro, A., Dreborg, S., Halken, S., Høst, A., Niggemann, B., Aalberse, R. *et al.* (2004). Dietary prevention of allergic diseases in infants and small children. Part III: Critical review of published peer-reviewed observational and interventional studies and final recommendations. *Pediatric Allergy and Immunology, 15*, 291–307.
National Institute for Health and Clinical Excellence. (2008). *Maternal and Child Nutrition* (No. PH011). London: National Institute for Clinical Excellence.

Nowak-Wegrzyn, A., Bloom, K. A., Sicherer, S. H., Shreffler, W. G., Noone, S., Wanich, N. *et al.* (2008). Tolerance to extensively heated milk in children with cow's milk allergy. *Journal of Allergy and Clinical Immunology, 122*(2), 342–347.

Ortolani, C., and Pastorello, E. A. (2006). Food allergies and food intolerances. *Best Practice and Research Clinical Gastroenterology, 20*(3), 467–483.

Ostblom, E., Egmar, A-C., Gardulf, A., Lilja, G., and Wickman, M. (2008). The impact of food hypersensitivity reported in 9-year-old children by their parents on health-related quality of life. *Allergy, 63*(2), 211–218.

Pereira, B., Venter, C., Grundy, J., Clayton, B., Hasan Arshad, S., and Dean, T. (2005). Prevalence of sensitization to food allergens, reported adverse reactions to foods, food avoidance, and food hypersensitivity among teenagers. *Journal of Allergy and Clinical Immunology, 116*(4), 884–892.

Primeau, M. N., Kagan, R., Joseph, L., Lim, H., Dufresne, C., Duffy, C. *et al.* (2000). The psychological burden of peanut allergy as perceived by adults with peanut allergy and the parents of peanut-allergic children. *Clinical and Experimental Allergy, 30*(8), 1135–1143.

Pumphrey, R. S. H. (2000). 'Lessons for management of anaphylaxis from a study of fatal reactions. *Clinical and Experimental Allergy, 30*(8), 1144–1150.

Pumphrey, R. S. H. (2004). 'Fatal anaphylaxis in the UK, 1992–2001.' In G. Bock and J. Goode (Eds.), *Anaphylaxis* (pp. 116–132). Chichester: Wiley.

Pumphrey, R. S. H., and Gowland, H. (2007). Further fatal allergic reactions to food in the United Kingdom, 1999–2006. *Journal of Allergy and Clinical Immunology, 119*(4), 1018–1019.

Sampson, H. A. (1999). Food allergy. Part 2: Diagnosis and management. *Journal of Allergy and Clinical Immunology, 103*(6), 981–989.

Sicherer, S. H., Noone, S. A., and Muñoz-Furlong, A. (2001). The impact of childhood food allergy on quality of life. *Annals of Allergy, Asthma and Immunology, 87*(6), 461–464.

Simons, E., Weiss, C. C., Furlong, T. J., and Sicherer, S. H. (2005). Impact of ingredient labelling practices on food allergic consumers. *Annals of Allergy, Asthma and Immunology, 95*(5), 426–428.

Venter, C., Arshad, S. H., Grundy, J., Pereira, B., Clayton, B., Voigt, K. *et al.* (2010). Time trends in the prevalence of peanut allergy: Three cohorts of children from the same geographical location in the UK. *Allergy, 65*(1), 103–108.

Venter, C., and Meyer, R. (2010). Symposium on 'Dietary management of disease'. Session 1: Allergic disease. The challenges of managing food hypersensitivity. *Proceedings of the Nutrition Society, 69*, 11–24.

Venter, C., Pereira, B., Grundy, J., Clayton, B., Arshad, S. H., and Dean, T. (2006). Prevalence of sensitization reported and objectively assessed food hypersensitivity amongst six-year-old children: A population-based study. *Pediatric Allergy and Immunology, 17*, 356–363.

Venter, C., Pereira, B., Voigt, K., Grundy, J., Clayton, C. B., Higgins, B., *et al.* (2008). Prevalence and cumulative incidence of food hypersensitivity in the first 3 years of life. *Allergy, 63*(3), 354–359.

Warner, J. O. (2005). European Food Labelling Legislation – A nightmare for food manufacturers and allergy sufferers alike. [Editorial]. *Pediatric Allergy and Immunology, 16*, 1–2.

Wood, R. A. (2003). The natural history of food allergy. *Pediatrics, 111*(6), 1631–1637.

Young, E., Stoneham, M. D., Petruckevitch, A., Barton, J., and Rona, R. (1994). A population study of food intolerance. *Lancet, 343*(8906), 1127–1130.

Yu, J. W., Pekeles, G., Legault, L., and McCusker, C. T. (2006). Milk allergy and vitamin D deficiency rickets: A common disorder associated with an uncommon disease. *Annals of Allergy, Asthma and Immunology, 96*, 615–619.

Part II

Children's food choices

6

Food promotion and food choice in children

E. J. Boyland and J. C. G. Halford, University of Liverpool, UK

Abstract: This chapter addresses food promotion aimed at children, and how such activity affects their food preferences, choices, intake, purchase-related behaviours as well as advertisement recall and recognition. We first review the extent, nature and effects of food promotion via television, new media and other avenues (e.g. print advertisements) including the advertising techniques used to make food products appeal to young people. We then describe the current state of regulation in the UK regarding broadcast and non-broadcast food advertising. This includes a discussion of the weaknesses in those regulations that should be addressed as part of efforts to reduce children's exposure to unhealthy food marketing and improve their diets and overall health.

Key words: television food advertising, food promotion, branding, food preference, food choice.

6.1 Introduction to food promotion aimed at children

Food promotion or advertising is marketing that involves the paid presentation and endorsement of food products by a sponsor (Kotler and Armstrong, 2004). Advertising is a multi-million dollar industry worldwide, and typically the products being promoted do not reflect the recommended diet. It has been estimated that for every US$1 the WHO spends on promoting healthy nutrition, US$500 is spent by the food industry promoting processed foods (Escalante de Cruz *et al.*, 2004). In the UK in 2003, Nestlé alone spent £43 million promoting breakfast cereals and chocolate, Kellogg spent £30 million promoting their cereals and Coca-Cola funded their soft drink advertising with £26 million (Escalante de Cruz *et al.*, 2004). Annually in the US, $1 billion is spent on youth-oriented media advertising, particularly on television (Story and French, 2004).

To communicate advertising messages to children, an ever increasing variety of media are used. However, television remains one of the most powerful sources of communication we have, both in terms of penetration into the home and universal usage (Abbatangelo-Gray *et al.*, 2008). It is perhaps unsurprising then that globally, television is still the primary medium used for advertising food and drink products (Hendersen and Kelly, 2005), comprising approximately 75% of all advertising spend in the UK in recent years (Hastings *et al.*, 2003).

In the UK, with the exception of the BBC, the vast majority of channels (whether via terrestrial broadcasting, digital transmission or via satellite systems) are commercial, i.e. they carry advertising, which typically includes food promotions. Other forms of advertising are more embedded into television content such as the use of programme sponsorship or product placement, which aim to achieve brand exposure without an evident distinction between programming and a direct advertisement (Institute of Medicine, 2005). However, marketers can also take advantage of a number of avenues in order to promote their products. Some of these are visible, and therefore can be tracked and potentially measured, including radio, magazine, and newspaper promotions. Technological innovation has also provided alternative means of reaching a specific target audience (such as young people) with advertising messages that are not so trackable or measurable, such as internet marketing and advergaming, mobile phone advertising, and viral advertising through social networking sites. However, what do we really know about the food promotion messages children are exposed to through the various forms of media?

6.2 The extent and nature of food promotion to children

6.2.1 Television food advertising

Numerous studies have investigated both the extent (frequency of advertising, proportion of overall advertisements (ads) for food products relative to other products/services) and the nature (types of food products promoted) of television food advertising. Although both the extent and nature of such advertising varies between countries, studies have shown that typically the majority of ads broadcast are for unhealthy products. In a 27.5 hour sample of US television, 49% of ads were for food, of which 91% were for foods or beverages containing high levels of fat, sodium or added sugars, or were low in nutrients (Batada *et al.*, 2008). Similarly, a recent study looking at Greek television found that 'healthy' food categories (for example cereals, fruits and vegetables) were the least advertised items and the less healthy options (dairy items and high sugar products) were the most advertised (Batrinou and Kanellou, 2009). During a 645 hour sample of Australian television,

81% of the food ads identified were also for unhealthy products, including fast food, takeaways, chocolate and confectionery items (Chapman *et al.*, 2006). A smaller study in New Zealand (60 hour sample) classified 66% of the food ads broadcast as being for high fat, high sugar and/or high salt foods (hereafter HFSS foods) (Jenkin *et al.*, 2008).

Other studies have specifically examined the television food advertising that children will be exposed to by focusing their analyses on certain time periods (e.g. after school viewing or Saturday morning programming), particular channels designed to appeal to children (dedicated children's channels) or around particular programmes popular with children. The timing of advertising within children's programming (breakfast, after school or weekend morning), children's peak viewing (evening weekday or weekend peak family viewing) or during programmes that specifically appeal to children during the schedule (family films or popular sporting events) is important. A US study found that food ads were more frequently broadcast during Saturday programming and on children's networks than on networks targeted at a general audience (Bell *et al.*, 2009). This study also reported that 70% of the food ads broadcast were for high sugar or high fat items, with few ads for fruit or vegetables evident (Bell *et al.*, 2009). Byrd-Bredbenner (2002) found that in and around the most popular Saturday morning programmes on children's channels, food was the most advertised category. Of the food ads broadcast, the vast majority were for breakfast cereals and foods that were high in fat and sugar, with only rare ads for produce, protein-rich foods or dairy products (Byrd-Bredbenner, 2002). Furthermore, a Bulgarian study showed that although 'only' 33.4% of ads broadcast during children's programmes were for food, 96.8% of those ads were for foods items containing high levels of fat, sugar and/or salt (Galcheva *et al.*, 2008). This study also found that ads for confectionery were mainly shown during movies directed at children, whereas snack food and soft drink ads were more likely to be associated with animation programmes or other children's shows (e.g. music or sports) (Galcheva *et al.*, 2008).

Some authors have studied trends in food advertising over time. Byrd-Bredbenner and Grasso (2000) observed that the number of ads broadcast (all categories, not just food) increased significantly between 1971 and 1998 but that the frequency of food ads broadcast did not change significantly over that time period. Kelly and colleagues examined food ads aimed at children on commercial Australian television between 2002 and 2006. Whilst overall levels of HFSS food advertising reduced over this time period, in 2006 the rate of HFSS food ads during children's viewing times was greater than that during adult viewing times, particularly in and around the most popular programmes for children (Kelly *et al.*, 2007).

Few studies have compared television food advertising between countries. However, an international comparative study was carried out by Consumers International in 1996, whereby television ads were monitored during approximately 20 hours of children's television in 13 countries (Australia,

Austria, Belgium, Denmark, Finland, France, Germany, Greece, Netherlands, Norway, Sweden, UK and the US). This study found that, in the vast majority of countries, food advertising comprised the largest category of advertised products to children. In addition, confectionery, breakfast cereals (usually with added sugar) and fast food restaurants accounted for over half of all food ads broadcast; whereas ads for fruits and vegetables were virtually non-existent (Dibb and Harris, 1996).

Recently, a more comprehensive international comparative study was completed which examined 192 hours of television from 13 countries (Australia, Brazil, Canada, China, Germany, Greece, Italy, Spain, Sweden, US and our own laboratory in the UK), for a total sample of 2496 hours broadcast between October 2007 and March 2008 (Kelly *et al.*, 2010). The three commercial channels most popular with children in each country were selected for inclusion, and the results indicated that, internationally, food ads (68 462 were assessed) accounted for between 11% and 29% of all ads broadcast, and overall, food was the second most frequently advertised product after channel promotions. Food items relatively high in undesirable nutrients and/or energy comprised 53% to 87% of all food advertisements shown, with fast food restaurant meals and chocolate/confectionery as the items most frequently advertised. It was also found that the rate of non-core food advertising was higher during children's peak viewing times (the broadcast periods where the highest numbers of children were watching) than during non-peak viewing times (with the UK data following this pattern) (Kelly *et al.*, 2010).

Given the importance of this topic, literature relating specifically to the UK is lacking. In 1998, Lewis and Hill found that during their 91h sample of UK television, 828 adverts were broadcast of which half were for food products (with food being the most heavily advertised product category). Of these food adverts, 60% were for breakfast cereals and confectionery/snacks (Lewis and Hill, 1998). With an oral health perspective, two further UK based studies were carried out by Chestnutt and Ashraf and Morgan and colleagues. Chestnutt and Ashraf (2002) found that during children's TV time, 73.4% of advertising was for products that are potentially harmful to teeth, whereas during primetime TV this fell to 18.6%. Morgan *et al.* (2008) studied 503 hours of UK children's television, during which 38.4% of food advertising time was devoted to high-sugar products (such as sweetened dairy items, e.g. yoghurts), confectionery, sugared cereals (breakfast cereals and snack bars), baked goods (cakes and biscuits) and drinks (sweetened hot chocolate and carbonated beverages). Given the rising prevalence of childhood obesity in the UK, the extent of unhealthy food promotion to children is worrying.

In addition, as part of their international study, Dibb and Harris (1996) completed a nutritional analysis of the foods advertised to children on UK television, and reported that over 60% were products high in fat, 50% were high in sugar and over 60% were high in salt. Overall, 95% of the UK food ads were for HFSS foods and, as the previously mentioned studies have suggested, this was a fairly consistent pattern found across the countries studied (Dibb and Harris, 1996). The UK sample from the Kelly *et al.* (2010) study comprised 9799 ads overall, of which 1461 (14.9%) were for food. Food and channel promotions were the most advertised product categories (each comprising 15% of all ads) followed by toys (9.5% of all ads). Of the food ads broadcast the most frequent items appearing were low fat dairy products, fast food items, high fat spreads and sauces, full cream dairy products, breakfast cereals with added sugar and/or low fibre and confectionery (Kelly *et al.*, 2010). Recently Sixsmith and Furnham (2010) reported that a far greater proportion of ads aimed at children were for unhealthy items than healthy items (77.1% v 22.9%) and that this was significantly different from the relative proportions of food types in ads not specifically aimed at children (55.8% unhealthy v 44.2% unhealthy).

Food ads aimed at children typically rely on fun, happiness, enhanced popularity, performance or mood, 'coolness', taste, flavour and almost never health. They are designed to grab attention through unusual sound effects, movement and fast pacing, fantasy, creative music, catchy jingles and repetition (Roberts and Pettigrew, 2007). The Hastings report concluded that 'the advertised diet contrasts sharply with that recommended by public health advisors, and themes of fun and fantasy or taste, rather than health and nutrition, are used to promote it to children. Meanwhile, the recommended diet gets little promotional support' (Hastings *et al.*, 2003).

Over the past few years a number of countries, including the UK, have adopted some form of regulatory approach to food promotion to children. However, the effects of food messages are cumulative and the patterns of food choice to which they have contributed may not readily be reversed. Moreover, as the most recent data demonstrate, even in countries with some regulatory code of practice in place, the extent of unhealthy food promotion to children remains surprising. Overall, it is clear that the foods advertised on television reflect a dietary pattern that would be associated with increased risk of obesity and are not in line with recommended nutritional guidelines (World Health Organisation, 2003). With the contribution of television advertising to childhood obesity being more closely scrutinised, and advertising being limited during child-specific programming (if not family viewing), marketers have looked to other media to promote products and brands. Although television remains the primary medium for food promotion, technological innovation has opened up a number of other avenues via which the food industry can promote their products.

6.2.2 Internet food advertising and 'advergaming'

As children spend increasing amounts of time on the internet, they are being increasingly targeted by online advertising. The internet is one of many 'emerging media' that have both expanded the number of advertising avenues available, and have also provided novel opportunities to target particular audiences – notably children (Moore, 2006). From a marketer's perspective, the internet has many advantages over television, not least regarding cost-effectiveness and audience-tracking capabilities (Moore, 2006). Online content requires attention to be focused, and whilst looking at online content, children's engrossment can be captured and maintained for extended periods of time (Kelly *et al.*, 2008A). In addition, internet advertising is not based on passive exposure as with television; children must actively seek the online content they require (Moore and Rideout, 2007) and therefore, whilst activity searching, those children are engaging with the media. Furthermore, the internet offers opportunities for advertisers to interact with children (Moore and Rideout, 2007) to generate engagement and interest in food promotion activities.

The vast majority of websites designed for children and adolescents permit advertising; indeed most rely on advertising as their primary source of revenue (Neuborne, 2001), and the use of 'advergames' is prevalent (Moore, 2006). The term 'advergames' refers to the phenomenon of video games present on commercially sponsored websites that contain embedded brand messages within entertaining animated puzzles or adventures (Moore and Rideout, 2007). The games offer the opportunity for children to play high energy games with high quality graphics for free, which has obvious appeal for young people (Neuborne, 2001). These games are created for the sole purpose of brand promotion (Neuborne, 2001), such as where 'Nestlé Push-up Frozen Treats are popping up all over the place and it's your job to bop 'em back down' (Moore, 2006, p. 5), with the product often very cleverly integrated into the game for continuous brand reinforcement (Moore, 2006)and although few authors have addressed this issue, there is some research evidence to suggest that playing advergames does have an effect on children's eating and eating-related behaviours.

Mallinckrodt and Mizerski (2007) found that after playing the advergame for a branded breakfast cereal, 8-year-old children reported significantly higher preferences for that cereal over other cereals and food types. In addition, Pempek and Calvert (2009) exposed 30 children aged 9–10 years to a healthy or a less healthy advergame; the children played the game twice and then chose and ate a snack. With only ten minutes' overall exposure to the advergame and embedded food promotion messages, children selected and consumed the type of snack being promoted in the game they had played (healthy or less healthy). As children who played the healthier version of the game chose and consumed a significantly greater number of healthy snacks than those who had played the less healthy game (Pempek and Calvert, 2009), this suggests that advergaming has potential for use in health promotion strategies.

However, if advergames are effective at altering food choice in children, this is a concern as typically the foods promoted on the internet are energy-dense foods not conducive to a healthy diet. Alvy and Calvert (2008) found that food promotion was present on seven out of ten popular children's websites, and the products being advertised were primarily sweets, cereal, fast food, and snack items. Similarly, Kelly and colleagues examined 196 popular children's websites and identified that food references on these sites were strongly skewed in favour of unhealthy foods compared to healthy foods (60.8% v 39.2%). It was also found that advergames were present on a majority of websites aimed at young children and adolescents, with games more likely to be featured on websites for high sugar drinks, ice-cream and chocolate/confectionery (Kelly *et al.*, 2008A).

6.2.3 Food promotion through other media

More and more companies are looking to promote their products via mobile devices such as Blackberry phones or Apple iPhones, to the extent that the mobile marketing industry was thought to be worth $229 million last year (Chordas, 2009). Promotions using mobile devices can take the form of advertising-supported applications, text messaging directing users to Web browsers or to text companies for entry to promotions or further information, and it has been suggested that ad recall is significantly higher following exposure on a mobile device compared to other avenues (Chordas, 2009). For example, Coca-Cola have launched a mobile phone application that requires the user to shake their phone to simulate shaking a bottle of Coca-Cola. Coca-Cola and Budweiser are also two corporations that have used a 'text2collect' system whereby consumers can text a code from the top of a can of the beverage to a certain number in order to enter a prize draw or to gain credits to be used on the company website. To date, no studies have investigated the effects of mobile food promotion on food choice.

There is also concern over children's exposure to printed ads in magazines. Children are believed to spend £250 million per year on comics and magazines (Childwise, 2004) and magazine advertising has been shown to be successful in terms of increased product awareness, sales and brand switching (King and Hill, 2008). The academic research in this area is extremely limited, but King and Hill did investigate the effects of exposure to printed ads for healthy, less healthy and non-food products on food choice and product recall in 309 children. Although food choice was not found to be affected by printed ad exposure, the children recalled significantly more of the less healthy food products (King and Hill, 2008).

Furthermore, in the US, many corporations are targeting children with food promotion messages via their school, with advertising opportunities including placing logos on school facilities, providing electronic equipment in exchange for advertising, providing branded educational materials and activities, participating in fund-raising activities, and sponsoring events (Graff, 2008). For example, in the US, numerous corporate-sponsored contests have taken place such as Pizza Hut's Book-It program and McDonald's McSpellIt Club (Story and French, 2004). In addition, around 20% of US high schools have branded food products available for purchase on the school site, such as Pizza Hut, Taco Bell or Subway (Story and French, 2004). As the school environment has been shown to have a powerful influence on how students eat, advertising energy-dense foods and beverages in schools could have a detrimental effect on children's dietary choices and overall health.

6.2.4 Advertising techniques

Advertisers are believed to use particular persuasive techniques to appeal to children and young people (such as the use of appeals, promotional characters, celebrity endorsement and giveaways), and such techniques do affect children's liking of ads (Nash *et al.*, 2009). Folta *et al.* (2006) noted that in food and beverage ads targeted at school-aged children, foods were typically associated with fun and good times (75% of food ads), pleasant taste (54.1%), being 'hip' or 'cool' (43.2%), and feelings of happiness (43.2%). Kelly *et al.* (2008B) found that premium offers and promotional characters were used in 21.4% and 7.3% of food ads respectively, but this was significantly higher during peak versus non-peak children's viewing times and the majority of ads using these techniques were for non-core foods.

Again, data emanating from the UK are limited. Lewis and Hill (1998) assessed the use of appeals in their study, investigating adverts broadcast on UK television during children's viewing times (weekday afternoons and weekend mornings) and classifying the appeals used into three categories; verbal appeals (e.g. 'tastes great'), product appeals (e.g. the product is presented as being superior to other brands), and emotional appeals (e.g. fun/happiness, peer acceptance). The findings indicated that food ads were significantly more likely to feature a number of these appeals than other categories of ad, namely animation, a story format, humour and the emotional appeal of fun/happiness/mood alteration (Lewis and Hill, 1998).

Branding is a critical aspect of advertising, particularly for children and young people; the majority of child-oriented food advertisements take a branding approach (Connor, 2006). Television advertising is thought to be very effective at building strong brands (Heath, 2009). The term 'brand' can be defined as 'a name, term, sign, symbol, design, or a combination of these, that identifies the goods or services of one seller or group of sellers and differentiates them from those of the competition' (Chang and Liu, 2009). Of all commodities, food is one of the most highly branded items, with over 80% of US grocery items being branded (Story and French, 2004). This level of branding of food products lends itself well to major advertising campaigns, and food manufacturers carry out advertising activity with the aim of building brand awareness and brand loyalty, as there is a belief that brand preference precedes purchase behaviour (Story and French, 2004).

Children are extremely important targets for branding activity; they have independent spending power but also exert considerable influence over family purchases. Food and drink purchases are the categories over which children have been shown to have particular influence (Søndergaard and Edelenbos,

2007). In addition, children are also seen as 'teenage and adult shoppers of the future' so, if brand loyalty can be fostered at a young age, this may reward the food company with a lifetime of sales, which could be worth in the region of $100 000 to the retailer (Escalante de Cruz *et al.*, 2004).

By the age of two years, children are already specifically targeted by cereal manufacturers in their television ads (McNeal and Ji, 2003). By mid-childhood, children have a very high level of recognition for brand logos (Kanner, 2006); in one study, 88% of 9–11 year olds were correctly able to recognise at least 16 out of 20 brand logos (Kopelman *et al.*, 2007). Between middle childhood and adolescence, understanding of branding develops; brands are no longer considered purely according to observable concrete aspects of a certain product but on a more abstract, conceptual level, whereby brand image relations to social status, prestige and group affiliation become more important (Chaplin and John, 2005).

Numerous types of food branding activities are used to appeal to children. Brand licensing is prevalent in children's programming, with the effect that children associate a programme or its characters with a particular brand and ultimately the programme itself becomes an advertisement for that food (Linn and Golin, 2006). This is not only the case with programming – the release of each new movie aimed at young people is typically accompanied by several product tie-ins. Fast food companies, in particular, often attract children by providing toy giveaways with meals for children, establishing playgrounds at their restaurants and opening restaurants in locations that are frequented by children (Sahud *et al.*, 2006).

Most brands aimed at children use characters and celebrities in their promotions and on product packaging, and their presence is thought to assist with generating brand identity and encouraging the development of a brand–consumer relationship (Lawrence, 2003). These characters can be either brand licensed characters (such as SpongeBob Squarepants™), whereby the character has been created for an animated programme or movie and is then licensed by brands to appear in their promotions; or brand equity characters that are created for the sole purpose of promoting a product or brand (Garretson and Niedrich, 2004). Many of these associations have been built up over generations; for example, Snap, Crackle and Pop™ have been used to promote Kellogg's Rice Krispies® since 1928, and Tony the Tiger™ has been the character for Kellogg's Frosties® since 1951 (Lawrence, 2003). Both children and adults report liking these characters and display trust and respect for them (Ülger, 2009).

A celebrity endorser is 'a famous person who uses public recognition to recommend or co-present with a product in an ad' (Lear *et al.*, 2009). The US Institute of Medicine notes that celebrity endorsements, such as Britney Spears advertising Pepsi® and Christina Aguilera endorsing Coca-Cola®, are often used in order to make the brand appeal to a certain age group or fan base (Institute of Medicine, 2005).

Behavioural outcomes, such as purchasing requests, are thought to be modified by advertising techniques such as premium offers (Hastings *et al.*, 2003). Children naturally focus their attention on techniques such as animation and visual effects, and emotional appeals do distract children from other aspects of ads, for example nutritional disclaimers or product information (Wicks *et al.*, 2009). As children enjoy watching ads and engage with them, it is likely that the marketing strategies stated above do have persuasive power (Hastings *et al.*, 2003). Given that we know the types of foods promoted via television, the internet and other media, it is important to address the effects that this marketing activity has on children's eating behaviours and consequently their diet and overall health.

6.3 The effects of food promotion to children

Several systematic reviews of the literature have summarised the existing evidence on this topic. The review of Hastings *et al.* (2003) came to the conclusion that food promotion 'is having an effect, particularly on children's preferences, purchase behaviour, and consumption'. It is important to note that the effect of food advertising is believed to be occurring at both a brand and category level (Hastings *et al.*, 2003). Therefore, food promotion does not only lead to individuals switching from one sweetened carbonated beverage brand to another; advertising activities are also thought to increase overall consumption of such beverages (Garde, 2008). However, food and marketing companies refute this point, claiming that only brand choices are affected by promotional activity (Harris *et al.*, 2009).

The World Health Organisation and the Food and Agriculture Organisation of the United Nations reported that the promotion of energy-dense foods is a 'probable' cause of increasing prevalence of overweight and obesity in children worldwide (WHO, 2003). In addition, the Institute of Medicine reviewed over 150 studies of food advertising and its effects on children, and their report concluded that exposure to television advertising is associated with adiposity in children aged 2–11 years (Institute of Medicine, 2005). The Office of Communications (Ofcom) stated that television advertising does have a 'modest direct effect, as well as a larger indirect effect, on children's food and drink preferences' (Ofcom, 2004). However, to attribute more than a 'modest direct effect' to food advertising is known to be extremely difficult, as it is virtually impossible to be able to identify and eliminate all other potential variables (Escalante de Cruz *et al.*, 2004).

Given the vast sums of money spent by food manufacturers on food promotion, it is logical to assume that they are an effective means of promoting sales (Henderson and Kelly, 2005). Exposure to advertising must, therefore, have an effect on behaviour. Specifically regarding children and young people, this behavioural change can be considered in terms of actual purchase behaviour, but also purchase-influencing behaviour (or 'pester power'). There is already a considerable amount of evidence to indicate that food preferences, choices and requests are modified by food advert exposure and branding, resulting in purchase or purchase-influencing behaviour being altered in favour of the advertised product (Resnik and Stern, 1977).

6.3.1 Effects on food preference and choice

In 2001, Borzekowski and Robinson showed preschool children a videotape of a cartoon either with or without embedded commercials. After viewing, the children were asked to identify their food preferences from pairs of similar products, one of which had been shown in the commercials and one had not. The children who had seen the videotape with the embedded commercials were significantly more likely to select the advertised product than children who had not seen the commercials.

Our own research has demonstrated that, following exposure to non-food advertisements, overweight and obese children showed a significantly greater preference for branded items than normal weight children; however, following food advertisements, these weight status differences were not apparent (Halford *et al.*, 2008A). This suggests that television food advertisement exposure is able to produce an 'obesogenic' food preference response in some children, so that normal weight children display food preference responses that are characteristic of overweight and obese children (Halford *et al.*, 2008A).

6.3.2 Effects on brand preference

It is often argued by marketers that advertising merely changes consumer preference between brands and has no overall effect on product popularity. In the literature it certainly seems like branding can have a potent effect on food choice. Existing, well established and well recognised logos can have powerful effects on young children's food choice, even when attached to products they are not normally associated with. A study by Robinson *et al.* (2007) found that when children were offered identical food and drink items, one in McDonalds branded packaging and the other in matched, but unbranded, packaging, the children reported preferring the taste of food and drink items if they thought they were from McDonalds. This effect was even seen for items that were not available for purchase at McDonalds at the time, such as carrot sticks (Robinson *et al.*, 2007). Food branding effects have been found to be particularly evident in overweight children (Forman *et al.*, 2009), which is consistent with our previous findings that link the effect of branding on food preferences with weight status (Halford *et al.*, 2008B).

Use of celebrity endorsement in food advertising is effective at increasing children's preferences for the product being promoted (Ross *et al.*, 1984). If the packaging includes a cartoon character, children are more likely to select that product over a similar product without the character (Ülger, 2009). Characters are believed to increase the persuasive appeal of an advert, and the use of characters has come under criticism for being a way of manipulating children's food choices (*Which?*, 2005). However, characters can also be used to help encourage healthier food choices. When Winnie the Pooh was featured in food promotion activities for satsumas, nationwide sales increased to 250 000 bags per week (*Which?*, 2007).

6.3.3 Effects on food intake

It is actual changes in consumption that link self-reported changes in food preference to changes in diet that would affect health. However, the impact of food promotion on energy intake and choice in scenarios with real food has, until recently, been little studied. In one of the earliest studies on the effects of television food advertising, Gorn and Goldberg (1982) found that children who viewed daily candy commercials were more likely to select candy rather than fruit as their choice of afternoon snack. However, this early study was limited in the range of food items offered (two fruit items and two confectionery items). Moreover, actual intake was not measured.

More recently, our own studies have used a paradigm whereby children are exposed to eight food or eight non-food advertisements, followed by the same cartoon in a within-participant, randomized study. Following advertising exposure, measurements were taken of children's snack food consumption (intake of sweet and savoury, high and low fat snack foods). Following food ad exposure, all children increased their food intake relative to the control (see Figures 6.1 and 6.2) (Halford *et al.*, 2004, 2007).

Further studies found that, not only did food advertising exposure produce a substantial and significant increase in caloric intake (of high fat and/or sweet energy-dense snacks) in all children, but also that this increase in intake was related to weight status (see Fig. 6.3) (Halford *et al.*, 2008B). The obese children increased their intake by the greatest amount following

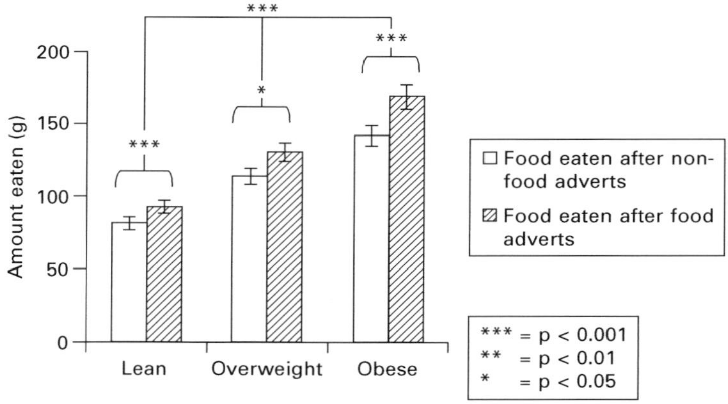

Fig. 6.1 Amount of food eaten after presentation of adverts.

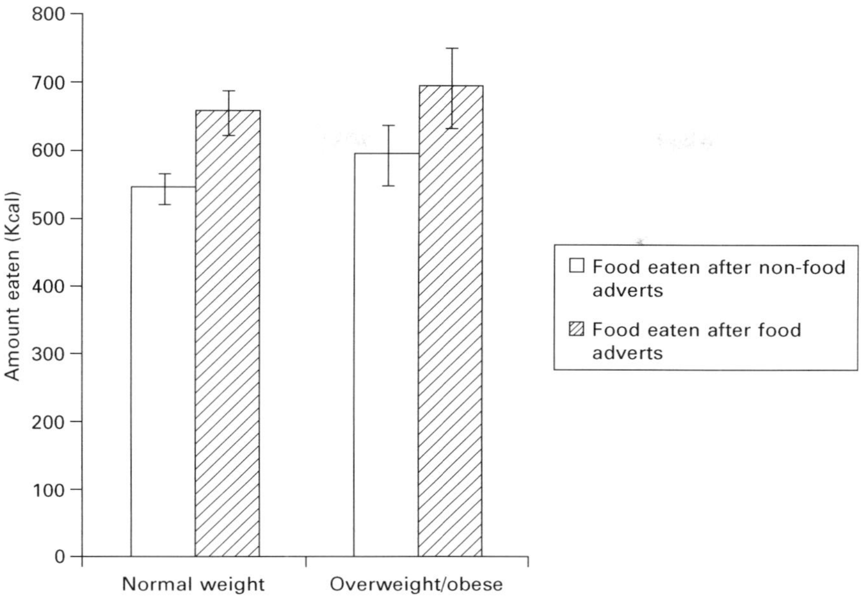

Fig. 6.2 Amount of food eaten after presentation of adverts.

the television food ad exposure. This suggests that overweight and obese children are more responsive to food promotion, and notably, in this study such promotion specifically stimulated the intake of energy-dense snack foods (Halford *et al.*, 2008B).

Furthermore, Buijzen *et al.* (2008) found that children's exposure to food advertising was significantly related to their consumption of both advertised brands and generic energy-dense product categories. However, studies have also shown that ads for healthier food products have an impact. Dixon *et al.* (2007) showed that exposing children to ads for nutritious foods positively improved attitudes and beliefs concerning these foods. In addition, Bannon and Schwartz (2006) found that if children were exposed to videos containing nutritional messages, they were more likely than children who had not seen the nutritional messages to select apples rather than crackers for a subsequent snack.

6.3.4 Effects on purchase requests/behaviour

Children are believed to independently spend over $6 billion annually for goods and services, and to directly influence another $130 billion of spending in family and household purchases, as well as possessing an indirect influence over an additional $130 billion spending (Macklin, 1994). Therefore, children are a lucrative market for advertisers to target, which is being increasingly

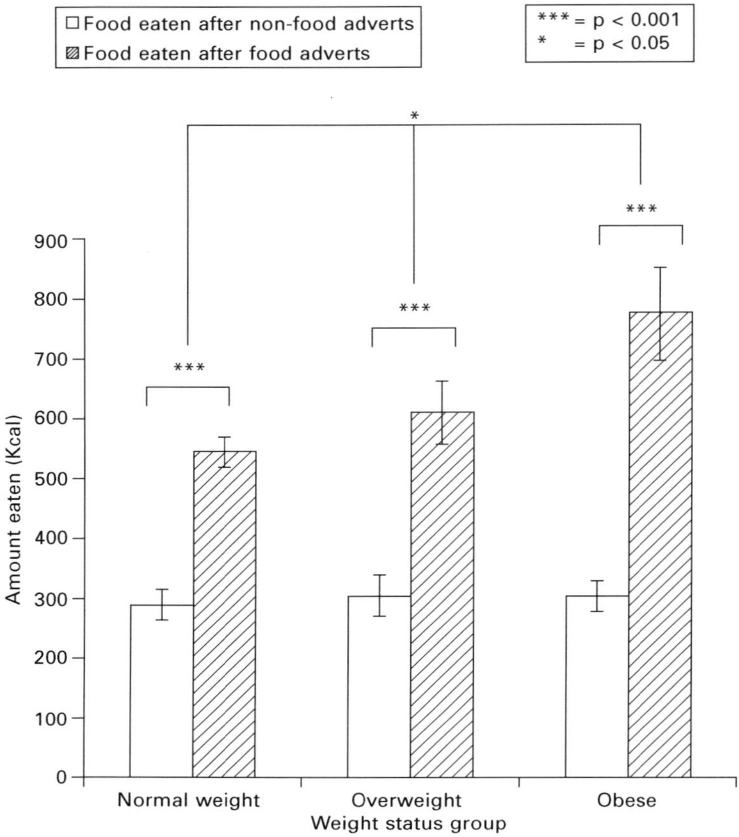

Fig. 6.3 Mean (± SEM) amount of food eaten by normal weight, overweight and obese children in the two advertisement conditions.

recognised. The largest product category for children's purchases is sweets, snacks and beverages (Schor and Ford, 2007). Furthermore, greater than 50% of parents interviewed for an international study reported that children are an important factor in influencing their purchasing decisions, and it was often stated that the 'child's demand' was their primary reason for buying a product (Escalante de Cruz *et al.*, 2004).

In a large review of the evidence, Hastings *et al.* (2003) agree that there is strong evidence that food promotion influences children's food purchase-related behaviour, defined as behaviour intended to influence parents' food purchases. As far back as 1976, it was first reported that there was a significant and positive correlation between the hours of commercial television children watched each week and the number of purchasing-influencing attempts made to their parent while food shopping (Galst and White, 1976). Subsequently, it was found that children who watched a cartoon embedded with food commercials made more requests for the advertised foods in a subsequent artificial shopping environment than the children who had watched the cartoon with no commercials (Brody *et al.*, 1981).

6.3.5 Advertising recall and recognition

Prior research indicates that at the age of two years, children have the capacity to recognise, classify and evaluate brand or product alternatives and actually express these preferences in letters to Santa (Macklin, 1994). Ability to recall and recognise brands is assumed to indicate positive attention and memory of advertising activity, and thus can imply that an ad or a brand has persuasive power (Curlo and Chamblee, 1998). Recall and recognition are different constructs, as 2–3 year old children were able to recall only one out of twelve brands, whereas when asked to select the correct brand from a number of given options (recognition), the success rate increased to eight out of twelve (Valkenburg and Buijzen, 2005). Recognition is thought to develop earlier than recall, perhaps due to less cognitive processing being required (Valkenburg and Buijzen, 2005). Both recall and recognition are thought to be required for sophisticated purchase decisions involving the brands being identified, evaluated and selected in varied retail environments and contexts (Valkenburg and Buijzen, 2005). Children do seem to develop relationships with brands, showing brand name recall and information retrieval about previous brand experiences, a relationship that is influenced (to varying and as yet unknown degrees) by both their peers and the mass media (Ji, 2002).

Our own research findings have demonstrated that following food ad exposure, correct recall of ads is significantly related to the subsequent number of food items selected on self-reported food preference measures (Halford *et al.*, 2008A). Furthermore, obese children correctly recognised more food ads than normal weight children (see Fig. 6.4), a recognition that

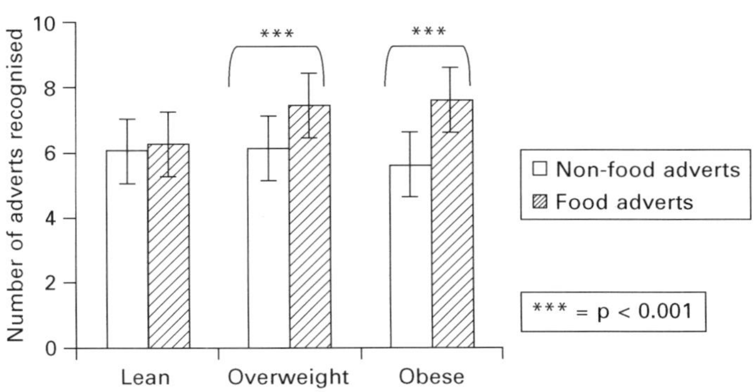

Fig. 6.4 Number of adverts recognised.

was positively correlated with the amount of food subsequently consumed (Halford *et al.*, 2004). Recognition of food ads was also related to body mass index in 5–7 year old children (Halford *et al.*, 2008B) which is consistent with the findings of other studies linking brand recognition and weight status (Arredondo *et al.*, 2009).

Previously, Hitchings and Moynihan (1998) interviewed 9–11 year old children to record their recall of food advertisements seen, and obtained three-day food diaries to determine consumption. The children's parents were also interviewed to find out what, if any, food requests had been received. A significant positive relationship was identified between the food ads recalled and the foods consumed, particularly regarding intake of soft drinks, crisps and savoury snacks. Interestingly, of the ten most requested food items, four were amongst the ten most frequently recalled television food ads (Hitchings and Moynihan, 1998).

6.3.6 Individual differences in food advertising response

Although, as discussed previously, the evidence exists to show that food advertising has an effect on children's preferences and choice, little is known about the mechanism for this effect and therefore how individual differences in response can be explained. It must be assumed that between ad exposure and purchase or purchase-influencing behaviour, there is a pathway featuring a number of factors that are not yet fully elucidated. This pathway occurs in, and is affected by, a child's context that supplies numerous potentially important variables, such as exposure to both advertised and novel products and brands in retail outlets, at home, school and in other settings, interactions with parents/siblings, exposure to other media sources and other advertising avenues among many other factors (Batada and Borzekowski, 2008). Such other factors may include the current physiological state of the individual, e.g. hunger/thirst levels or even mood (Mela, 2001), but also other long-term intrinsic (e.g. genotype, eating style) and extrinsic (parental control, food availability, peer influence) mediating factors.

Few researchers have addressed the issue of individual differences in response; however the roles of cue responsiveness and media literacy are purported to have a potential role in mediating between ad exposure and food preference, brand preference and eating behaviours in children.

Food ads are thought to act as cues for food intake, so that exposure to such cues may act to promote food consumption and related behaviours (Harris *et al.*, 2009). Indeed, external stimuli are able to provoke eating even in the absence of nutritional need (Rogers, 1999) and this explanation could at least partially account for differential effects of food ads on children's preferences and choice, due to individual variations in food cue responsiveness (Carnell *et al.*, 2008). For example, Schacter's externality theory of obesity (Schacter, 1971) asserts that obese individuals are more influenced by external stimuli than lean people are. Indeed, in several studies, obese individuals have been found to have more appetitive responses to food cues. It has been found that adiposity in 3–5 year old children was positively related to scores on the subscale of the Child Eating Behaviour Questionnaire that measures 'food cue responsiveness' (Carnell and Wardle, 2008). Further, in response to food cues, it has been found that obese children increase their food intake by more than normal weight children (Jansen *et al.*, 2003). Food cues are highly salient stimuli, and responsiveness could be one potential mediating factor in the relationship between food ad exposure and effects on food preference and choice.

In addition, the degree of media literacy a child has may partially mediate their response to food advertising. It has been purported that younger children may have increased susceptibility to advertising when compared with older children, adolescents or adults because they do not possess the cognitive development necessary to be able to understand the persuasive intent of ads and therefore cannot critically judge the advertising messages (Oates *et al.*, 2003). There is much debate over the age at which children are able to distinguish between advertising and programming content, thought to be a crucial aspect of media literacy. One author contends that 5–8 year olds can (in a majority of cases) recognise the distinction between programming and advertising if the response format is non-verbal (Bijmolt *et al.*, 1998). Other authors believe that younger children may be able to make the distinction, although they may be basing their assessment on factors such as the length of the advert compared to a programme. The younger children may also be more easily confused by the appearance of a cartoon character which acts to blur the line between ad and programme content, and they also may find it more difficult to verbalise their understanding (Pine, 2003).

It is also not fully elucidated whether even an understanding of the intent of advertising actually provides children with the supposed 'cognitive defences' required to counteract or resist the persuasive nature of the messages (Livingstone and Helsper, 2006). However, findings have indicated that once an older child (10–12 years) has attributed a degree of persuasive intent to an ad, that a child is less likely to believe the claims, reports reduced liking of the ad, and is less likely to desire the products advertised (Rozendaal *et al.*, 2009). Some media literacy programmes have been carried out across the globe, but have not been sufficiently evaluated as to their effect on children's critical understanding of advertising (Matthews, 2007).

To summarise, research evidence to date indicates that the majority of foods promoted to children are energy-dense and low in nutrients, and the promotion of these foods has a detrimental effect on children's food intake, food preferences, food choices, and purchase requests. Concerns over food advertising and the health consequences for children have led campaigners to call for regulatory changes regarding such advertising, particularly regarding the commercial messages to which children are exposed.

6.4 Implications for the food industry, healthcare professionals and policy makers: regulation of food marketing activity

6.4.1 Regulatory changes to television food advertising in the UK

The UK has recently implemented new legislation designed to limit the advertising of high fat, sugar and/or salt (HFSS) foods to children. As of January 2009, the advertising of HFSS foods is banned on dedicated children's channels (Ofcom, 2007). Advertising of such foods is also prohibited in and around programming of particular appeal to children on all channels, regardless of when these programmes are scheduled (Ofcom, 2007). However, the effectiveness of such regulations at reducing children's exposure to HFSS advertising is yet to be critically evaluated and the new rules have come in for much criticism. Particular concerns have been raised regarding the way programmes are deemed to be 'of particular appeal to children', using the proportion of children in the audience as opposed to the overall viewing figure; therefore, if a programme is also watched by adults it is unlikely to be covered by the restrictions even if over a million children are watching (*Which?*, 2006). Indeed, one survey found that there is a clear discrepancy between the programmes most watched by children and the programmes covered by the restrictions; out of the 30 most popular programmes with 4–15 year olds, the first programme to be included in the restrictions is the 27th most popular programme in the list (SpongeBob Squarepants) – HFSS advertising would be free to continue around the 26 more popular programmes before this (*Which?*, 2006).

Although the negative effects of 'junk food' advertising has provoked considerable debate, very little attention has been devoted to potential strategies to increase healthy food advertising to encourage healthy eating amongst children. This is despite evidence that such 'counter-advertising' can be an effective strategy for promoting healthy behaviour, either through ensuring that television channels must broadcast 'anti-junk food' messages or requiring a greater proportion of healthy food than unhealthy food advertisements be shown (Dixon *et al.*, 2007).

6.4.2 Non-broadcast advertising regulation

In the UK, advertising (other than on television) is either regulated using voluntary codes or is not regulated at all. The Committee of Advertising Practice (CAP) is responsible for the UK's advertising codes covering printed ads, posters and other promotional media in public places, cinema and DVD ads, online ads, viewdata ads (i.e. Teletext), marketing databases, sales promotions and ad promotions (CAP, 2010). The CAP code is enforced by the Advertising Standards Authority (ASA), who are a self-regulating body set up by the advertising industry to deal with issues of compliance with the rules (Children's Food Campaign, 2008). However, concerns have been raised that the current regulations do not cover product packaging, the colour and shape of foods, new media (website content, commercial emails, mobile phone text messaging, marketing activity originating outside of the UK, product placement e.g. in computer games), brand equity characters (e.g. Tony the Tiger™ for Kellogg's Frosties®), sponsorship, point-of-sale marketing, or the placement of print ads, despite evidence suggesting these factors do have an effect on children's choices (Children's Food Campaign, 2008).

6.5 Summary

In summary, amid the current obesity epidemic, questions have been raised about the influence of food advertising on children's food-related behaviours and consequently their habitual diets and overall health. Considerable research evidence has been assimilated to demonstrate effects of exposure to food advertising on children's brand preferences, food preferences, food intake and the number of requests children make to parents for products they have seen advertised. These effects are not product or brand specific but rather before brand and may sustain unhealthy eating patterns as they still predominantly promote a diet that is far from healthy. Even with food promotion during children's programming being restricted in some countries, the extent of food promotion to which children are exposed via television remains extensive. Although television continues to be the primary medium for food promotion, new media (such as the internet and mobile phones) provide opportunities for novel, targeted and often interactive food branding and advertising. It is clear that the extent and sophistication of these activities are ever increasing. However, the viral and often 'underground' nature of some of these promotional phenomena make it difficult to identify and effectively monitor them, gauge their spread, or examine their impact. Neither the effects of such innovative promotional activity nor the effectiveness of recent restrictions regarding television advertising of energy-dense foods has yet to be fully elucidated, but certainly empirical evidence suggests that interventions to limit exposure to high fat, sugar and/or salt foods and to increase the media promotion of healthy, nutritious food groups could be beneficial in encouraging children to make better dietary choices.

6.6 References

Abbatangelo-Gray J, Byrd-Bredbenner C and Austin SB (2008), 'Health and Nutrient Content Claims in Food Advertisements on Hispanic and Mainstream Prime-time Television', *J Nut Ed Behav*, 40(6), 348–354.

Alvy LM and Calvert SL (2008), 'Food marketing on popular children's web sites: A content analysis', *JADA*, 108, 710–713.

Arredondo E, Castaneda D, Elder JP, Slymen D and Dozier D (2009), 'Brand name logo recognition of fast food and healthy food among children' *J Community Health*, 34, 73–78.

Bannon K and Schwartz MB (2006), 'Impact of nutrition messages on children's food choice: Pilot study', *Appetite*, 46, 124–129.

Batada A and Borzekowski DL (2008), 'Snap! Crackle! What? Recognition of cereal advertisements and understanding of commercials' persuasive intent among urban, minority children in the US', *J Children and Media*, 2(1), 19–36.

Batada A, Seitz MD, Wootan MG and Story M (2008), 'Nine out of 10 food advertisements shown during Saturday morning children's television programming are for foods high in fat, sodium, or added sugars, or low in nutrients', *JADA*, 108, 673–678.

Batrinou AM, and Kanellou A (2009), 'Healthy food options and advertising in Greece', *Nutr Food Sci*, 39(5), 511–519.

Bell RA, Cassady D, Culp J and Alcalay R (2009), 'Frequency and Types of Foods Advertised on Saturday Morning and Weekday Afternoon English- and Spanish-language American Television Programs', *J Nutr Ed Behav*, 41(6), 406–413.

Bijmolt THA, Claassen W and Brus B (1998), 'Children's understanding of TV advertising: Effects of age, gender, and parental influence', *J Con Pol*, 21, 171–194.

Borzekowski DLG and Robinson TN (2001), 'The 30-second effect: an experiment revealing the impact of television commercials on food preferences of pre-schoolers', *JADA*, 101(1), 42–46.

Brody GH, Stoneman Z, Lane S and Sanders AK (1981), 'Television food commercials aimed at children, family grocery shopping, and mother–child interactions', *Fam Relat*, 30(3), 436–439.

Buijzen M, Schuurman J and Bomhof E (2008), 'Associations between children's television advertising exposure and their food consumption patterns: A household diary-survey', *Appetite*, 50, 231–239.

Byrd-Bredbenner C (2002), 'Saturday morning children's television advertising: A longitudinal content analysis', *Fam Con Sci Res J*, 30(3), 382–403.

Byrd-Bredbenner C and Grasso D (2000), 'Trends in US prime-time television food advertising across three decades', *Nutr Food Sci*, 30(2), 59–66.

Carnell S, Haworth CMA, Plomin R and Wardle J (2008), 'Genetic influences on appetite in children', *Int J Obes*, 32, 1468–1473.

Carnell S and Wardle J (2008), 'Appetite and adiposity in children: Evidence for a behavioral susceptibility theory of obesity', *Am J Clin Nutr*, 88(1), 22–29.

Chang HH and Liu YM (2009), 'The impact of brand equity on brand preference and purchase intentions in the service industries', *Service Ind J*, 29(12), 1687–1706.

Chaplin LN and John DR (2005), 'The development of self-brand connections in children and adolescents', *J Con Res*, 32, 119–129.

Chapman K, Nicholas P and Supramaniam R (2006), 'How much food advertising is there on Australian television?', *Health Promot Int*, 21(3), 172–180.

Chestnutt IG and Ashraf FJ (2002), 'Television advertising of foodstuffs potentially detrimental to oral health – a content analysis and comparison of children's and primetime broadcasts', *Commun Dental Health*, 19, 86–89.

Children's Food Campaign (2008), *Protecting children from unhealthy food marketing*. ISBN: 978-1-903060-45-2. http://www.sustainweb.org/publications.

Childwise (2004), *A concise overview of tracking kids' media and purchasing habits from 1994-2002 by the experts in child research*, www.childwise.co.uk/trends.htm.

Chordas L (2009), 'On the go: Mobile devices are becoming new marketing and advertising platforms for some carriers' brands' *Mobile Marketing, Best's Review*, August 2009.

Committee of Advertising Practice (2010), *The UK code of non-broadcast advertising, sales promotion, and direct marketing* (12th Edition). London: TSO. Available from: http://www.cap.org.uk/The-Codes/New-Advertising-Codes.aspx [Accessed 5 April 2010].

Connor SM (2006), 'Food-related advertising on preschool television: Building brand recognition in young viewers', *Pediatrics*, 118(4), 1478–1485.

Curlo E and Chamblee R (1998), 'Ad processing and persuasion: The role of brand identification', *Psychol and Marketing*, 15(3), 279–299.

Dibb S and Harris L (1996), *A spoonful of sugar. Television food advertising aimed at children: An international comparative study*, Consumers International.

Dixon HG, Scully ML, Wakefield MA, White VM and Crawford DA (2007), 'The effects of television advertisements for junk food versus nutritious food on children's food attitudes and preferences', *Social Sci and Med*, 65, 1311–1323.

Escalante de Cruz A, Phillips S, Visch M and Saunders DB (2004), *The Junk Food Generation: A multi-country survey of the influence of television advertisements on children*, Consumers International.

Folta SC, Goldberg JP, Economos C, Bell R and Meltzer R (2006), 'Food advertising targeted at school-age children: A content analysis', *J Nutr Ed Behav*, 38, 244–248.

Forman J, Halford JCG, Summe H, MacDougall M and Keller KL (2009), 'Food branding influences ad libitum intake differently in children depending on weight status. Results of a pilot study', *Appetite*, 53, 76–83.

Galcheva SV, Iotova VM, Stratev VK (2008), 'Television food advertising directed towards Bulgarian children', *Arch Dis Child*, 93, 857–861.

Galst JP and White MA (1976), 'The unhealthy persuader: The reinforcing value of television and children's purchase-influencing attempts at the supermarket', *Child Dev*, 47(4), 1089–1096.

Garde A (2008), 'Food advertising and obesity prevention: What role for the European Union?', *J Con Pol*, 31, 25–44.

Garretson JA and Niedrich RW (2004), 'Spokes-characters', *J Advertising*, 33(2), 25–36.

Gorn GJ and Goldberg ME (1982), 'Behavioral evidence of the effects of televised food messages on children', *J Con Res*, 9, 200–205.

Graff SK (2008), 'First amendment implications of restricting food and beverage marketing in schools', *Ann Am Acad Pol Soc Sci*, 615, 157–177.

Halford JCG, Boyland EJ, Cooper GD, Dovey TM, Smith CJ, Williams N, Lawton CL and Blundell JE (2008A), 'Children's food preferences: Effects of weight status, food type, branding and television food advertisements (commercials)', *Int J Pediatric Obes*, 3, 31–38.

Halford JCG, Boyland EJ, Hughes GM, Oliveira LP and Dovey TM (2007a), 'Beyond-brand effect of television (TV) food advertisements/commercials on caloric intake and food choice of 5–7-year-old children', *Appetite*, 49, 263–267.

Halford JCG, Boyland EJ, Hughes GM, Stacey L, McKean S and Dovey TM (2008B), 'Beyond-brand effect of television (TV) food advertisements on food choice in children: The effects of weight status', *Public Health Nutr*, 11(9), 897–904.

Halford JCG, Gillespie J, Brown V, Pontin EE and Dovey TM (2004), 'Effect of television advertisements for foods on food consumption in children', *Appetite*, 42, 221–225.

Harris JL, Pomeranz JL, Lobstein T and Brownell KD (2009), 'A Crisis in the Marketplace: How Food Marketing Contributes to Childhood Obesity and What Can Be Done', *Ann Rev Pub Health*, 30, 211–225.

Hastings G, Stead M, McDermott L, Forsyth A, MacKintosh AM and Rayner M (2003), *Review of research on the effects of food promotion to children*, Centre for Social Marketing, The University of Strathclyde, UK.

Heath R (2009), 'Emotional engagement: How television builds big brands at low attention', *J Advertising Res*, 49(1), 62–73.

Henderson VR and Kelly B (2005), 'Food Advertising in the Age of Obesity: Content Analysis of Food Advertising on General Market and African American Television', *J Nutr Ed Behav*, 37(4), 191–196.

Hitchings E and Moynihan PJ (1998), 'The relationship between television food advertisements recalled and actual foods consumed by children', *J Human Nutr Diet*, 11, 511–517.

Institute of Medicine (2005), *Food Marketing to Children and Youth: Threat or Opportunity?* Washington DC, The National Academies Press.

Jansen A, Theunissen N, Slechten K, Nederkoorn C, Boon B, Mulkens S and Roefs A (2003), 'Overweight children overeat after exposure to food cues', *Eating Behav*, 4(2), 197–209.

Jenkin G, Wilson N and Hermanson N (2008), 'Identifying "unhealthy" food advertising on television: A case study applying the UK Nutrient Profile Model', *Public Health Nutr*, 12(5), 614–623.

Ji MF (2002), 'Children's relationships with brands: 'True love' or 'One-night' stand?' *Psychology and Marketing*, 19(4), 369–387.

Kanner AD (2006), 'The corporatized child', *The California Psychologist* 39(1).

Kelly B, Bochynska K, Kornman K, Chapman K (2008A), 'Internet food marketing on popular children's websites and food product websites in Australia', *Public Health Nutr*, 11(11), 1180–1187.

Kelly B, Hattersley L, King L and Flood V (2008B), 'Persuasive food marketing to children: Use of cartoons and competitions in Australian commercial television advertisements', *Health Promot Int*, 23(4), 337–344.

Kelly B, Smith B, King L, Flood V and Bauman A (2007), 'Television food advertising to children: The extent and nature of exposure', *Public Health Nutr*, 10(11), 1234–1240.

Kelly B, Halford JCG, Boyland EJ, Chapman K, Bautista-Castaño I, Berg C, Caroli M, Cook B, Coutinho JG, Effertz T, Grammatikaki E, Keller K, Leung R, Manios Y, Monteiro R, Pedley R, Prell H, Raine K, Recine E, Serra-Majem L, Singh S, Summerbell C (2010), 'Television food advertising to children: A global perspective', *Am J Public Health*, 100(9), 1730–1736.

King L, Hill AJ (2008), 'Magazine adverts for healthy and less healthy foods: Effects on recall but not hunger or food choice by pre-adolescent children', *Appetite*, 51, 194–197.

Kopelman CA, Roberts LM and Adab R (2007), 'Advertising of food to children: Is brand logo recognition related to their food knowledge, eating behaviours and food preferences?', *J Public Health*, 29(4), 358–367.

Kotler P and Armstrong G (2004), *Principles of Marketing*, Upper Saddle River, NJ: Pearson Education/Prentice Hall.

Lawrence D (2003), 'The role of characters in kids marketing', *Young Consumers*, 4(3), 43–48.

Lear KE, Runyan RC and Whitaker WH (2009), 'Sports celebrity endorsements in retail products advertising', *Int J Retail and Distribution Man*, 37(4), 308–321.

Lewis MK and Hill AJ (1998), 'Food advertising on British children's television: A content analysis and experimental study with nine-year olds', *Int J Obes*, 22, 206–214.

Linn S and Golin J (2006), 'Beyond commercials: How food marketers target children', *Loyola of Los Angeles Law Review*, 39(13), 13–32.

Livingstone S and Helsper EJ (2006), 'Does advertising literacy mediate the effects of advertising on children? A critical examination of two linked research literatures in relation to obesity and food choice', *J Comm*, 56, 560–584.

Macklin MC (1994), 'The Impact of Audiovisual Information on Children's Product-related Recall', *J Con Res*, 21(1), 154.

Mallinckrodt V and Mizerski D (2007), 'The effects of playing an advergame on young children's perceptions, preferences and requests', *J Advertising*, 36(2), 87–100.

Matthews AE (2007), 'Children and obesity: a pan-European project examining the role of food marketing', *Eur J Public Health*, 18, 7–11.

McNeal JU and Ji MF (2003), 'Children's visual memory of packaging', *J Con Marketing*, 20(5), 400–427.

Mela DJ (2001), 'Determinants of food choice: Relationships with obesity and weight control', *Obes Res*, 9(4), 249s–255s.
Moore ES (2006), *It's child's play: Advergaming and the online marketing of food to children*, Kaiser Family Foundation, Menlo Park, CA.
Moore ES, Rideout VJ (2007), 'The online marketing of food to children: Is it just fun and games?', *J Pub Pol and Marketing*, 26(2), 202–220.
Morgan M, Fairchild R, Phillips A, Stewart K and Hunter L (2008), 'A content analysis of children's television advertising: Focus on food and oral health', *Public Health Nutr*, 12(6), 748–755.
Nash A, Pine KJ and Messer DJ (2009), 'Television alcohol advertising: Do children really mean what they say?', *Br J Dev Psychol*, 27, 85–104.
Neuborne E (2001), 'For kids on the web, it's an ad, ad, ad, ad world', *Business Week*, 3475, August 13, 108–109.
Oates C, Blades M, Gunter B and Don J (2003), 'Children's understanding of television advertising: A qualitative approach', *J Marketing Comm*, 9(59), 59–71.
Ofcom (2004), *Childhood obesity: Food advertising in context*.
Ofcom (2007), *Television advertising of food and drink products to children: Final statement*.
Pempek TA, Calvert SL (2009), 'Tipping the balance: Use of advergames to promote consumption of nutritious foods and beverages by low-income African American children', *Arch Pediatr Adolesc Med*, 163(7), 633–637.
Pine KJ (2003), 'Conceptualising and assessing young children's knowledge of television advertising within a framework of implicit and explicit knowledge', *J Marketing Man*, 19, 459–473.
Resnik A and Stern BL (1977), 'Children's television advertising and brand choice: A laboratory experiment', *J Advertising*, 6(3), 11–17.
Roberts M and Pettigrew S (2007), 'A thematic content analysis of children's food advertising', *Int J Advertising*, 26(3), 357–367.
Robinson TN, Borzekowski DLG, Matheson DM and Kraemer HC (2007), 'Effects of fast food branding on young children's taste preferences', *Arch Pediatr Adolesc Med*, 161(8), 792–797.
Rogers PJ (1999), 'Eating habits and appetite control: A psychobiological perspective', *Proc Nutr Soc*, 58, 59–67.
Ross RP, Campbell T, Wright JC, Huston AC, Rice ML and Turk P (1984), 'When celebrities talk, children listen: An experimental analysis of children's responses to TV ads with celebrity endorsement', *J App Dev Psychol*, 5, 185–202.
Rozendaal E, Buijzen M, Valkenburg PM (2009), 'Do children's cognitive defenses reduce advertised product desire?', *Communications*, 34, 287–303.
Sahud HB, Binns HJ, Meadow WL and Tanz RR (2006), 'Marketing fast food: Impact of fast food restaurants in children's hospitals', *Pediatr*, 118(6), 2290–2297.
Schacter S (1971), *Emotions, obesity and crime*, New York, Academic Press.
Schor JB and Ford M (2007), 'From tastes great to cool: Children's food marketing and the rise of the symbolic', *J Law, Med and Ethics*, 35(1), 10–21.
Sixsmith R and Furnham A (2010), 'A content analysis of British food advertisements aimed at children and adults', *Health Promotion Int*, 25(1), 24–32.
Søndergaard HA and Edelenbos M (2007), 'What parents prefer and children like – Investigating choice of vegetable-based food for children', *Food Qual Pref*, 18, 949–962.
Story M and French S (2004), 'Food advertising and marketing directed at children and adolescents in the US', *Int J Behav Nutr Physical Activity*, 1, 3.
Ülger B (2009), 'Packages with cartoon trade characters versus advertising: An empirical examination of preschoolers' food preferences', *J Food Prod Marketing*, 15, 104–117.

Valkenburg PM and Buijzen M (2005), 'Identifying determinants of young children's brand awareness: Television, parents and peers', *App Dev Psychol*, 26, 456–468.
Which? (2005), *Shark tales and incredible endorsements*, February.
Which? (2006), *Television advertising of food and drink products to children: Further consultation*, December.
Which? (2007), *Cartoon heroes and villains*, August.
Wicks J, Warren R, Fosu I and Wicks R (2009), 'Dual-modality disclaimers, emotional appeals, and production techniques in food advertising airing during programs rated for children', *J Advertising*, 38(4), 93–105.
World Health Organisation (2003), *Diet, Nutrition and Prevention of Chronic Diseases*. WHO Technical Report Series 916. Geneva, Switzerland.

7

Increasing children's food choices: strategies based upon research and practice

K. E. Williams, Penn State Hershey Medical Center, USA

Abstract: Children's food choices have a variety of implications for their health and well-being. Strategies for modifying food choices have been documented by studies in the basic and clinical research literatures. This chapter discusses several methods of promoting diet changes, including repeated exposure, modifying foods, and reinforcing acceptance of novel foods. In addition to a review of the empirical literature, possible applications of these methods are discussed. The role of family influences on food selection are also reviewed and strategies for moderating or adapting these influences are discussed. In addition, in each of the sections of this chapter, the empirical literature pertaining to these methods is reviewed and possible applications of the various methods for food selection are discussed.

Key words: taste preference, food selection, repeated exposure, food choice.

7.1 Introduction

Children's food preferences and their intake are controlled by the interplay of a range of biological and environmental factors. Some of these factors influence food selection early in the course of development, with both the taste and olfactory systems functioning even before birth (Ganchrow and Mennella, 2003). Children use these sensory systems to experience the flavors of their mother's diet through amniotic fluid and this experience can lead to increased preference for these flavors at birth (Mennella *et al.*, 2001). While children's diets initially consist only of milk from their mothers, they also experience flavors from their mother's diet through breast milk and this experience has been shown to affect children's fruit and vegetable consumption (Mennella *et al.*, 2001). While early learning affects food selection, there is also evidence that children are born with a preference for sweet tastes (Steiner, 1977).

Even though early learning can increase children's preference to a wider range of foods, a developmental milestone that occurs in young children has been called food neophobia, or an avoidance of novel foods (Cooke, 2007). Emerging between 18–24 months of age, neophobia limits the development of diet variety, with research showing that childen with a greater degree of neophobia have narrower diets (Falciglia *et al.*, 2000; Skinner *et al.*, 2002). While neophobia is described as a phase, there is no evidence that the course of normal development automatically leads to a varied and balanced diet for all children. In fact, research has demonstrated that children report preferences for foods of questionable nutritional benefit, causing both caregivers and clinicians to have a great interest in modifying their preferences. American children reported liking French fries, potato chips, and chocolate chip cookies. They also reported disliking broccoli and cucumber (Skinner *et al.*, 2002). Unfortunately, the finding that children like foods high in fat and sugar, but dislike vegetables is not unique to American children, but has been replicated in children from France (Bellisle *et al.*, 2000), Great Britain (Cooke and Wardle, 2005), Germany (Diehl, 1999), and Spain (Perez-Rodrigo *et al.*, 2003; Serra-Majem *et al.*, 2001). As food preferences have been shown to be related to food selection (Drewnowski, 1997), children's food preferences have many implications for a child's health, development, and well-being.

While many children may prefer foods of limited nutritional value, there is a subset of children whose limited food selection is the target of clinical intervention. Food selectivity by type, defined as eating a narrow range of food that is nutritionally inappropriate, was identified in 74 of 349 children referred to a feeding program (Field *et al.*, 2003), and 134 of 234 children in a subsequent sample of children referred to the same program (Williams *et al.*, 2009). For these, children a range of interventions has been used to increase diet variety, some of which will be discussed here.

The factors involved in the development of children's food preferences and their selection of foods have been extensively researched. In addition to a number of laboratory studies, there are some studies which have occurred in natural settings such as preschools, and a growing body of clinical research involves children with a range of feeding problems. This chapter will provide a brief overview of this literature, with a focus on interventions that have been used to modify or change diet preferences and increase intake of novel foods. Possible applications of these interventions for influencing food selection will also be discussed. The family influences children's food selection in multiple ways. Some of these influences will also be examined.

7.2 The role of exposure in the development of taste preferences in children

7.2.1 A review of the literature

The mere exposure effect holds that simply exposing a person to an unfamiliar stimulus leads the person to rate the stimulus more favorably (Zajonc, 1968). Various research methodologies have demonstrated repeated exposure to novel foods increases preference for those foods. A survey involving 564 mothers of preschool children found the early introduction of fruits and vegetables during weaning was associated with increased consumption of these foods during later childhood (Cooke *et al.*, 2004). Laboratory studies involving children have shown that increased exposure to novel foods increases the preference for those foods (Birch and Marlin, 1982; Sullivan and Birch, 1994). Further, this research has found that tasting, and not looking, at novel foods is required to increase preference (Birch *et al.*, 1987). Birch and her colleagues have conducted numerous studies involving repeated taste exposure and have found that the exposure does indeed require repetition, with studies showing five and ten exposures (Birch and Marlin, 1982), and up to 15 exposures (Sullivan and Birch, 1990), were required to change children's preferences and intake.

Further research conducted in natural settings has also demonstrated repeated taste exposure can increase diet variety. In a home-based study, parents were asked to have their children taste vegetables daily over a 14-day period (Wardle *et al.*, 2003a). Wardle and her colleagues found that children exposed to the novel food reported liking this food more than children in control groups who only received either nutritional information about the food or no intervention. It is noteworthy that parents in the exposure group also reported that the daily tastes increased their children's willingness to try other novel foods that were not part of the research. In a second study conducted by Wardle and her colleagues, the effects of repeated exposure and repeated exposure plus reward were used in a school-setting (Wardle *et al.*, 2003b). Children in the exposure only condition were asked to taste a novel food (red peppers) daily for ten days while children in the exposure plus reward condition were asked to taste the novel food and then given a reward (a sticker) for tasting the food. Children in the control condition were not offered daily tastes. Children in both the exposure only condition and exposure plus reward conditions reported a greater change in liking the novel food and ate more of the food than controls. Repeated exposure was also used with infants in the home setting to increase consumption of disliked vegetables (Maier *et al.*, 2007). While this study also demonstrated that repeated exposure increased acceptance of the target food, in this case, a pureed vegetable, it also demonstrated that acceptance of the vegetable was maintained over a period of nine months.

These studies show promise in the use of repeated exposure as a method of increasing diet variety but there are limitations to their use. In Wardle and colleagues' home-based study, 14 of 48 parents in the exposure group failed to offer the target vegetable more than nine times, thus it may be difficult to get parents to provide enough exposures to make preference change possible. There is also evidence that the 5 to 15 exposures generally discussed in the research by Birch and colleagues are not enough for all foods, and possibly all age groups. In one study using two groups of school-aged children, 7–9 and 10–12 year olds, up to 20 exposures were used and willingness to try novel foods was achieved only in the older group (Loewen and Pliner, 1999). In most of the research involving repeated exposure in children, foods that would be generally considered appealing, such as fruits, cheeses, and juice, were often used. While Wardle and colleagues' use of red pepper and Maier *et al.*'s inclusion of pureed vegetable were exceptions, there is still little basic research showing that repeated exposure is effective in getting children to eat vegetables or foods considered by children to be less appealing. A wider range of foods, however, has been introduced in the clinical studies that have included repeated taste exposure as a component in interventions for food selectivity (Paul *et al.*, 2007; Pizzo *et al.*, 2009). One intervention combined repeated taste exposure with escape prevention, which involved continuing to present a bite of food until it was consumed by the child. This intervention was implemented by Paul and colleagues in a feeding program to treat two children with autism with extreme food selectivity who had failed community-based treatment. One child, a 3.5-year-old boy consumed almost exclusively milk, hot dogs, and grilled cheese sandwiches, and the second child, a 5-year-old girl, ate nothing and was dependent upon gastrostomy tube feedings. The children were presented with foods from all food groups chosen by the parents from a list of 139 common foods. Across the course of treatment, brief probe meals were offered to evaluate which foods the children would eat, and measure progress. During these probe meals, the children were praised for eating, but were not required to do so. The children were introduced to novel foods in taste sessions. In each taste session, a pea-sized bite of food was presented and the session was terminated as soon as the bite was consumed. As the child was eating a particular food, within 30 seconds in a taste session the bite size was systematically increased to full spoonfuls. A particular food was considered as successfully eaten when the child ate at least three full teaspoons of that food in a probe meal. Across the course of treatment, the number of bites eaten in probe meals continued to increase. After 15 days of intensive treatment, the boy was eating 65 foods and after 13 days of intensive treatment, the girl was eating 49 foods and she no longer needed tube feedings. At three month follow-up, the boy's parents reported he was eating 53 foods and the girl's parents reported she was eating 47 foods and continued to thrive without tube feedings. While successful, the study was conducted in an intensive feeding program and most of the treatment was conducted by therapists, although parents were successfully trained to continue treatment in the home setting after discharge. In a subsequent study, the same intervention was utilized with a briefer clinic-based phase and a focus on rapidly transferring the treatment to the home setting (Pizzo *et al.*, 2009). Pizzo and her associates worked with three boys with food selectivity, a five-year-old boy with a history of gastroesophageal reflux who predominantly ate smooth foods and milk, a nine-year-old boy with attention deficit hyperactivity disorder who ate mainly starches and milk products, and a four-year-old boy with autism whose diet consisted largely of the same five foods. The clinic-based treatment lasted five days for one boy, and four days for the other two boys and the children's parents were successfully trained to implement the intervention in the home setting. The outcomes showed that each boy continued to make progress at home after the brief intensive treatment, with each of the boys adding more than 30 new foods to their diets at the end of one month (Pizzo *et al.*, 2009). Together, these studies suggest that repeated taste exposure can be used as a clinical tool for increasing food selection of children with significant limitations in diet variety. These studies also showed that, if conducted consistently and intensively, foods from all groups could be successfully added to the children's diets.

One of the important pieces of information derived from the laboratory studies on taste exposure was the need for exposure to be repeated, with 10–15 exposures being commonly recommended to parents. This information was derived from studies involving groups of children offered only a limited number of foods. It was not clear if this recommendation, derived mainly from the Birch studies discussed previously, applies to an individual child across time as multiple foods are added to the child's diet. One study using a clinical sample attempted to examine this issue with the goal of determining if the number of exposures needed to modify food preferences would decrease as a child's dietary variety increased. Again using the Paul *et al.* methodology described earlier, the data were analyzed for six children being treated in a feeding program for extreme food selectivity (Williams *et al.*, 2008). Using a longitudinal approach, these researchers counted the number of taste exposures required before a novel food was eaten in a meal and found that, as more novel foods were added to a child's diet, the number of taste exposures required for subsequent novel foods to be eaten in meals decreased. This study, entitled 'Practice Makes Perfect', suggests that eating novel foods becomes more likely as diet variety increases. Thus, if a child becomes used to eating novel foods and is regularly exposed to novel foods, the number of exposures required before a child eats portions of a novel food may be less than the often suggested 10 to 15 exposures.

7.2.2 Rationale for using taste exposure

Taste exposure has not only been shown to be an effective tool in increasing diet variety, but it has been shown to work for all ages of children. The size of the taste used in several studies was pea-sized, making the effort required by the child very low. The use of repeated exposure is conceptually simple; thus it could be used by parents, teachers, and other individuals in the child's natural environment. While the exposures for a particular novel food do need to occur repeatedly, an exposure-based intervention could be easily integrated into the child's daily schedule. If the child was exposed only to a single bite of a novel food daily during snack time at preschool, the number of exposures would quickly accumulate. In several studies involving taste exposure just reviewed, the exposures occurred in a neutral setting outside of the home (e.g. preschool, university laboratory, clinic). There are several possible reasons why children may be more likely to taste novel foods in other settings. It might be easier to induce children to taste new foods in an environment where same-aged peers who have less suspicion of the novel foods are present and are also trying the foods. The home setting may be associated with eating a narrow range of foods, and the child has already learned that tasting new foods is not required. It is also possible that children may be more likely to taste novel foods for therapists, teachers, or researchers than for caregivers, because these persons do not have the same learning history with the child who may have already learned to associate the caregiver with eating certain foods while avoiding other foods.

Even though we know that repeated exposure to novel foods can increase diet variety, we also know that parents often do not provide the number of repeated exposures required and fail to offer foods that are rejected by their children. In one study, the average number of exposures provided before mothers decided their children liked or disliked a food was less than three (Carruth *et al.*, 1998). In examining a large sample of children with feeding problems, we have found a significant inverse relationship between the caregiver's willingness to offer foods to their children other than those served during family meals and the number of foods reported eaten by their children (Hendy *et al.*, 2009b). This finding, that children who reject foods eaten by the family and are offered alternative foods eat a narrower variety of foods than children not offered alternative foods, is related to our discussion of repeated taste exposure. Children who are offered alternative meals that typically consist only of preferred foods, never have the opportunity to taste novel foods (since novel foods are not offered), thus these children never develop preferences for novel foods.

7.3 Modifying foods to improve their acceptance and consumption by children

7.3.1 A review of the literature

In both laboratory and clinical studies, acceptance of particular foods has been influenced by various modifications to the food. One of these methods has been to combine preferred and novel tastes or foods. Using a procedure described as 'conditioned enhancement', researchers offered college students various flavors of herbal tea, with some teas being sweetened with sucrose while others were left unsweetened (Zeller *et al.*, 1983). The students provided hedonic rating for each flavor of tea, with the sweetened teas receiving higher ratings than the unsweetened teas. The researchers suggested that this provided evidence of flavor–flavor conditioning and that the liking of neutral flavors or tastes could be enhanced if paired with a hedonically positive taste, such as sugar (Zeller *et al.*, 1983). In other example of flavor–flavor conditioning, Pliner and Stallberg-White (2000) compared children's willingness to taste unfamiliar chips alone, with a familiar dip, or with an unfamiliar dip. As the researchers predicted, the addition of the familiar dip increased the children's willingness to taste unfamiliar chips. Clinical studies have also utilized the pairing of foods as one component in a treatment package. In order to increase consumption of vegetables in a 14-year-old boy with autism and food selectivity, the vegetables were covered with a preferred condiment, namely catsup (Ahearn, 2003). The blending of preferred and novel foods has also been used as a treatment for food refusal by Mueller *et al.* (2004). In this study, foods were blended at ratios of 10% novel to 90% preferred and 20% novel to 80% preferred. The results showed that the blended foods increased the probability that novel foods would later be eaten without being blended with preferred foods. An analogous procedure was also used to increase milk consumption in a four-year-old child in a preschool setting (Tiger and Hanley, 2006). In this case study, a child who consistently refused to drink milk was presented with milk mixed with chocolate syrup, a preferred condiment. After the child was consistently drinking the chocolate milk, the chocolate was systematically faded out of the milk until the child was drinking only milk. In these studies, the flavor of the foods targeted for consumption (the novel foods) was altered either by being mixed with a condiment or by being blended with a preferred food. In another study, the simultaneous presentation of a novel food and a preferred food was used in the treatment of a seven-year-old boy with autism (Kern and Marder, 1996). In this study, the child was presented with a novel food (e.g. a small piece of vegetable) that was placed on top of a preferred food (e.g. a corn chip). While this form of simultaneous presentation may not alter the flavor of the novel food, one would expect when covered with a condiment or blended together with a preferred food, the simultaneous presentation of a novel and preferred food did serve to increase acceptance of the novel food.

As an alternative to combining preferred and novel foods, the consumption of novel foods has also been increased by modifying the amount of the food being presented. In working with children who exhibit problems with eating, clinicians have commonly discussed modifying the volume or texture of foods in order to decrease the response effort required of the child. In the treatment of children with food refusal, one study evaluated the acceptance bites of food which varied in size (Kerwin *et al.*, 1995). The results showed that acceptance was highest for the smallest bite size. In the previously discussed clinical interventions which utilized repeated exposure studies, bites of novel foods the size of a pea were initially presented, with the size of the bite for a particular food increasing only after a child was eating that food within a specific time criterion and without exhibiting inappropriate behaviors. In addition to manipulating the bite size to increase the probability of acceptance, other studies have modified other aspects of the foods offered. In two studies, children who ate only lower textures were taught to accept higher textures by systematically increasing the texture of the food (Shore *et al.*, 1998; Luiselli and Gleason, 1987).

7.3.2 Possible applications of modifying foods

Modifying foods to increase their consumption has become widespread in recent years, with food companies and manufacturers now blending vegetables into pasta meals, pasta sauces, juices, and even meat products. Recent popular press books have described how to improve children's diets by suggesting methods of either mixing fruits and vegetables into other food dishes, or masking the fruits and vegetables. Although this trend will no doubt continue and will increase consumption of more foods deemed as healthy, e.g. vegetables, it is not clear that by serving a particular food in some modified form it will increase consumption of that food if offered in its original form. For example, if a child eats pasta sauce containing blended cauliflower, his consumption of cauliflower will increase, but if presented with only cauliflower it is not clear that eating the sauce will increase the probability that the child will consume the cauliflower presented alone. The use of stimulus fading does, however, provide a method of transitioning from eating a food that has been modified in some way (e.g. blended into another food, mixed with a condiment) to eating that food alone. In a study conducted by Piazza and her colleagues, preferred and novel foods were blended together, with the initial mixture consisting of only 10% novel food. Across the course of the intervention, the percentage of preferred food was systematically decreased as the percentage of novel food was increased, until the child was eating only the novel food. This type of fading procedure does take time, but can be a very successful method of establishing new foods in a child's diet.

Studies which initially offered pea-sized bites of a food, then systematically increased the bite size based upon the child's acceptance of that particular food, demonstrate the use of another form of fading that could be incorporated into many interventions. The gradual increase in volume has been used with success, even with children having severe feeding problems, and no doubt could be used as a tool to introduce novel tastes or types of food. It is interesting that a recent study found that the shape of a snack food influenced long-term liking, with small-shaped snack foods remaining stable in liking and large-shaped snack foods decreasing in liking over repeated consumptions (Liem and Zandstra, 2009). It is possible that this finding is due to the fact that the children perceive a lower response effort in eating smaller pieces of snack food which translates into more liking for the smaller food.

7.4 Reinforcement-based interventions used for increasing acceptance of novel foods by children

7.4.1 A review of the literature

The use of reinforcement or rewards for eating has been controversial. It has been suggested that by providing reinforcement for eating a particular food, the intrinsic motivation for that food decreases. The evidence to support this view is largely based upon two studies conducted by Birch and her colleagues. In the initial study, the preferences for seven fruit juices and seven play activities were measured for twelve children in baseline sessions (Birch *et al.*, 1982). The children were told that, in order to gain access to a play activity, they were required to drink a specific amount of a fruit juice. The results showed that the juices the children were required to drink in order to gain access to play activities decreased in preference while the juices that were offered, but which they were not required to drink, did not decrease in preference. This has been cited as evidence of the 'overjustification effect' that occurs when an extrinsic reward is offered (e.g. the play activity) and the child discounts the instrumental activity (e.g. drinking the required fruit juice) as a means to an end. Since the children were required to drink more of the juice to access the play activity than they had spontaneously consumed in baseline sessions, an alternative explanation would be that because the children were required to drink more than the amount they had taken spontaneously, the juice became aversive. A subsequent study involved 45 children and was conducted in a preschool at a regularly scheduled snack time (Birch *et al.*, 1984). The children were assigned to one of six conditions, two control conditions and four instrumental eating conditions, in which they would be either praised or given tickets for a movie for drinking a milk drink. While the children in the control groups showed no decreased preference for the milk drink they were offered at snacks, the children in the four instrumental groups did show a decreased preference. Although the data from this study are widely cited as evidence that extrinsic rewards (e.g. praise, movies) decrease preference for the food that had to be consumed to earn the reward, Birch and her colleagues stated that the results of the study could have alternatively resulted from the children drinking more of the milk drink than they would have drank without the contingency being in effect (Birch *et al.*, 1984).

While parents have been warned against rewarding consumption of foods that are healthy, but may not be preferred, (e.g. 'eat all of your broccoli and you may have a toy') (Benton, 2004), the use of positive reinforcement has been used with success in a variety of contexts related to children's food choice and consumption. An intervention designed to increase healthy food choices in eight preschoolers involving the use of praise and stickers as a reward for choosing a healthy snack was formulated by Stark *et al.* (1986). In this study, children were trained to discriminate between 'red' foods (e.g. potato chips, cookies, cheese puffs) and 'green' foods (e.g. various fresh fruits and vegetables), with the reward delivered contingent on choosing a 'green' food. The results showed that five of the children chose healthy snacks (i.e. 'green' foods) in the maintenance phase of the intervention even though no nutritional instructions, feedback, or stickers were given and only praise continued (Stark *et al.*, 1986). This provides some evidence for the use of rewards to improve food selection with no evidence of the overjustification effect. The use of positive reinforcement is wide-spread in the treatment literature involving children's feeding problems. Working with children who exhibit little or no interest in eating, clinicians have commonly included positive reinforcement as a component in their interventions. In a recent review of food refusal, a severe feeding problem defined as a child's refusal to eat all or most foods presented, resulting in the child either failing to meet caloric needs or being dependent on supplemental tube feedings, positive reinforcement was used in 37 of the 38 intervention studies reviewed (Williams *et al.*, in press). The type of reinforcement used ranged widely, with some studies using only praise and others using tangible rewards or access to preferred activities. The extensive utilization of reinforcement as a component in interventions for feeding and eating problems in children is not unique to food refusal. Both a recent review of eating problems in children with autism spectrum disorders (Williams and Seiverling, 2010) and a book on the treatment of eating problems in children with special needs (Williams and Foxx, 2007) describe numerous studies involving interventions including some form of reinforcement.

7.4.2 Applications of reinforcement-based interventions

While a pair of laboratory studies have suggested the use of rewards can be detrimental, a large number of clinical studies have demonstrated the utility of reinforcement as a component in interventions for children with feeding and eating problems. The Birch studies showed that preference for a particular food decreased when a child was required to consume a specific amount in order to gain access to a reinforcer. This may provide an important caution in the use of reinforcement for eating. In the Birch studies, it appeared that the children were required to eat more than they would have typically eaten, in order to gain access to the reinforcer, possibly eating past the point of satiety. The use of reinforcement in modifying food selection would not necessarily involve eating large amounts of a particular food, but rather could be used as a consequence for tasting a novel food. If this were the case, rather than a decrease in food preference as found in the Birch studies, one would predict an increase in preference as the child is repeatedly exposed to the novel food. The clinical literature describing positive reinforcement as a component in interventions for feeding problems is extensive, suggesting that, when used appropriately, reinforcement can be an effective tool in modifying food selection and consumption. In clinical settings, the children referred there have already demonstrated deficits in developing appropriate eating behaviors and diet variety. Reinforcement is a tool that has been successfully used to both help these children improve their nutritional status and develop age-appropriate skills. When using reinforcement, the goal is to change the behavior identified as the target of treatment and then systematically eliminate the use of not only the reinforcement, but all intervention procedures.

7.5 Family influences on children's food choice

7.5.1 A review of the literature

Caregivers play a critical role in their children's food choices and influence their food choices in several ways. Caregivers eat in front of their children, with the children observing and often imitating the caregivers' behavior. Modeling eating behavior is thus one of the most prominent ways in which caregivers can influence their children's food selection. The importance of modeling by caregivers has been demonstrated in several studies, with one study showing that children were more likely to eat a particular food if an adult tasted that food prior to offering the food, rather than just offering the food (Harper and Sanders, 1975). A similar outcome was found in another study in which children were more likely to eat a new food if an adult ate the same type of food than if the adult ate a different food or ate no food (Addressi *et al.*, 2005). Indirect evidence of modeling comes from a survey of 427 families which revealed that children who ate with parents, siblings, or parents and siblings, ate more foods from the basic food groups (Stanek *et al.*, 1990) than children who did not. The effects of modeling extends to liquids as well, and in a study based upon maternal reports, mothers who drank more milk, frequently had daughters who drank more milk and less soda (Fisher *et al.*, 2004).

Caregivers, most often mothers, are responsible for their children's nutrition in that they purchase, prepare, and serve the foods offered to their children. Not only are caregivers responsible for which foods are offered to their children, caregivers also determine when foods are offered, the portion size of the food offered, and how often a particular food is offered. The availability of the foods offered by caregivers has been a focus of nutrition research. Several studies have found the availability of foods has been related to their consumption, with child-reported availability of fruits and vegetables predicting higher consumption of these foods (Cullen *et al.*, 2003; Kratt *et al.*, 2000, Wind *et al.*, 2006). Parents of 2008 children were asked to complete extensive questionnaires concerning various aspects of children's nutrition and parent mealtime actions (Hendy *et al.*, 2009a). The results showed that the largest predictor of fruit and vegetable consumption was the daily availability of fruits and vegetables. Children have further demonstrated a preference for healthier foods when they are readily available at home (Baranowski *et al.*, 1999; Story *et al.*, 2002). It is also known that when specific foods (e.g. high-calorie snack foods) are not available, people will shift their preferences to other foods (Smith and Epstein, 1991).

In addition to modeling the consumption of foods and controlling access to foods, caregivers also provide information about the food in terms of health benefits (e.g. 'eat your carrots, they will make you see better') or palatability (e.g. 'here, try this, it tastes delicious'). Research has shown that this information, especially information about the taste of the food, increases the probability that the child will accept the food when it is offered (Lumeng *et al.*, 2008).

7.5.2 Applications related to family influences

While caregivers provide a powerful influence on the development of children's food preferences, it is important that caregivers fully understand their significant role and what actions they can take to ensure their children learn to accept the foods required for a well-balanced diet. With children more likely to eat familiar foods, caregivers must realize they have the ability to increase the familiarity of foods by offering them consistently at meals and modeling their consumption.

7.6 Conclusion

There are multiple strategies supported by empirical research that can be used to modify children's food selections. These strategies, including those discussed in this chapter, can produce changes in a child's diet selection, but all take time and consistent application. As a clinician who works daily with children having feeding or eating problems and their families, I see caregivers who, well-meaning, but often inadvertently, prevent their children from making positive changes. While many caregivers want their children to eat well-balanced diets, they are prone to believing that their children's eating habits are fixed and relatively resistant to change, so they continue eating routines that prevent improvements in food choice. As discussed earlier, caregivers are quick to stop offering foods their children have rejected, reducing the possible exposures the children will have to novel foods. While it should be the case that 'children eat what their parents serve', our clinical experience tells us that, 'parents serve what their children eat'. This may result in the child being offered a narrow variety of foods and in some cases a selection that is not well-balanced. The lack of variety leads some parents to provide their children with supplements, often high-calorie beverages, which in turn can adversely affect food selection because the child is satiated from consuming the calorically-dense supplements. While there are challenges to the modification of children's diet selection, as discussed in this chapter, there are numerous methods and interventions that can be used to modify children's food choices.

7.7 References

Addressi E, Galloway AT, Visalberghi E, and Birch LL (2005) Specific social influences on the acceptance of novel foods in 2–5 year-old-children, *Appetite,* 45, 264–271.

Ahearn WH (2003) Using simultaneous presentation to increase vegetable consumption in a mildly selective child with autism, *J Appl Behav Anal*, 36, 361–365.

Baranowski T, Cullen KW, Baranowski J (1999) Psychosocial correlates of dietary intake: Advancing dietary intervention, *Annu Rev Nutr,* 19, 17–40.

Bellisle F, Rolland-Cachera MF, and Kellogg Scientific Advisory Committee 'Child and Nutrition' (2000) Three consecutive (1993, 1995, 1997) surveys of food intake, nutritional attitudes and knowledge, and lifestyle in 1000 French children, aged 9–11 years, *J Human Nutr Diet*, 13, 101–111.

Benton D (2004) Role of parents in the determination of the food preferences of children and the development of obesity. *International Journal of Obesity*, 28, 858–869.

Birch LL, Birch D, Marlin DW, and Kramer L (1982) Effects of instrumental consumption on children's food preference, *Appetite,* 3, 125–134.

Birch LL and Marlin DW (1982) I don't like it; never tried it: Effects of exposure on two-year-old children's food preferences, *Appetite,* 3, 353–360.

Birch LL, Marlin DW, and Rotter J (1984) Eating as the 'means' activity in a contingency: Effects on young children's food preference. *Child Dev,* 55, 532–539.

Birch LL, McPhee L, Shoba BC, Pirok E, and Steinburg L (1987) What kind of exposure reduces children's food neophobia? *Appetite,* 9, 171–178.

Carruth BR, Skinner J, Houck K, Moran, J, Coletta F, Ott, D (1998) The Phenomenon of 'Picky Eater': A Behavioral Marker in Eating Patterns of Toddlers, *J Am Coll Nutr* 17, 180–186.

Cooke L (2007) The importance of exposure for healthy eating in childhood: A review, *J Hum Nutr Diet*, 20, 294–301.

Cooke LJ and Wardle J (2005) Age and gender differences in children's food preferences, *Br J Nutr,* 93, 741–746.

Cooke LJ, Wardle J, Gibson EL, Sapochnik M, Sheiham A and Lawson M (2004) Demographic, familial and trait predictors of fruit and vegetable consumption by preschool children, *Public Health Nutr*, 7, 295–302.

Cullen KW, Baranowski T, Owens E, Marsh T, Rittenberry L, and de Moor C (2003) Availability, accessibility, and preferences for fruit, 100% fruit juice, and vegetables influence children's dietary behavior, *Health Educ Behav*, 30, 615–626.

Diehl JM (1999) Food preferences of 10- to 14-year-old boys and girls, *Schweiz Med Wochenschr,* 129, 151–161.

Drewnowski A (1997) Taste preferences and food intake, *Annu Rev Nutr*, 17, 237–253.

Falciglia GA, Couch SC, Gribble LS, Pabst SM, Frank R (2000) Food neophobia in childhood affects dietary variety, *J Am Diet Ass,* 100, 1474–81.

Field D, Garland M, Williams K (2003) Correlates of Specific Childhood Feeding Problems, *J Paediatr Child Health*, 39, 299–304.

Fisher JO, Mitchell DC, Smiciklas-Wright H, Mannino M, and Birch LL (2004) Meeting calcium recommendations from ages 5–9 reflects mother-daughter beverage choices and predicts bone mineral status. *Am J Clin Nutr, 79,* 698–706.

Ganchrow JR and Mennella JA (2003) The ontogeny of human flavor perception. In Doty RL, editor. *Handbook of Olfaction and Gustation.* 2nd edn. Marcel Dekker; New York, 823–946.

Harper LV and Sanders KM (1975) The effects of adults' eating on young children's acceptance of unfamiliar foods, *J Exp Child Psychol*, 20, 206–214.

Hendy HM, Williams KE, Camise TS, Eckman N, and Hedemann A (2009a) The parent mealtime action scale: Development and association with children's diet and weight, *Appetite*, 52, 328–339.

Hendy HM, Williams KE, Riegel K, and Paul C (2009b) Parent mealtime actions that mediate associations between children's fussy-eating and their weight and diet, *Appetite,* 54, 191–195.

Kern L, Marder TJ (1996) A comparison of simultaneous and delayed reinforcement as treatments for food selectivity, *J Appl Behav Anal*, 29, 243–246.

Kerwin ML, Ahearn WH, Eicher PS, and Burd DM (1995) The costs of eating: A behavioral economic analysis of food refusal, *J App Behav Anal*, 28, 245–260.

Kratt P, Reynolds K, and Shewchuk R (2000) The role of availability as a moderator of family fruit and vegetable consumption, *Health Educ Behav,* 27, 471–482.

Liem DG and Zandstra EH (2009) Children's liking and wanting of snack products: Influence of shape and flavour. *Int J Behav Nutr Phys Act*, 6, 38.

Loewen R and Pliner P (1999) Effects of prior exposure to palatable and unpalatable novel foods on children's willingness to taste other novel foods, *Appetite,* 32, 351–366.

Luiselli JK, Gleason DJ (1987) combining sensory reinforcement and texture fading procedures to overcome chronic food refusal, *J Behav Ther Exp Psych*, 18, 149–155.

Lumeng JC, Cardinal TM, Jankowski M, Kaciroti N, and Gelman SA (2008) Children's use of adult testimony to guide food selection, *Appetite,* 51, 302–310.

Maier A, Chabanet C, Schaal B, Issanchou S, Leathwood P (2007) Effects of repeated exposure on acceptance of initially disliked vegetables in 7-month old infants. *Food Qual Pref,* 18, 1023–1032.

Mennella JA, Jagnow CP, and Beauchamp, GK (2001) Prenatal and postnatal flavor learning by human infants, *Pediatr*, 107, E88.

Mueller MM, Piazza CC, Patel MR, Kelley ME, and Pruett A (2004) Increasing variety of foods consumed by blending nonpreferred foods into preferred foods, *J Appl Behav Anal,* 37, 159–170.

Paul C, Williams KE, Riegel K, Gibbons B (2007) Combining repeated taste exposure and escape extinction, *Appetite*, 49, 708–711.

Perez-Rodrigo C, Rivas L, Serra-Majem L, and Aranceta J (2003) Food preferences of Spanish children and young people: The enKid study. *European Journal of Clinical Nutrition*, 57, Suppl 1:S45–8.

Pizzo B, Williams KE, Paul C, and Riegel K (2009) Jump start exit criterion: Exploring a new model of service delivery for the treatment of childhood feeding problems, *Behav Inter,* 24, 195–203.

Pliner P and Stallberg-White C (2000) 'Pass the ketchup, please': Familiar flavors increase children's willingness to taste novel foods, *Appetite,* 34, 95–103.

Serra-Majem L, García-Closas R, Ribas L, Pérez-Rodrigo C, and Aranceta J (2001) Food patterns of Spanish schoolchildren and adolescents: The enKid study, *Public Health Nutr*, 4, 1433–1438.

Shore BA, Babbitt RL, Williams KE, Coe DA, Snyder A (1998) Use of texture fading in the treatment of food selectivity, *J Appl Behav Anal*, 31, 621–633.

Skinner JD, Caruth BR, Bounds W, Ziegler P, and Reidy K (2002) Do food-related experiences in the first 2 years of life predict dietary variety in school-aged children? *J Nutr Educ Behav*, 34, 310–315.

Smith JA and Epstein LH (1991) Behavioral economic analysis of food choice in obese children, *Appetite,* 17, 91–95.
Stanek K, Abbott D, and Cramer, S. (1990) Diet quality and the eating environment of preschool children. *J Am Diet Ass*, 90, 1582–1584.
Stark LJ, Collins FL, Osnes PG, and Stokes TF (1986) Using reinforcement and cueing to increase healthy snack food choices in preschoolers, *J Appl Behav Anal*, 19, 367–380.
Steiner JE (1977) Facial expressions of the neonate infant indicating the hedonics of food-related chemical stimuli. In J. M. Weiffenbach (Ed.), *Taste and Development* (pp. 173–189). Bethesda, MD: US Department of Health, Education, and Welfare.
Story M, Neumark-Sztainer D, and French S (2002) Individual and environmental influences on adolescent eating behaviors, *J Am Diet Assoc, 102(supplement),* S40–51.
Sullivan SA and Birch LL (1990) Pass the sugar, pass the salt, *Dev Psychol*, 26, 546–551.
Sullivan SA and Birch LL (1994) Infant dietary experience and acceptance of solid foods, *Pediatr,* 93, 271–277.
Tiger JH and Hanley GP (2006) Using reinforcer pairing and fading to increase the milk consumption of a preschool child, *J Appl Behav Anal,* 39, 399–403.
Wardle J, Cooke L, Gibson EL, Sapochnik M, Sheilham A, and Lawson M (2003a) Increasing children's acceptance of vegetables: A randomized trial of guidance to parents. *Appetite,* 40, 155–162.
Wardle J, Herrera ML, Cooke L, and Gibson EL (2003b) Modifying children's food preferences: The effects of exposure and reward on acceptance of an unfamiliar vegetable. *Eur J of Clin Nutr,* 57, 341–348.
Williams KE, Field DG, and Seiverling L (in press) Food refusal in children: A review of the literature, *Res Dev Disabil.*
Williams KE and Foxx RM (2007) *Treating eating problems of children with autism spectrum disorders and developmental disabilities,* Austin, TX, Pro-Ed.
Williams KE, Paul C, Pizzo B, Riegel K (2008) Practice does make perfect: A longitudinal look at repeated taste exposure, *Appetite*, 51, 739–742.
Williams KE, Riegel K, and Kerwin ML (2009) Feeding disorder in infancy and early childhood: How often is it seen? *Child Healthcare,* 38, 123–136.
Williams KE and Seiverling L (2010) Eating problems in children with autism spectrum disorders, *Top Clin Nutr*, 25, 27–37.
Wind M, de Bourdeaudhuij I, Velde SJT, Sandvik C, Due P, Krepp KI, and Brug J (2006) Correlates of fruit and vegetable consumption among 11-year-old Belgian-Flemish and Dutch schoolchildren, *J Nutr Educ Behav*, 38, 211–221.
Zajonc RB (1968) Attitudinal effects of mere exposure, *J Per Soc Psychol*, 9, Monograph supplement No. 2, Part 2.
Zeller DA, Rozin P, Aron M, and Kulish C (1983) Conditioned enhancement of human's liking for flavor by pairing with sweetness, *Learning and Motivation*, 14, 338–350.

8

School-based interventions to improve children's food choices: the Kid's Choice Program

H. M. Hendy, Penn State University, USA

Abstract: This chapter briefly reviews problems faced by children who have overeating and/or fussy-eating patterns, and the benefits of school-based interventions to encourage them to make healthy food choices. Program components suggested by past theory and research are reviewed, then a more focused review is provided for the Kid's Choice Program, which was designed as an easy-to-use, cost-effective school–home partnership to encourage children to develop healthy behaviors in their everyday environments. The chapter describes the new features included in the Kid's Choice Program that are not typically included in other available school-based interventions, and the simple school procedures used in the Kid's Choice Program are outlined. Documentation is provided for the program's effectiveness for increasing children's fruit and vegetable consumption and choice of low-fat and low-sugar healthy drinks for both children eating school-provided lunches and home-packed lunches, as well as the program's effectiveness for improving food choices and weight status for overweight children embedded within the sample. Program acceptability ratings by children, parents, and school staff are described, program costs per child per month of application are estimated, and documentation is given for the effectiveness of the Kid's Choice Program when delivered by small teams of four parent volunteers.

Key words: school programs, child food choices, fruits and vegetables.

8.1 Introduction

8.1.1 The problem of overeating and fussy-eating patterns in children

Children may face a number of problems due to their poor eating patterns, with overeating and fussy-eating patterns being perhaps the most common patterns. For example, over 30% of school-aged children in the United States are now overweight or obese (Hedley *et al.*, 2004), and they face a number of health, social, and psychological problems. Health problems associated with child obesity include diabetes, high blood pressure, gallstones, sleep apnea, orthopedic abnormalities such as bowed legs and back problems, hirsutism, and menstrual irregularities (Must and Strauss, 1999). Social problems include peer teasing, rejection, and being stereotyped as lazy, stupid, ugly, and worthless (Davison and Birch, 2001; Latner and Stunkard, 2003; Turnbull *et al.*, 2000). Psychological problems include poor body image, low self-esteem, depression, anxiety disorders, and quality of life self-rated as poor as that of children with cancer (Schwimmer *et al.*, 2003; Williams *et al.*, 1999). Children with fussy-eating patterns typically accept only a limited variety of foods and they are often underweight (Carruth *et al.*, 2004; Dovey *et al.*, 2008; Galloway *et al.*, 2005). Surprisingly, children with fussy-eating patterns severe enough to be treated in hospital feeding clinics may often show normal weight status (Williams *et al.*, 2005), perhaps because they eat mostly starches and high-calorie foods (Schreck *et al.*, 2004), and because parents often add nutritional supplements to their diets (Lockner *et al.*, 2008). Whether underweight or overweight, when fussy-eating patterns are left untreated in childhood, they may result in diet and health problems that last into adolescence and adulthood (Falciglia *et al.*, 2000; Timimi *et al.*, 1997).

To avoid these risks associated with overeating and fussy-eating patterns in children, the Centers for Disease Control and Prevention (CDCP, 2000) in the United States have recommended that children be encouraged to develop eating habits that include consumption of a variety of foods from all food groups (especially more fruits and vegetables because they are high in nutrients and low in calories), portion control to manage total daily calories, and selection of healthy drinks that are low-fat and low-sugar. Unfortunately, fruits and vegetables (FV) tend to be the foods most rejected by children (ADA, 2000; Gleason and Suitor, 2000), and both overweight and fussy-eating, children may have difficulty choosing FV and practicing portion control in the 'supersize-me' American food environment, with its prevalence of ready-made snack foods and fast-food restaurants offering a wide variety of palatable foods in large portions that are high-fat, high-sugar, and high-salt (Rozin *et al.*, 2006). Encouraging children to eat small amounts of fruits and vegetables during the first part of their meals may be a realistic goal that offers two advantages: (i) It may serve as a portion control strategy because it has been found to reduce total mealtime calorie consumption in adults by 12% (Rolls *et al.*, 2004), and (ii) it may enhance the palatability and acceptability of FV by children because these foods are eaten at the beginning of the meal when children are most hungry.

8.1.2 Benefits of school-based programs to change children's food choices

The healthy food choices recommended by the CDCP (e.g. eating a greater variety of foods, and especially fruits and vegetables, learning portion control, choosing foods and drinks that are low-fat, low-sugar, and low-salt) are often the focus of clinical programs available in hospitals for overweight children or for fussy-eating children. However, such clinical programs typically take place in special settings away from children's everyday life, so the skills learned there may not always generalize to their everyday settings, and the children may feel singled out from their peers when required to participate in these special programs. Most children in the United States have lunch at school five days a week (James *et al.*, 1996), and the school-provided lunch is often their most frequent exposure to fruits and vegetables (Baranowski *et al.*, 1997; Burchett, 2003), which makes school lunch a unique opportunity to encourage children to learn healthy food choices in their everyday environment and while in the company of their peers.

8.2 School-based interventions to improve children's food choices: components suggested by theory and past research

8.2.1 Nutrition education

Suggestions for components that might be included in effective school-based interventions come from a number of sources that include theory, past research with average-developing children, and clinical observations of children with severe feeding problems (Benton, 2004; Faith *et al.*, 2004; Patrick and Nicklas, 2005). For example, past research with average-developing children suggests that school programs focusing on nutrition education alone are rarely successful in changing children's food consumption patterns (Burchett, 2003; Contento *et al.*, 1995). A number of successful school-based intervention programs have included a nutrition education component (Blanchette and Brug, 2005; Howerton *et al.*, 2007; Knai *et al.*, 2006), but because these programs also included other intervention components (see below), the effectiveness of the nutrition education component alone remains doubtful. Additions of nutrition curriculum might also face the problem of poor acceptance by busy teachers and other school staff, especially if research suggests that nutrition education alone can improve only children's knowledge about healthy foods, but not their consumption of them.

8.2.2 Repeated taste exposure

Social Cognitive Theory (Bandura, 1997) would suggest that children's confidence to eat healthy foods would be enhanced by providing them with repeated taste experiences of the foods. Mere exposure to foods without tasting them does not appear sufficient for children to learn to like them (Birch *et al.*, 1987), and a number of studies have documented that children need approximately 8 to 10 taste experiences over time to learn to enjoy a specific food (Birch and Marlin, 1982; Birch *et al.*, 1987; Wardle *et al.*, 2003). To get these taste experiences started, pairing the new taste with a familiar taste has been found effective for increasing children's consumption of the new taste (Pliner, 2008). However, each taste exposure should avoid the aversive effects of satiation, which can result if children are pushed to consume a large amount of a food at one time (Rolls *et al.*, 1981).

8.2.3 Availability of food choices

Self Determination Theory (Deci and Ryan, 1985) would suggest that intrinsic motivation for any behavior (including choosing healthy foods) would be enhanced by perceived choices surrounding the behavior. Food choice during school lunch has also been recommended by children themselves during focus group interviews to determine factors associated with children's willingness to try new lunch foods (James *et al.*, 1996; Marples and Spillman, 1995). In addition, experimental research has documented that offering children choices during school lunch can increase their consumption of fruits and vegetables (Hendy, 1999; Perry *et al.*, 2004). However, other research suggests that offering children food choices may have complex effects on their food consumption and preference ratings, with these effects depending on the details of how such 'choices' are presented. For example, one experimental study found that offering children the choice of whether or not to eat novel foods served during school lunch (e.g. 'Do you want any of this mango?') increased their consumption of these foods above that seen with mere exposure (Hendy, 1999). On the other hand, questionnaire research with average-developing children as well as children with extreme fussy-eating patterns suggests that if parents become too permissive, allow excessive food choices, and even make special meals for their children that are different from the shared family meals, these children may develop such restricted food selection patterns that it may harm their diet quality and weight status (Hendy *et al.*, 2009a, 2010b; Timimi *et al.*, 1997). At the other extreme, forcing them to eat foods by threats of punishment may push food consumption beyond the point of satiation and make foods aversive to them, perhaps for a lifetime (Batsell *et al.*, 2002; Galloway *et al.*, 2006; Rolls *et al.*, 1981; Rozin, 1986; Sanders *et al.*, 1993). Forbidding children to eat some of their favorite high-fat, high-sugar, and high-salt snack foods may also backfire and result in over-consumption of these foods later when children have the opportunity (Baughcum *et al.*, 2001; Birch *et al.*, 2001; Fisher and Birch, 1999).

Another approach that takes the middle ground between extremely permissive and extremely punitive and restrictive approaches is offered by

Social Cognitive Theory (Bandura, 1997), which suggests that if children receive gentle and positive 'verbal persuasion' to sample small amounts of healthy foods during meals (e.g. 'Just try one bite.'), their self-efficacy or confidence to eat these foods would be strengthened. Over time, such repeated taste experiences would also help children reach the apparent threshold of 8 to 10 tastes they need to begin to enjoy the foods (Birch and Marlin, 1982; Birch *et al.*, 1987; Wardle *et al.*, 2003). In support of this approach, past research has found that children's consumption of fruits and vegetables was greater if their parents often used such positive 'verbal persuasion' to encourage their children to sample the mealtime food choices presented to them (Hendy *et al.*, 2009; Orrell-Valente *et al.*, 2007).

8.2.4 Offers of reinforcement for eating

Social Cognitive Theory (Bandura, 1997) would also suggest that children's healthy food choices could be improved by offering them reinforcements as an incentive to give these foods a try. However, past research indicates that the use of reinforcement during meals may have complex effects on children's food consumption and preference ratings, depending on the details of how the rewards are used. For example, many studies have demonstrated that offering children reinforcement will increase their consumption of fruits and vegetables (Baranowski *et al.*, 2000; Davis *et al.*, 2000; Hendy, 1999; Horne *et al.*, 1995; Perry *et al.*, 1998; Reynolds *et al.*, 2000a,b; Stark *et al.*, 1986; Story *et al.*, 2000). However, other studies suggest that when the reinforcement offered is also a food, children's later preference ratings tend to be increased for the food offered as the reinforcement and decreased for the food they had to eat to earn that reinforcement (Birch *et al.*, 1982, 1984; Newman and Taylor, 1992). These drops in children's later preferences for foods they must eat to earn reinforcement have been called 'discounting effects' or 'over-justification effects' (Lepper *et al.*, 1973) and they have been explained in two ways. A cognitive explanation suggests children come to think that if they must be offered reinforcement to eat a food, the food must taste bad and they do not like it (Newman and Layton, 1984; Newman and Taylor, 1992). A satiation explanation suggests that if the offer of reinforcement pushes food consumption past the point of satiation, children will begin to dislike that food (Hendy *et al.*, 2005). Fortunately, such 'over-justification' drops in food preference ratings may be avoided if children are required to eat only small amounts of the food to earn the reinforcement, and if only small and delayed reinforcement is offered for such food consumption (Eisenberger and Cameron, 1996; Hendy *et al.*, 2005, 2007; Horne *et al.*, 1995). The use of small and delayed reinforcement is often accomplished by offering children small tokens immediately after they eat the healthy foods, then later allowing them to trade their tokens for small prizes or favorite activities (but not including favorite foods). Such token reinforcement programs may be effective for improving food consumption and preference ratings because they avoid food satiation effects, they make reinforcement less prominent on a daily basis, and they provide time for children to discover pleasant properties of the foods themselves (Hitt *et al.*, 1992; Newman and Layton, 1984).

8.2.5 Peer modeling

Group Socialization Theory (Harris, 1995) and Social Cognitive Theory (Bandura, 1997) would both emphasize the importance of peer models for the development of any new behavior in children, including making healthy food choices. Past research has also documented the effectiveness of peer models for increasing fruit and vegetable consumption in children during school lunch (Hendy, 2002; Hendy and Raudenbush, 2000; Horne *et al.*, 1995). In some of these school programs, scripted peer-modeling has been used, in which the trained peer model says prearranged food-acceptance phrases (e.g., 'Mmmm! I love mangos!') before eating the food described. Even though the children listening to these phases may come to mimic them ('OK, we know you love mangos.'), the intervention remains effective (Hendy, 2002). School-based programs that provide more naturalistic and incidental peer-modeling might be expected to be even more effective to encourage other children to try healthier food choices. For example, when a young child who usually rejects fruits and vegetables during school lunch finds that he/she is surrounded by nearly 100 peers who are trying small bites of fruits and vegetables and spontaneously making comments about them (e.g. 'These baby carrots are crunchy and sweet!'), the observing child may not be cognitively sophisticated enough to dismiss the other children's food consumption as 'just to get a prize on Friday,' so only the powerful impact of peer modeling remains.

8.2.6 Support from school staff and parents

Prevention and intervention programs to improve children's healthy food choices might be expected to be most effective if they involve a school–home partnership because these are the two environments where children spend most of their time. Unfortunately, even school programs with documented effectiveness for improving children's food choices are not always well accepted by busy school staff or parents, which reduces the probability that the school would continue the programs in long-term applications (Baranowski *et al.*, 2000; Contento *et al.*, 1995; Bauer *et al.*, 2004; Burchett, 2003; Horne *et al.*, 1995; Perry *et al.*, 1998; Reynolds *et al.*, 2000a,b). Some of the roles asked of school staff and parents have included teachers and school nurses adding nutrition curriculum or special presentations, cafeteria staff providing more fruit and vegetable choices for children during school lunches, cafeteria aides monitoring and rewarding children's healthy food choices, and parents completing healthy food activities with their children at home. Objections raised by school staff have included the belief that their present nutrition curriculum is adequate to encourage children's healthy food choices, reluctance to invest the time and costs necessary to present the program's components, doubt that offers of rewards can be effective for improving children's healthy food choices, and/or frustration that their efforts to improve children's nutrition are thwarted by parents who send their children to school with home-packed lunches filled with high-fat, high-sugar, and high-salt foods (Bauer *et al.*, 2004; Cullen *et al.*, 2000). Objections raised by parents may include the belief that their children's diet and weight are mostly genetically determined so that any program is unlikely to produce changes, the belief that their children's diet and weight problems are only a stage and they will 'grow out of it' on their own without intervention, reluctance to invest the time and costs for any home components of the program (e.g. serving more fruits and vegetables during meals, allowing children to help with food choices and preparation, recording children's food consumption), and hesitancy to improve their own eating habits in order to provide their children with good models for healthy food choices.

8.2.7 Multi-component school programs available

Reviews are available for the many school-based intervention programs now available to improve children's healthy food choices (Blanchette and Brug, 2005; Howerton *et al.*, 2007; Knai *et al.*, 2006), often with a focus on fruit and vegetable consumption. These programs include the 'Gimme-5' program by Baranowski and colleagues (2000), the 'Food Dudes' program by Horne and colleagues (1995), the '5-a-Day-Power-Plus' program by Perry and colleagues (1998, 2004), the 'Know Your Body' program by Resnicow and colleagues (1992), the 'High-5' program by Reynolds and colleagues (2000a,b), and the 'Kid's Choice Program' (Hendy *et al.*, 2005, 2007, 2009b, 2010a). Unfortunately, any improvements in children's healthy food choices that are produced by these school-based programs typically last only as long as the programs are in place. More long-term adoption of a school-based intervention for healthy food choices in children would certainly be influenced by the program's cost and acceptability by children, school staff, and parents (Baranowski *et al.*, 2000; Bauer *et al.*, 2004; Perry *et al.*, 1998; Reynolds *et al.*, 2000a,b), but little research documents such program costs or acceptability ratings. The ideal school-based program for long-term adoption would appear to be one that can be demonstrated to be effective for improving children's healthy food choices, and one that is simple in design, low in cost, and high in acceptability to those involved.

8.3 Focused review of school-based interventions to improve children's food choices: the Kid's Choice Program

8.3.1 New features of the Kid's Choice Program

The Kid's Choice Program was designed to be an easy to use, cost-effective, school-based program to encourage children to develop weight management behaviors while in their everyday environment. As described in more detail in sections below, the development of the program has included a number of features rarely included in other available school-based interventions (Blanchette and Brug, 2005; Howerton *et al.*, 2007; Knai *et al.*, 2006). For example, the Kid's Choice Program uses simple school procedures to enhance its acceptability by children, parents, and school staff. The program's effectiveness has been evaluated using direct measures of changes in the targeted behaviors (e.g. eating fruits and vegetables first during the meal, choosing low-fat and low-sugar healthy drinks, exercising) rather than relying on more indirect measures such as parent or child reports, which are more subject to social desirability effects. The Kid's Choice Program has been evaluated for whether it is effective in improving healthy food choices in both average-developing and overweight children, and for whether it is effective for improving weight status of overweight children embedded within the sample without singling them out in any way from their peers. The program has been evaluated for whether any increases in healthy food choices produced by the token reinforcement used in the Kid's Choice Program also produced 'over-justification' drops in the children's preference ratings for these healthy food choices (Birch *et al.*, 1982, 1984; Lepper *et al.*, 1973; Newman and Layton, 1984; Newman and Taylor, 1992). The program has been evaluated for its acceptability by children, parents, and school staff, which is important for any school-based program intended for long-term applications. The program costs have been calculated per child per month, which may allow school leaders to plan expenses for long-term application of the program, including the development of formal and informal sources of funds. Finally, the Kid's Choice Program has been evaluated for whether it can be effectively applied by small teams of parent volunteers rather than by large teams of university researchers, which is also important for school leaders in making their decision for long-term application of the program for their school.

8.3.2 Simple school procedures of the Kid's Choice Program

The Kid's Choice Program includes three simple school procedures:

(i) Children wear nametag necklaces during school lunch and recess three days each week.
(ii) Star-shaped holes are punched into the nametags as token reinforcement when children show specific small amounts of the targeted weight

management behaviors, with at least two choices being available for each behavior.

(iii) Reward Days are presented once each week for children to trade their stars for small prizes.

Each procedure used in the Kid's Choice Program was guided by theory and past research (as described above). For example, the small and delayed reinforcement offered to children (with stars given daily as token reinforcement, but with prizes available only weekly as back-up reinforcement) was chosen as part of the Kid's Choice Program procedures to remove the daily focus from prizes so that children have an opportunity to discover pleasing properties of the weight management behaviors themselves (Hitt *et al.*, 1992). The availability of at least two choices for each target behavior was chosen for the Kid's Choice Program to reduce the risk of satiation effects (Rolls *et al.*, 1981), as were the small daily expectations for each behavior (such as requiring that children eat only 1/8 cup of FV to earn a star). Small daily expectations were also chosen so that children could gradually accumulate the repeated taste experiences that appear necessary in order to learn to enjoy a new food (Birch and Marlin, 1982; Wardle *et al.*, 2003). Finally, the presentation of the Kid's Choice Program during school lunch was chosen to make incidental peer modeling available for the target behaviors, which may be even more powerful than the use of trained peer models (Hendy, 2002; Hendy and Raudenbush, 2000).

8.3.3 Effectiveness and acceptability of the Kid's Choice Program

The first evaluation of the effectiveness of the Kid's Choice Program focused on whether it could increase children's FV consumption during school lunch (Hendy *et al.*, 2005). Throughout its one-month application, the program was found to be effective in increasing children's consumption of fruit if they received the star-shaped holes punched into their nametags for eating fruit, and for increasing children's consumption of vegetables if they received the holes in their nametags for eating vegetables, with once-weekly Reward Days offered when the children could trade their stars for small prizes. (See Figs 8.1 and 8.2 from Hendy *et al.*, 2005.) FV consumption was measured by trained lunch observers, who recorded whether or not children ate at least 1/8 cup of FV during school lunch. This first evaluation of the Kid's Choice Program was also shown to be equally effective for increasing FV consumption of average-weight and overweight children embedded within the large sample of school-age children. (See Fig. 8.3 from Hendy *et al.*, 2007). Finally, interviews with children before and after the month-long application of the Kid's Choice Program found that these improvements in FV consumption were accomplished without any sign of the 'over-justification effects' that might have reduced children's preferences for the rewarded foods (Hendy *et al.*, 2005, 2007).

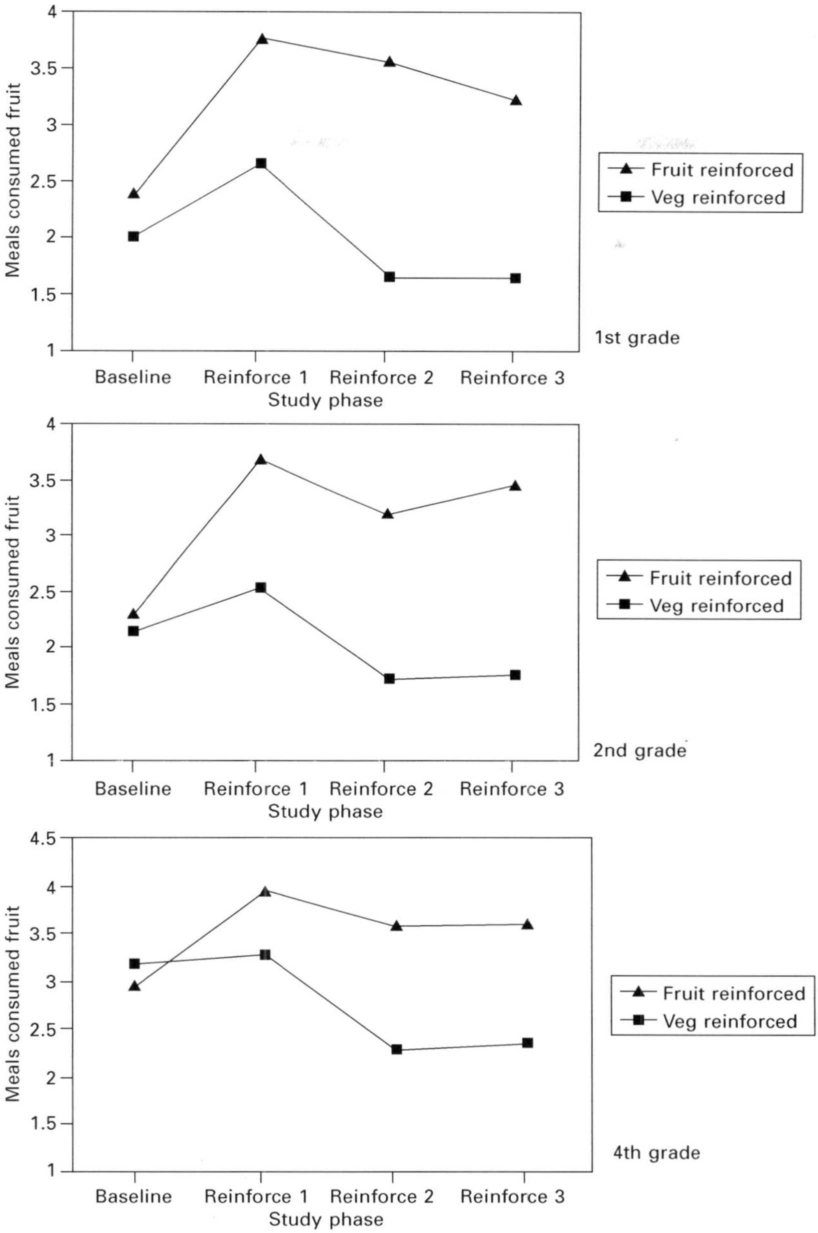

Fig. 8.1 Changes in *fruit* consumption across four study phases (one four-meal block under baseline, three four-meal blocks under token reinforcement in the Kid's Choice Program) for children who received reinforcement for eating either fruit or vegetables. Fruit consumption was scored as the number of four meals in which 1/8 cup of fruit was consumed, with significant and lasting increases seen only for children reinforced for fruit ($p < 0.001$). Graphs are shown for 60 1st graders (29 reinforced for fruit, 31 for vegetables), 61 2nd graders (33 reinforced for fruit, 28 for vegetables), 67 4th graders (34 reinforced for fruit, 33 for vegetables). (Figure is from Hendy *et al.*, 2005).

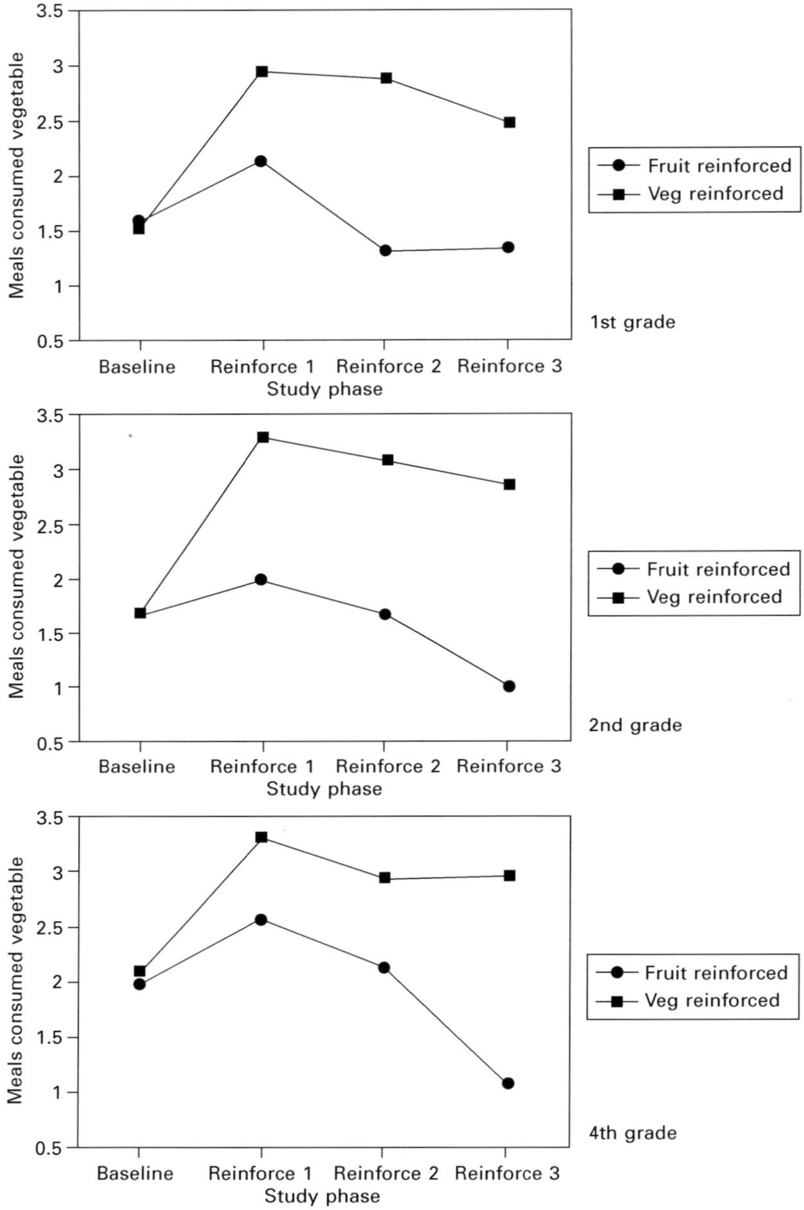

Fig. 8.2 Changes in *vegetable* consumption across four study phases (one four-meal block under baseline, three four-meal blocks under token reinforcement in the Kid's Choice Program) for children who received reinforcement for eating fruit or vegetables. Vegetable consumption was scored as the number of four meals in which 1/8 cup of vegetables was consumed, with significant and lasting increases seen only for children reinforced for vegetables ($p < 0.001$) Graphs are for 60 1st graders (29 reinforced for fruit, 31 for vegetables), 61 2nd graders (33 reinforced for fruit, 28 for vegetables), 67 4th graders (34 reinforced for fruit, 33 for vegetables). (Figure is from Hendy *et al.*, 2005.).

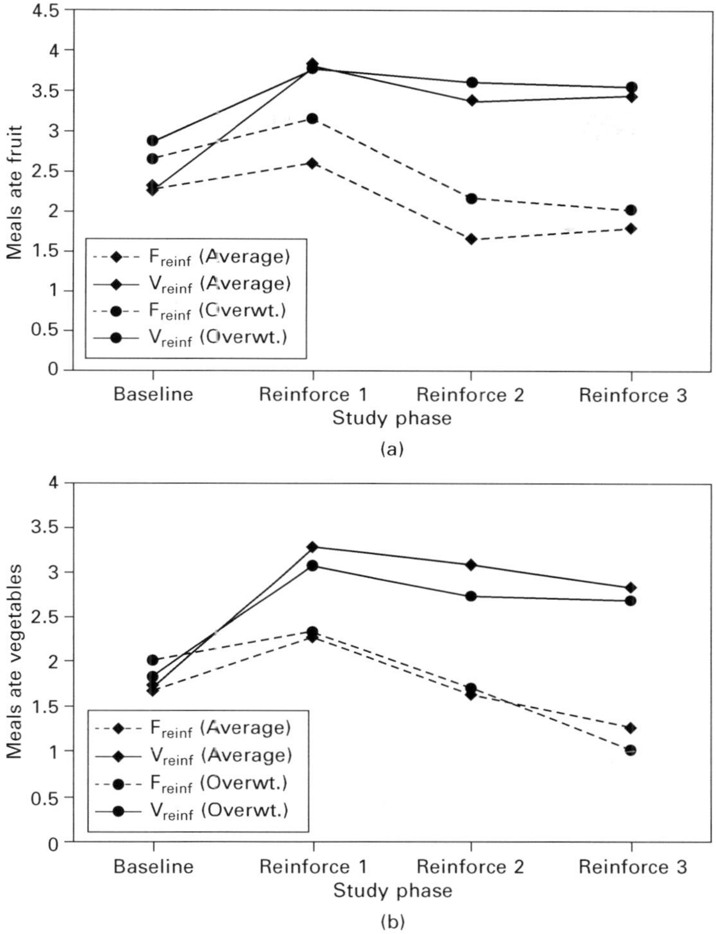

Fig. 8.3 (a) Changes in *fruit* consumption across four study phases of the Kid's Choice Program (one four-meal block under baseline conditions, three four-meal blocks under reinforcement conditions) by children who received reinforcement either for eating fruit or for eating vegetables, and by children who were either average-weight or overweight. (Of 99 average-weight children, 51 were reinforced for eating fruit and 48 for eating vegetables. Of 55 overweight children, 22 were reinforced for eating fruit and 33 for eating vegetables.) Fruit consumption was defined as the number of four meals 1/8 cup was eaten. Both average-weight and overweight children reinforced for eating fruit showed significant increases in fruit consumption ($p < 0.001$). (b) Changes in *vegetable* consumption across four study phases of the Kid's Choice Program (one four-meal block under baseline conditions, three four-meal blocks under reinforcement conditions) by children who received reinforcement either for eating fruit or for eating vegetables, and by children who were either average-weight or overweight. (Sample sizes are described above.) Vegetable consumption was defined as the number of four meals 1/8 cup was eaten. Both average-weight and overweight children reinforced for eating vegetables showed significant increases in vegetable consumption ($p < 0.001$). (Figure is from Hendy *et al.*, 2007).

The second evaluation of the effectiveness of the Kid's Choice Program was conducted three days a week for one month in a different school from that used during the first application, but with similar success (Hendy *et al.*, 2009b). Results demonstrated that the program produced increases in children's healthy food choices (eating FV first during lunch, choosing low-fat and low-sugar healthy drinks), with these improvements lasting throughout the one-month application of the program. Interviews with the children and questionnaires from their parents also documented that the Kid's Choice Program was well accepted, with the children giving a mean acceptability rating of 2.9 (SD = 0.3) using their three-point scale, and with the parents giving a mean acceptability rating of 4.4 (SD = 0.9) using their five-point scale.

The third application of the Kid's Choice Program was again conducted on three days each week in another school, but this time for three months, this time targeting three weight management behaviors (eating 1/8 cup fruit or vegetables first during the meals, choosing low-fat and low-sugar healthy drinks, and exercising many steps daily as measured with a pedometer), and this time including a home component in which parents were given cards to record five days per week whether or not their children showed the three target behaviors in their home environments (Hendy *et al.*, 2010a). The three-month application of the program produced improvements in all three target behaviors that lasted throughout the application of the program, it was effective for increasing the healthy food choices for both children who ate the school-provided lunch and those who ate home-packed lunches, and it reduced the body mass index percentile (BMI%) of overweight children embedded within the sample without singling them out from their peers. Interviews with children and questionnaires from parents again documented that the program had high acceptability ratings. Questionnaires were also used to evaluate which specific procedures used in this application of the Kid's Choice Program were most and least acceptable to school staff. School staff supported the use of nametags, holes punched into them for token reinforcement, small prizes available during Reward Days, and the focus on weight management behaviors (eating fruits and vegetables, choosing healthy drinks, exercising). School staff disliked the use of pedometers to record exercise because of their frequency of being lost and broken; they preferred instead that observers record children's exercise during recess, and they recommended that parent volunteers deliver the Kid's Choice Program rather than school staff. Although parents gave the Kid's Choice Program high acceptability ratings for school applications, only 20% of the parents completed Parent Records of whether their children showed the three weight management behaviors in the home environment. Parents explained that they were too busy to record the behaviors, that they believed their children's behavior and weight problems were only a stage and they would 'grow out of it' on their own, that serving more fruits and vegetables and healthy drinks was costly, and that they were not ready to improve their own weight management behaviors to serve as a good model for their children.

The fourth application of the Kid's Choice Program was conducted at the same school as the third application, but during the next school year, and this time with the program delivered three days a week entirely by a team of four parent volunteers (Hendy *et al.*, 2010a). Training of the parent volunteers required approximately five minutes, during which time they were each given a one-page description of the goals and procedures of the Kid's Choice Program, they were each given a star-shaped hole-puncher, and they were given an orange ping-pong ball as a visual reminder of the amount of fruit or vegetable the children were required to eat (1/8 cup) to earn a star punched into their nametags. Each parent volunteer was assigned two rows of 25 children seated at the long school lunch tables, and then ten minutes into their lunch period, the parent volunteer walked along the row to deliver one star-shaped hole to children's nametags for each of the three target behaviors: eating 1/8 cup fruit or vegetables during this first ten minutes of lunch, choosing low-fat and low-sugar drinks, and exercising 1000 steps. (n.b. Here, children's exercising behavior was recorded in steps on pedometers, but in a later application of the Kid's Choice Program by a team of parent volunteers, the parents simply observed recess for ten minutes and gave children token reinforcement if they had been moving around during that time.) This application of the Kid's Choice Program delivered entirely by four parent volunteers was found successful for increasing all three weight-management behaviors, both for children eating the school-provided lunch and for those eating home-packed lunches.

8.3.4 Materials and costs for the Kid's Choice Program

Costs for the Kid's Choice Program per child per month were calculated in both the second and third applications described above used to evaluate the program (Hendy *et al.*, 2009b, 2010a). The program was found to cost approximately two US dollars per child per month of application. Unless more high-quality nametags are desired (e.g. made with laminated cover-weight and neon-colored paper, attached to durable ¾ inch cloth lanyards), the children's nametag necklaces can easily be produced from supplies readily available at most schools (e.g. sturdy paper and string). Similarly, although star-shaped hole-punchers deliver token reinforcement that is more attractive and more difficult to counterfeit, the simple round-shaped hole-punchers that can be found in most schools are adequate. The primary expense of the Kid's Choice Program is the small prizes offered during the weekly Reward Days as back-up reinforcement for which children trade in the 'stars' in their nametags they earned for their healthy behavior choices. These small prizes may include purchased items (e.g. fancy pencils, notebooks, puzzles, crayons, balls, stuffed animals, silly hats, cards), but they may also include donated items from local businesses or access to special privileges or activities favored by the children (e.g. coupons for grocery store purchases, movies, extra recess time, being first in line at school lunch), which can greatly reduce the costs of the Kid's Choice Program if the school and parents are creative and resourceful.

8.3.5 Future applications of the Kid's Choice Program

The Kid's Choice Program shows promise for long-term adoption by schools for a number of reasons:

- it is simple in design with children wearing nametag necklaces during school lunch, with stars punched into nametags when children choose healthy behaviors, and with Reward Days presented once a week for children to trade their stars for small prizes,
- it has documented its effectiveness for improving recommended weight management behaviors in school children while in their everyday environments,
- it has documented its effectiveness for improving weight status of overweight children embedded within the school sample and without singling them out from their peers,
- it receives good acceptability ratings from children, parents, and school staff (with the exception of the use of pedometers to record exercise),
- it can be effectively delivered by small teams of parent volunteers so that it does not add to the workload of busy school staff, and
- it is relatively low in cost at two US dollars per child per month of application. The nametag necklaces and the hole-punchers used to deliver token reinforcement in the Kid's Choice Program are readily available with typical school supplies. The small prizes used by the Kid's Choice Program during Reward Days are the greatest expense of the program, but they are readily available in bulk from a variety of vendors. Costs may be reduced further by community-donated prizes, by school fund-drives, or by applications for state-sponsored wellness grants.

Because the Kid's Choice Program was developed with applications in small-town elementary schools in eastern Pennsylvania with mostly Caucasian children, future applications of the program should be evaluated in schools with more regional and ethnic diversity. Further research should also consider the ideal age at which to present the Kid's Choice Program for maximum impact on lasting healthy behaviors of children. Past research suggests that even children in preschool may respond to many components included in the Kid's Choice Program that was developed for elementary school-age children, including offers of reinforcement and availability of peer models (Hendy, 1999, 2003; Hendy and Raudenbush, 2000), and some research suggests that two to five years of age may serve as a sensitive period in the development of children's food acceptance patterns (Cashdan, 1994).

Finally, to encourage the Kid's Choice Program to be a true school–home partnership, future applications of the program should make greater efforts to encourage parents to record their children's healthy behaviors in the home environment. To reduce the perceived burden for busy parents, perhaps simplified Parent Records could be used that reduce the number of days of recording children's healthy behaviors from five to three. Perhaps parent volunteers could develop easy-to-use and low-cost 'Idea Lists' for each targeted behavior with suggestions for how parents might encourage these behaviors in the home environment. For example, recent research suggests that children are more likely to make healthy food choices if parents regularly practice a number of specific mealtime actions (Birch *et al.*, 2001; Hendy *et al.*, 2009, 1010c; Hughes *et al.*, 2008; Lumeng *et al.*, 2008): parents make fruits and vegetables available daily for their children, parents model daily fruit and vegetable consumption, parents often use positive persuasion in which they describe the good taste of the foods offered for meals, parents set mealtime expectations that the child taste mealtime foods offered, parents infrequently model consumption of high-fat or high-sugar or high-salt snack foods, parents avoid complete restriction of children's favorite foods, and parents avoid making 'special meals' for their children that are different than the shared family meal. Ideas for parents might also include recipes for preparations of fruits and vegetables and healthy drinks that are well accepted by children and made from low-cost and locally-available ingredients, neighborhood locations of low-cost but high-quality fresh produce, family food-tasting or exercising parties in neighborhood homes or parks, and other creative and cost-effective plans to make it easier for busy parents to encourage their children to extend the healthy behaviors learned from the school-based Kid's Choice Program to their other everyday environments.

8.4 References

American Dietetic Association (2000). Local support for nutrition integrity in schools. *Journal of the American Dietetic Association*, 100, 108–111.

Bandura, A. (1997). *Self-efficacy: The Exercise of Control*. New York: Freeman and Company.

Baranowski, T., Davis, M., Resnicow, K., Baranowski, J., Doyle, C., Lin, L. S., Smith, M., and Wang, D. T. (2000). Gimme 5 fruit, juice and vegetables for fun and health: Outcome evaluation. *Health Education and Behavior*, 27, 96–111.

Baranowski, T., Smith, M., Hearn, M. D., Lin, L. S., Baranowski, J., Doyle, C., Resnicow, K., and Wang, D. T. (1997). Patterns in children's fruit and vegetable consumption by meal and day of the week. *Journal of American College Nutrition*, 16, 216–223.

Batsell, W. R., Brown, A. S., Ansfield, M. E., and Paschall, G. Y. (2002). 'You will eat all of that!': A retrospective analysis of forced consumption episodes. *Appetite*, 38, 211–219.

Bauer, K. W., Yang, Y. W., and Austin, S. B. (2004). 'How can we stay healthy when you're throwing all of this in front of us?' Findings from focus groups and interviews in middle schools on environmental influences on nutrition and physical activity. *Health Education and Behavior*, 31, 34–36.

Baughcum, A. E., Powers, S. W., Johnson, S. B., Chamberlin, L. A., Deeks, C. M.,

Jain, A., and Whitaker, R. C. (2001). Maternal feeding practices and beliefs and their relationships to overweight in early childhood. *Journal of Developmental and Behavioral Pediatrics*, 22, 391–408.
Benton, D. (2004). Role of parents in the determination of the food preferences of children and the development of obesity. *International Journal of Obesity*, 28, 858–869.
Birch, L. L., Birch, D., Marlin, D., and Kramer, L. (1982). Effects of instrumental eating on children's food preferences. *Appetite*, 3, 125–134.
Birch, L. L., Fisher, J. O., Grimm-Thomas, K., Markey, C. N., Sawyer, R., and Johnson, S. L. (2001). Confirmatory factor analysis of the child feeding questionnaire: A measure of parental attitudes, beliefs and practices about child feeding and obesity proneness. *Appetite*, 36, 201–210.
Birch, L. L., and Marlin, D. W. (1982). I don't like it; I never tried it. Effects of exposure on two-year-old children's food preference. *Appetite*, 3, 353–360.
Birch, L. L., Marlin, D. W., and Rotter, J. (1984). Eating as the 'means' activity in a contingency: Effects on young children's food preferences. *Child Development*, 55, 432–439.
Birch, L, L., McPhee, L., Shoba, B. C., Pirok, E., and Stineberg, L. (1987). What kind of exposure reduces children's food neophobia: Looking vs. tasting? *Appetite*, 9, 171–178.
Blanchette, L., and Brug, J. (2005). Determinants of fruit and vegetable consumption among 6–12-year old children and effective interventions to increase consumption. *Journal of Human Nutrition and Diet*, 18, 431–43.
Burchett, H. (2003). Increasing fruit and vegetable consumption among British primary schoolchildren: A review. *Health Education*, 103, 99–109.
Carruth, B. R., Ziegler, P. J., Gordon, A., and Barr, S. I. (2004). Prevalence of 'picky/fussy' eaters among infants and toddlers and their caregivers' decision about offering new food. *Journal of the American Dietetic Association*, 104, S57–S64.
Cashdan, E. (1994). A sensitive period for learning about food. *Human Nature*, 5, 279–291.
Centers for Disease Control and Prevention. (2000). *School health index for physical activity and healthy eating: A self-assessment and planning guide*. Atlanta, GA, CDCP.
Contento, I. R., Balch, G. I., and Bronner, Y. L. (1995). The effectiveness of nutrition education and implications for nutrition education, policy, programs, and research: A review of research. *Journal of Nutrition Education*, 27, 277–418.
Cullen, K. W., Eagan, J., and Baranowski, T. *et al.* (2000). Effect of a la carte and snack bar foods at school on children's lunchtime intake of fruits and vegetables. *Journal of the American Dietetic Association*, 100, 1482–1486.
Davis, M., Baranowski, T., Resnicow, K., Baranowski, J., Doyle, C., Smith, M., Wang, D. T., Yaroch, A., and Hebert, D. (2000). Gimme 5 fruit and vegetables for fun and health: Process evaluation. *Health Education and Behavior*, 27, 167–176.
Davison, K. K., and Birch, L. L. (2001). Weight status, parent reaction, and self-concept in five year-old girls. *Pediatrics*, 107, 46–53.
Deci, E. L., and Ryan, R. M. (1985). *Intrinsic Motivation and Self Determination in Human Behavior*. New York: Plenum.
Dovey, T. M., Staples, P. A., Gibson, E. L., and Halford, J. C. G. (2008). Food neophobia and 'picky/fussy' eating in children: A review. *Appetite*, 50, 181–193.
Eisenberger, R., and Cameron, J. (1996). Detrimental effects of reward. *American Psychologist*, 51, 1153–1166.
Faith, M. S., Scanlon, K. S., Birch, L. L., Francis, L. A., and Sherry, B. (2004). Parent–child feeding strategies and their relationships to child eating and weight status. *Obesity Research*, 12, 1711–1722.
Falciglia, G. A., Couch, S. C., Gribble, L. S., Pabst, S. M., and Frank, R. (2000). Food neophobia in childhood affects dietary variety. *Journal of the American Dietetic Association*, 100, 1474–1481.

Fisher, J. O., and Birch, L. L. (1999). Restricting access to foods and children's eating. *Appetite*, 32, 405–419.
Galloway, A. T., Fiorito, L. M., Francis, L. A., and Birch, L. L. (2006). 'Finish your soup': Counterproductive effects of pressuring children to eat on intake and affect. *Appetite*, 46, 318–323.
Galloway, A. T., Fiorito, L. M., Lee, Y., and Birch, L. L. (2005). Parental pressure, dietary patterns and weight status among girls who are 'picky/fussy' eaters. *Journal of the American Dietetic Association*, 103, 692–698.
Gleason, P., and Suitor, C. (2000). *Changes in Children's Diets: 1989–91 to 1994–96*. Washington, DC: United States Department of Agriculture.
Harris, J. R. (1995). Where is the child's environment? A group socialization theory of development. *Psychological Review*, 102, 458–489.
Hedley, A. A., Ogden, C. L., Johnson, C. L., Carroll, M. D., Curtin, L. R., and Flegal, K. M. (2004). Prevalence of overweight and obesity among US children, adolescents, and adults, 1999–2002. *Journal of the American Medical Association*, 29, 2847–2850.
Hendy, H. M. (1999). Comparison of five teacher actions to encourage children's new food acceptance. *Annals of Behavioral Medicine*, 21, 20–26.
Hendy, H. M. (2002). Effectiveness of trained peer models to encourage food acceptance in preschool children. *Appetite*, 39, 217–225.
Hendy, H. M., and Raudenbush, B. (2000). Effectiveness of teacher modeling to encourage food acceptance in preschool children. *Appetite*, 33, 61–76.
Hendy, H. M., Williams, K. E., and Camise, T. S. (2005). 'Kids Choice' school lunch program increases children's fruit and vegetable acceptance. *Appetite*, 45, 250–263.
Hendy, H. M., Williams, K. E., and Camise, T. S. (2010a). Kid's Choice Program improves weight management behaviors and weight status of school children. *Unpublished manuscript*.
Hendy, H. M., Williams, K. E., Camise, T. S., Alderman, S., Ivy, J., and Reed, J. (2007). Overweight and average-weight children equally responsive to 'Kids Choice Program' to increase fruit and vegetable consumption. *Appetite*, 49, 683–686.
Hendy, H. M., Williams, K. E., Camise, T. S., Eckman, N., and Hedemann, A. (2009a). The Parent Mealtime Action Scale (PMAS): Development and association with children's diet and weight. *Appetite*, 52, 328–339.
Hendy, H. M., Williams, K. E., Camise, T. S., Rahn, D., Costigan, C., Gaskins, S., and Moyer, C. (2009). Kid's Choice Program improves two weight management behaviors in school children. In A. Papareschi and H. Eppolito (Eds) *Fruit and Vegetable Consumption and Health*. Hauppauge, NY: Nova Science Publishers.
Hendy, H. M., Williams, K. E., Riegel, K., and Paul, C. (2010b). Parent mealtime actions that mediate associations between children's fussy eating and their weight and diet. *Appetite*, 54, 191–195.
Hitt, D. D., Marriott, R. G., and Esser, J. K. (1992). Effects of delayed rewards and task interest on intrinsic motivation. *Basic and Applied Social Psychology*, 13, 405–414.
Horne, P. J., Fergus-Lowe, C. F., Fleming, P. F. J., and Dowey, A. J. (1995). An effective procedure for changing food preferences in five to seven year old children. *Proceedings of the Nutrition Society*, 54, 441–452.
Howerton, M. W., Bell, B. S., Dodd, K. W., Berrigan, D., Stozenberg-Solomon, R., and Nebeling, L. (2007). School-based nutrition programs produced a moderate increase in fruit and vegetable consumption: Meta and pooling analyses from seven studies. *Journal of Nutrition Education and Behavior*, 39, 186–196.
Hughes, S. O., Shewchuk, R. M., Baskin, M. L., Nicklas, T. A., and Qu, H. (2008). Indulgent feeding style and children's weight status in preschool. *Journal of Developmental and Behavioral Pediatrics*, 29, 403–410.
James, D., Rienzo, B., and Franzee, C. (1996). Using focus group interviews to understand school meal choices. *Journal of School Health*, 66, 128–131.

Knai, C., Pomerlau, J., Lock, K., and McKee, M. (2006). Getting children to eat more fruit and vegetables: A systematic review. *Preventive Medicine*, 42, 85–95.

Latner, J. D., and Stunkard, A. J. (2003). Getting worse: The stigmatization of obese children. *Obesity Research*, 11, 452–456.

Lepper, M. R., Green, D., and Nisbett, R. E. (1973). Undermining children's intrinsic interest with extrinsic reward: A test of the 'overjustification' hypothesis. *Journal of Personality and Social Psychology*, 28, 129–137.

Lockner, D. W., Crowe, T. K., and Skipper, B. J. (2008). Dietary intake and parent's perception of mealtime behaviors in preschool-age children with autism spectrum disorder and in typically developing children. *Journal of the American Dietetic Association*, 108, 1360–1363.

Lumeng, J. C., Cardinal, T. M., Jankowski, M., Kaciroti, N., and Gelman, S. A. (2008). Children's use of adult testimony to guide food selection. *Appetite*, 51, 302–310.

Marples, C. A., and Spillman, D. (1995). Factors affecting students' participation in the Cincinnati public school lunch program. *Adolescence*, 30, 745–754.

Must, A., and Strauss, R. S. (1999). Risks and consequences of childhood and adolescent obesity. *International Journal of Obesity and Related Metabolic Disorders*, 23 (Suppl. 2), S2–S11.

Newman, J., and Layton, B. D. (1984). Overjustification: A self-perception perspective. *Personality and Social Psychology Bulletin*, 10, 419–425.

Newman, J., and Taylor, A. (1992). Effect of a means–end contingency on young children's food preferences. *Journal of Experimental Child Psychology*, 55, 431–439.

Orrell-Valente, J.K., Hill, L.G., Brechwald, W.A., Dodge, K.A., Pettit, G.S., and Bates, J.E. (2007). 'Just three more bites': An observational analysis of parents' socialization of children's eating at mealtime. *Appetite*, 48, 37–45.

Patrick, H., and Nicklas, T. A. (2005). A review of family and social determinants of children's eating patterns and diet quality. *Journal of the American College of Nutrition*, 24, 83–92.

Perry, C. L., Bishop, D. B., Taylor, G. L., Davis, M., Story, M., Gray, C., Bishop, S. C., Mays, R. A. W., Lytle, L. A., and Harnack, L. (2004). A randomized school trial of environmental strategies to encourage fruit and vegetable consumption among children. *Health Education and Behavior*, 31, 65–76.

Perry, C. L., Bishop, D. B., Taylor, G., Murray, D. M., Mays, R. W., Dudovitz, B. S., Smyth, M., and Story, M. (1998). Changing fruit and vegetable consumption among children: The 5-a-Day Power Plus program in St Paul, Minnesota. *American Journal of Public Health*, 88, 603–609.

Pliner, P. (2008). Cognitive schemas: How can we use them to improve children's acceptance of diverse and unfamiliar foods? *British Journal of Nutrition*, 99, S2–S6.

Resnicow, K., Cohn, L., Reinhardt, J., Cross, D., Futterman, R., Kirschner, E., Wynder, E. L., and Allegrante, J. P. (1992). A three-year evaluation of the Know Your Body program in inner-city schoolchildren. *Health Education Quarterly*, 19, 463–480.

Reynolds, K. D., Franklin, F. A., Binkley, D., Raczynski, J. M., Harrington, K. F., Kirk, K. A., and Person, S. (2000a). Increasing the fruit and vegetable consumption of fourth-graders: Results from the High-5 project. *Preventive Medicine*, 30, 309–319.

Reynolds, K. D., Franklin, F. A., Leviton, L. C., Maloy, J., Harrington, K. T., Yaroch, A. L., Person, S., and Jester, P. (2000b). Methods, results, and lessons learned from process evaluation of the High 5 school-based nutrition intervention. *Health Education and Behaviors*, 27, 177–186.

Rolls, B. J., Roe, L. S., and Meengs, J. S. (2004). Salad and satiety: Energy density and portion size of a first-course salad affect energy intake at lunch. *Journal of the American Dietetic Association*, 104, 1570–1576.

Rolls, B. J., Rolls, E. T., Rowe, E. A., and Sweeney, K. (1981). Sensory specific satiety in man. *Physiology and Behavior*, 27, 137–142.

Rozin, P. (1986). One-trial acquired likes and dislikes in humans: Disgust as a US food predominance, and negative learning predominance. *Learning and Motivation*, 17, 180–189.

Rozin, P., Fischler, C., Shields, C., and Masson, E. (2006). Attitudes towards large numbers of choices in the food domain: A cross-cultural study of five countries in Europe and the USA. *Appetite*, 46, 304–308.

Sanders, M.R., Patel, R.K., LeGrice, B., and Shepard, R.W. (1993). Children with persistent feeding difficulties: An observational analysis of the feeding interactions of problem and non-problems eaters. *Health Psychology*, 12, 64–73.

Schreck, K. A., Williams, K. E., and Smith, A. F. (2004). A comparison of eating behaviors between children with and without autism. *Journal of Autism and Developmental Disorders*, 34, 433–438.

Schwimmer, J. B., Burwinkle, T. M., and Varni, J. W. (2003). Health-related quality of life of severely obese children and adolescents. *Journal of the American Medical Association*, 289, 1813–1819.

Stark, L. J., Collins, F. L., Osnes, P. G., and Stokes, T. F. (1986). Using reinforcement and cueing to increase health snack food choices in preschoolers. *Journal of Applied Behavior Analysis*, 19, 367–380.

Story, M., Mays, R. W., Bishop, D. B., Perry, C. L., Taylor, G., Smyth, M., and Gray, C. (2000). 5- a-Day Power Plus: Process evaluation of a multi-component elementary school program to increase fruit and vegetable consumption. *Health Education and Behavior*, 27, 187–200.

Timimi, S., Douglas, J., and Tsiftssopoulou, K. (1997). Selective eaters: A retrospective case note study. *Child: Care, Health and Development*, 23, 265–278

Turnbull, I. D., Heaslip, S., and McLeod, H. A. (2000). Preschool children's attitudes to fat and normal male and female stimulus figures. *International Journal of Obesity and Related Metabolic Disorders*, 24, 1705–1706.

Wardle, J., Herrera, M. L., Cooke, L., and Gibson, E. L. (2003). Modifying children's food preferences: The effects of exposure and reward on acceptance of an unfamiliar vegetable. *European Journal of Clinical Nutrition*, 57, 341–348.

Williams, C. L., Bulli, M. T., and Deckelbaum, R. J. (2001). Prevention and treatment of childhood obesity. *Current Atherosclerosis Reports*, 3, 486–497.

Williams, K. E., Gibbons, B., and Schreck, K. (2005). Comparing selective eaters with and without developmental disabilities. *Journal of Developmental and Physical Disabilities*, 17, 299–309.

Part III

Design of food and drink products for children

9

Consumer testing of food products using children

R. Popper and J. J. Kroll, Peryam and Kroll Research Corporation, USA

Abstract: Children represent a large segment of the food and beverage market, and for products to be successful in this competitive market they must appeal to the consumer, namely the child. It is important to understand how children may differ from adults, with respect to both sensory perception and preference. In conducting research with children, it is critical to select methods that are within the children's linguistic, cognitive and motor capabilities. Particularly important in consumer testing is the choice of method for measuring food acceptability. With the right research tools, consumer testing with children can make a valuable contribution to the development and optimization of products for this segment.

Key words: children, sensory perception, consumer testing, food preference, hedonic scaling.

Note: This chapter was originally published as Chapter 16 'Consumer testing of food products using children' by R. Popper and J. J. Kroll in *Consumer-led food product development*, ed. H. MacFie, Woodhead Publishing Limited, 2007, ISBN: 978-1-84569-072-4.

9.1 Introduction

Nearly one-third of the world's population is under the age of 15. In the United States alone, there are over 50 million consumers in that age group, accounting for a youth market in excess of $300 billion, with food and beverage representing as much as 60% of that market.

The size of the business opportunity has resulted in a highly competitive environment for food manufacturers as they try to gain and maintain their share of the youth market. While parents serve an important gatekeeper function in determining which products are purchased, the 'pester' power and influence of even young children on food purchase decisions continues to rise. Today's children have more choices and more influence over their parents' purchase decisions than ever before. Children are also making many more of their own purchase decisions, with ever greater sums of money under their direct disposal. Therefore, no manufacturer can succeed in the youth market place today without optimizing products for their consumer target – the child. By successfully appealing to children, marketers also stand a chance of building long-term brand loyalty, as early exposure to products and brands may form the basis for brand choices later in life.

Successfully developing and optimizing foods and beverages for children requires involving children in the product development process. Children's needs and wants differ from those of adults, and product development must be guided by insights into what uniquely motivates and appeals to them. For new products, input from children may be needed at every stage of product development, from early idea exploration and prototype screening on through product and package optimization, as well as advertising copy development. For products undergoing reformulation, either for the purpose of cost reduction or product improvement, research may be needed to confirm that the product change is not detrimental to acceptability or does indeed improve the product.

In conducting research with children, it is important that the methods employed take into consideration the physical, emotional, and cognitive development of the children being asked to participate in the study. The assumption that methods appropriate for adults can be used with little or no modification in a study involving children is almost certain to lead to disappointing results. Furthermore, it is important to consider the specific age of the child in deciding what methods to employ, since motor skills, language skills, and reasoning abilities develop rapidly during childhood.

The primary focus of this chapter is on methods appropriate for quantitative testing of product acceptability with children who are between the ages of 6 and 12. Methods for testing pre-school-age children are also briefly considered. Infants and toddlers require methods grounded in behavioral observation, which are outside the scope of this chapter. Children who are above the age of 12 are capable of using many of the same research tools as adults. The chapter begins with a review of what is known about children's sensory perception and how food preferences develop, areas that can have important implications for product design as well as testing methodology. The chapter then reviews the techniques for quantitative consumer testing and provides examples of the types of questions and scales appropriate for testing with children of different ages.

9.2 Sensory perception: sensitivity and perceived intensity

Are children more or less sensitive than adults to taste or olfactory stimulation? Studies of taste thresholds present a confusing picture, with some studies suggesting that children as young as 5–7 years of age have similar detection thresholds as adults, others finding that children of this age have poorer sensitivity than adults (Guinard, 2001). Various methodological differences among the studies have been suggested as the source of these inconsistencies (James *et al.*, 1997). In their study, James *et al.* tested 8–9-year-old children and young adults of both sexes under the same experimental conditions, determining detection thresholds for sucrose, sodium chloride, citric acid, and caffeine. A two-alternative forced-choice procedure was used, in which respondents had to indicate which sample 'tasted stronger' (one of the samples contained only water, the other the taste stimulus). The fact that the thresholds did not differ across two replications was indicative of the reliability of the procedure. Girls had detection thresholds similar to the adults; boys, on the other hand, proved to be somewhat less sensitive than adults, especially in the case of citric acid.

Greater differences in sensitivity between children and adults are evident as the task increases in complexity. Oram *et al.* (2001) compared 8–9-year-old children to adults in terms of their ability to recognize a particular taste (e.g. sweet) in a mixture of two tastes (e.g. sweet and sour). While children were able to correctly identify a taste as sweet, sour, or salty when it was the only taste present, they performed markedly poorer than adults in correctly identifying the components of a binary taste mixture. Children tended to recognize only one of the components, the adults recognized both. These differences could be due to differences in taste perception, in cognitive ability (e.g. ability to separately process two sensations), or in response strategy (e.g. children may have focused on the more intense or more appealing taste quality).

Children and young adults tend not to differ much with respect to olfactory thresholds (Lehrner *et al.*, 1999). However, while children's olfactory sensitivity is very similar to that of adults, children are less likely than young adults to correctly identify (name) an odor or to recognize it as one that had been presented earlier in the experiment (Lehrner *et al.*, 1999; Lehrner and Walla, 2002). The fact that children perform less well at identifying odors than young adults is not surprising. Children also perform less well than young adults in picture identification (Cain *et al.*, 1995). Children have the olfactory sensitivity but lack odor-specific knowledge, which accumulates slowly over time. Odors may be unfamiliar to children; and, even if familiar, may not have been become strongly associated with verbal descriptors. Semantic encoding (that is, the association of smells with words) is a key component in odor memory (Rabin and Cain, 1984), especially in children (Lehrner *et al.*, 1999; Lumeng *et al.*, 2005). Cain *et al.* showed that when given the opportunity to learn odor names in a paired association task, children improve quickly in performance, although the learning curve is much attenuated when the odors are novel to begin with.

Another measure of sensory sensitivity, separate from detection threshold, is supra-threshold intensity perception. Compared with adults, children appear to perform less well at ranking the sweetness of beverages varying in amount of sucrose (Kimmel *et al.*, 1994; De Graaf and Zandstra, 1999; Liem *et al.*, 2004a). The rate at which perceived intensity changes with stimulus concentration may also differ between children and adults. Zandstra and De Graaf (1998) varied the concentration of sucrose in orange drink and found that for children aged 6–12 sweetness increased less rapidly as a function of sucrose than it did for adolescents or adults. Using a category scaling procedure, the children rated the low sucrose concentrations as sweeter than did the adults, but rated the high sucrose concentrations as less sweet. In a second study, De Graaf and Zandstra (1999) replicated these results for orange drink, but found that in water the sweetness functions for adults and children were similar (as was also reported by James *et al.*, 2003). Thus, food context may affect children and adults differently. This conclusion is supported by James *et al.* (1999), who used the method of magnitude estimation to scale sweetness, and by Temple *et al.* (2002), who used a computer-based time-intensity scaling procedure. Both studies found that sweetness increased in a similar fashion for both adults and children in response to increases of sucrose in water, but increased more slowly in orange drink and some other food applications. In the case of these more complex stimuli, children may have found it difficult to attend exclusively to sweetness and may have been influenced in their sweetness ratings by other sensory characteristics.

While sweetness is the sensory characteristic most frequently studied with children, a number of studies have been reported on supra-threshold sourness perception. These studies indicate that adults and children rate sourness similarly in response to variations in citric acid, both in orange drink (Zandstra and De Graaf, 1998) and in gelatin dessert (Liem and Mannella, 2003).

Much remains unknown with regard to differences between adults and children in sensory perception, especially in modalities other than olfaction and taste (for the few examples of research on texture perception in children, see Szczesniak, 1972; Oram, 1998; Narain, 2005). Adults and children show many similarities in sensory sensitivity, both in terms of detection thresholds and super-threshold intensity perception. In cases where differences have been reported, it is important to consider the possible sources for the findings. Any determination of threshold sensitivity or supra-threshold perception in children is complicated by the fact that measuring sensory perception in children is difficult – differences between adults and children in sensory perception may reflect, in part at least, differences in how children interpret the question they are asked and how they use the scales on which the research is based. Liem *et al.* (2004a) provide an example of how important the question is to the experimental outcome. In their study, 4-year-old children were not able to reliably discriminate the intensity of beverages differing in sweetness, using either a two-alternative forced choice or a ranking procedure. However, when asked to state their preference, the children consistently preferred the sweeter of two formulations in a pair and were able to rank order beverages from least to most preferred. Obviously, the children could indeed discriminate among the sweetness levels, but did not understand the intensity scaling instructions.

A number of the studies on intensity scaling cited above included control conditions in which children and adults rate simple visual stimuli for appearance characteristics (such as darkness or length) using the scaling procedures used to rate taste intensity. Children and adults usually perform identically on scaling such visual characteristics, suggesting that performance differences in perception of taste intensity are not solely a result of the scaling methodology. Whether the observed differences in taste sensitivity reflect maturational differences in the sensory systems of children and adults or developmental differences in attention and cognition has yet to be fully sorted out. The fact that differences between children and adults are more likely to reveal themselves with complex rather than simple taste stimuli (e.g. with taste mixtures and real foods rather than simple aqueous solutions) suggests that higher mental processing plays at least some part in accounting for the age difference in performance.

One practical implication of these findings is that to the extent to which children and adults differ in their sensory perception, children may not notice changes in product formulation to the same degree as adults. Ingredient substitutions and reformulations such as a reduction in sodium or a removal of trans fatty acids need to be tested with children in order to determine whether children notice a difference. Of course, whether a difference in sensory perception is of a magnitude to result in a difference in food acceptability is a separate, and usually more critical, question.

9.3 The origin of food preferences

Humans are born with an innate liking for sweet and an aversion to bitter, as has been shown by studies of reflexive facial expressions and food intake in newborns (see Birch, 1999, for a review). These genetic predispositions make evolutionary sense, since sweet foods (e.g. certain fruits) tend to be nutritious and high in energy, whereas bitter foods can be poisonous. Sour tastes are also rejected by newborns. A genetic predisposition towards liking of salt has not been so clearly established; newborns are indifferent to salt, but infants at 4 months show a liking for moderate levels of salt, possibly the result of a natural maturation process (Beauchamp *et al.*, 1986).

Humans are also genetically predisposed to avoid unfamiliar foods (Birch, 1999). In human evolution, this food neophobia served a protective function, since unfamiliar foods could cause illness or death. However, an infant's early experience with foods begins to counteract this neophobic response. While basic tastes such as sweetness and bitterness are intrinsically pleasant and unpleasant, the preferences for specific foods are largely learned, and the diversity of world cuisines attests to the role of culture and environment in shaping food preferences and overcoming the neophobic response (Rozin, 1984).

Many food preferences are learned based on the positive physiological consequences that follow consumption, such as feeling of satiety (Birch *et al.*, 1999). However preferences are acquired even in the absence of such positive physiological reinforcement, based on repeated exposure to a food alone. Zajonc (1968) was the first to identify the 'mere exposure effect' across a variety of stimulus domains, demonstrating that simply the repeated exposure to a stimulus, such as a sound or shape, can enhance liking. The role of early experience in food preferences has been demonstrated in a variety of studies. What the mother eats during pregnancy and lactation can affect an infant's flavor preferences (Birch, 1999), because of flavor cues contained in amniotic fluid or breast milk. Beauchamp and Moran (1984) showed that infants who were routinely fed sweetened water during the first months of life showed a greater preference for sweetened water at 2 years of age. Even bitter-tasting foods are subject to early learning effects. Protein hydrosolate infant formula (recommended for infants that do not tolerate cow's milk) tastes bitter as well as sour and is not well accepted by infants. Mennella and Beauchamp (2005) showed that exposure to these formulas starting shortly after birth leads to greater acceptance (as measured by intake) in infants aged 5–11 months. Early experience with protein hydrosolate formulas also has consequences for food preferences later during childhood. According to Liem and Menella (2002), children who experienced protein hydrosolate formulas early in life showed a preference at age 4–7 for higher levels of citric acid in juice (i.e. preferred a more sour taste) than did infants with no such experience.

The effect of exposure seems to be proportional to the amount of repetition. In a study conducted by Birch and Marlin (1982), 2-year-old children were exposed to initially unfamiliar foods with varying frequency (from zero to 20 times) over a period of several weeks. Preference for foods at the end of the study was almost perfectly correlated with exposure frequency: the more frequently a child was exposed to the food, the more the child liked it.

Food preference is also subject to social influences. Birch (1980) showed that 4-year-old children were influenced in their preferences by their peers who sat next to them during lunch. For example, children who initially did not like a vegetable grew to like it after repeatedly observing a peer consume that vegetable. This change in preference was relatively long lasting, persisting for several weeks and in the absence of the peers. In general (see Birch, 1999), older children are more effective role models than younger ones, mothers are more effective than strangers, and, for older preschoolers, adult heroes are more effective than ordinary adults.

There are several implications – for marketers, product developers, and researchers alike – of the way food preferences are acquired. Children's neophobia is likely to affect their willingness and response to novel foods in a research setting. Loewen and Pliner (2000) developed a questionnaire for assessing individual differences in neophobia in children that might be a useful attitudinal measurement for helping to explain children's response to novel foods in test situations.

Marketers and product developers need to balance children's desire for novelty with their propensity to prefer the familiar. The success of green colored ketchup in the United States, which combines a familiar flavor with an unfamiliar color, is a good example of this principle. In a laboratory context, Pliner and Stallberg-White (2000) demonstrated a similar phenomenon, showing that 10–12-year-old children were far more willing to try an unfamiliar chip when it was combined with a familiar dip than when it was presented with an unfamiliar dip.

The effect of repeated exposure on food acceptance among children suggests that product sampling and other strategies that encourage repeat consumption may help build acceptance of a new product. The learning effect also has implications for how to test novel foods with children. The limited exposure typical in taste tests may lead product development to underestimate the potential for unfamiliar flavors or textures. Finally, the demonstrated effects of social role models on food acceptance provides marketers with a continued reason to attempt to leverage peer influence through advertising or grass-roots marketing campaigns.

9.4 Difference between children and adults in food preferences

Perhaps the most widely documented difference in preference between children and adults is that children prefer a greater intensity of sweetness than adults. The heightened preference for sweetness among children was first reported by Desor *et al.* (1975) and was subsequently confirmed by Desor and Beauchamp (1986) in a longitudinal study, in which the same respondents were tested at two points in time – at age 11–15 and ten years later. The heightened preference for sweetness, which was reflected in the percentage of respondents who chose the sweetest of four sucrose concentration, decreased from the first test to the second, demonstrating that this preference declines with age. Using ranking or scaling methods instead of choice procedures, a number of other studies have also found that the optimal level of sweetness is higher for children than adults (Zandstra and De Graaf, 1998; De Graaf and Zandstra, 1999; Liem *et al.*, 2004a). Children also prefer higher levels of salt than adults, as has been demonstrated both with 9–11-year-old children (Desor *et al.*, 1975) as well as pre-schoolers (Beauchamp and Cowart, 1990). The reasons for this heightened preference for sweet or salty are not fully understood, but are believed to be rooted in development rather than the result of environmental influences.

Work by Liem and colleagues has revealed a segment of children with a preference for extreme sour tastes. Across a number of studies (Liem and Mennella, 2003; Liem *et al.*, 2004b), the researchers found that about one-third of children aged 5–12 showed a preference for an extreme sour taste, in contrast to adults as well as other children who preferred lower levels of sourness. All children, regardless of their preference, were equally able to discriminate among different levels of sourness, and showed the same level of discrimination as adults. Thus, the preference for extreme sour cannot be attributed to differences in sensory perception. The 'sour-loving' children did differ from the other children with respect to a number of other factors: they were less neophobic, had a greater preference for bright colors, tended to experience a wider variety of fruits, and tended to like other sour foods (sour candies, lemons), behaviors that may be examples of 'thrill seeking' among these children.

Whether the preference for extreme sour extends to preferences for other extreme tastes has not been investigated so far, and no longitudinal studies have yet been conducted to determine how this sour preference changes with age. It is also unclear whether the preference for extreme sour is the result or the cause of the observed differences in food habits.

Adults and children differ not only in their preferred intensity for certain basic tastes. Moncrieff (1966) studied olfactory preferences among adults and children and concluded that children aged 10–14 prefer fruity over floral smells, whereas the opposite was true for adults. With respect to food texture, children seem to prefer simple, smooth textures (Urbick, 2002) and, in bread products, dislike crunchy or chewy textures, especially at a young age where chewing efficiency is lower (Narain, 2005). The preference for simple textures may be an example of children's preference for foods with low 'complexity' (Ringel, 2005).

Children and adults may also differ in the relative importance they place on the appearance, taste and texture in assessing overall acceptability. Moskowitz (1994) cites a case study on ice cream in which children were found to place the same importance on appearance, flavor and texture, contrary to adults, who placed more emphasis on flavor and texture than appearance. Tuorila-Ollikainen *et al.* (1984) found that children put more emphasis on sweetness in soft drinks than on any other attribute, consistent with the demonstrated liking for sweet taste among children. Comparing children of different ages with respect to liking of meats, Rose *et al.* (2004a,b) found that taste and smell were of predominant importance to older children (aged 10–11), whereas texture and mouth feel characteristics were more likely to influence acceptability in the younger children (aged 6–7), as Chambers and Bowers (1993) showed was the case for adults.

In summary, the results of published research (as well as those of unpublished industrial studies) demonstrate the importance of optimizing products for children based on their distinct preferences. A product that is optimal for children is likely to differ from one that is optimal for adults – and may also differ from one that adults *think* would be optimal for children (Moskowitz, 1994).

9.5 Research methods for consumer testing of food products for children

The research task and measurement technique employed in a study involving children must be age appropriate, since language, cognitive, and motor skills vary significantly by age. The Swiss psychologist Jean Piaget is well known for his description of the stages of a child's cognitive and linguistic development. For example, Piaget distinguishes the 'pre-operational' stage (aged 2–6) from the 'concrete-operational' stage (aged 7–12). In the pre-operational stage, children are more likely to focus on a single aspect of a stimulus, whereas concrete-operational children have the ability to perceive stimuli multidimensionally.

Gollick (2002) describes some of the limitations of children that may affect their ability to answer questions in a research study. Very young children, for example, have difficulty with concept formation (e.g. sweetness) and classification (e.g. like/dislike). Even when they understand the principles, their attention span may limit their ability to perform the task. For example, $3^1/_2$-year-old children may understand a sorting task, but only about half the children may have the attention span to remember the assignment and therefore successfully complete the task.

'Seriation,' the ability to rank things in order of magnitude, is not fully mastered until age 7, according to Gollick, and this has implications for the reliability of any scaling results from younger children. In addition, children have limited memory skills, which may affect their ability to remember a succession of flavors presented for evaluation in a sensory test. Gollick also notes the difficulty that children aged 6 and under have in attending to more than one aspect of a stimulus at one time, as Piaget's theory suggests. As a consequence, young children may attend to only one dimension of a food, unlike older children, who may be able to base their reaction on a simultaneous consideration of multiple aspects.

Unfortunately, the child's age is far from being a perfect predictor of a child's ability to participate in research. There is tremendous variation in skills among children of the same age. Gollick's experience with cognitive testing has shown that the age at which 10% of children can master a particular task, compared with the age at which 90% of children can do so, varies by as much as 4 years. Thus, assumptions regarding what a particular age group can do are often going to be true only approximately, and researchers need to take into account the considerable variation in children's abilities, even at similar ages. As Chambers (2005) has pointed out, particular caution is needed with respect to children in the 'cusp' years, i.e. those that are transitioning from one developmental stage to another. For example, children age 6–7 are at the border of the pre-operational and the concrete-operational stages of development, and this age group is likely to be quite variable with respect to their cognitive abilities.

Guinard (2001) has summarized published studies with regard to children's abilities to perform a variety of sensory testing methods at different ages (see also ASTM, 2003). As one would expect, the younger the age group, the more challenging it is to devise valid, reliable test methods. These reviews conclude that children 2–3 years old are capable of expressing preference between two choices, but not much else. Children aged 4–5 are, in addition, capable of performing attribute-based paired comparison tasks ('which is sweeter?'), ranking products in terms of preference, and rating products on simple hedonic scales. Children aged 6–7 are capable of more complex scaling tasks (e.g. intensity) and performing certain discrimination tests (e.g. triangle tests). By age 8, children are capable of performing virtually any kind of standard sensory test. By this age, children are also capable of self-administering many tests with only occasional assistance from the interviewer or experimenter. At younger ages, one-on-one interviews are usually required.

When products are expected to appeal to a wide age range, it is often convenient to test older children (8 and above), who are subject to fewer limitations regarding the appropriate research technique and who can self-administer the tests (which is less costly and time consuming than one-on-one interviewing). However, when the core target age for the product is specifically younger children, it may not be appropriate to focus exclusively on the older age group.

9.6 Hedonic testing with children

9.6.1 Hedonic scales

Being able to determine the level of a child's liking for a product has obvious importance to product development. A number of hedonic scales for children have been proposed, some using pictures (often faces), some using words, and some a combination of pictures and words (see ASTM, 2003). Three examples of pictorial scales, two of which are also verbally anchored, are shown in Fig. 9.1.

Kroll (1990) introduced a verbal liking scale for testing children (see Table 9.1), which has become known as the Peryam & Kroll (P&K) or the super good/ super bad scale. The scale is similar to the traditional 9-point hedonic scale, except that the verbal anchors associated with the scale are more child-friendly – instead of using terms such as 'like extremely' and 'dislike extremely,' for example, it employs the terms 'super good' and 'super bad.' Testing children in the range of 5–10 years old, Kroll compared several scale variations, including

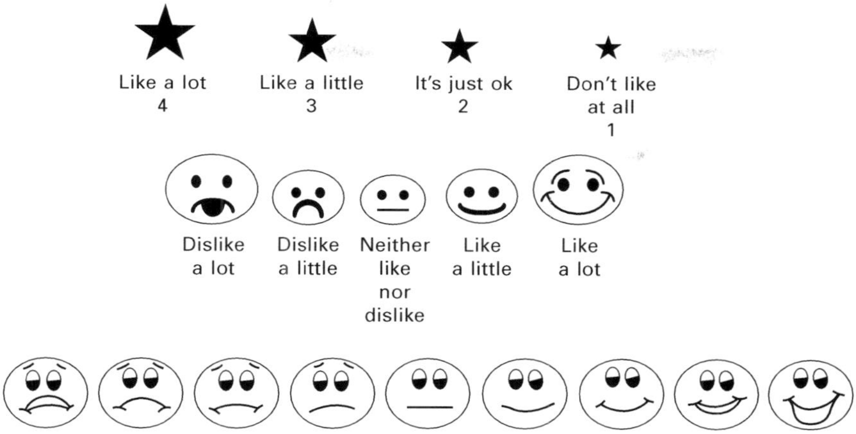

Fig. 9.1 Examples of pictorial hedonic scales for children.

Table 9.1 The traditional adult hedonic scale and the P&K hedonic scale for children

Traditional adult hedonic scale	P&K hedonic scale for children
Like extremely	Super good
Like very much	Really good
Like moderately	Good
Like slightly	Just a little good
Neither like nor dislike	Maybe good or maybe bad
Dislike slightly	Just a little bad
Dislike moderately	Bad
Dislike very much	Really bad
Dislike extremely	Super bad

the traditional 9-point scale, the 9-point P&K scale, and a 9-point face scale (similar to the one shown at the bottom of Fig. 9.1). Kroll also tested 7-point versions of these same three scales. Scales were compared on the basis of their ability to discriminate between two beverages (which paired preference tests showed were differentially preferred). All scales found a significant difference in liking between the two beverages, but with the P&K scale the difference was more highly significant than for the face scale and the traditional scale. Across scale types, the 9-point scales discriminated better than the 7-point scales, even among 5–7-year-old children.

These results challenged two prevailing assumptions, namely that face scales were superior to verbal scales when testing children, and that shorter scales were better than longer scales. Spaeth *et al.* (1992), working with 8–10-year-old children, confirmed Kroll's conclusions in a study comparing 3-point, 5-point, and 9-point versions of three scale types: the traditional hedonic scale, a face scale without verbal anchors, and a box scale verbally anchored only at the endpoints. The authors concluded that children do not use face scales better than purely verbally anchored scales and do not use short scales better than longer ones. Also, anchoring the 9-point scale only at the end-points yields the same results as the traditional hedonic scale.

Face scales may actually be detrimental by introducing unintended bias or confusing the child. A face intended to show a degree of 'dislike' can be interpreted by a child as conveying anger, a face intended to show 'liking' may suggest 'happiness.' Children may choose the 'happy' face because they like it better, rather than because it represents their opinion about the food they taste. Cooper (2002) has found that the eyes and the mouth are particularly important to the interpretation of the facial expression and are more likely than other elements to lead to misinterpretations of the scale unless carefully chosen. She also indicates that there are cultural differences with respect to the interpretation of facial expression. Certain expressions are appropriate in some cultures, but not in others.

While children 8–10-years-old can effectively use verbal 9-point scales, their ratings, compared with adults, are often higher. Figure 9.2 compares the distribution of ratings for adults and children rating the same products, with children using the 9-point P&K scale, and adults using the standard hedonic scale. The children most frequently responded with the top-most category of the scale, 'super good,' unlike the adults, who responded less positively. Other studies show that younger children will give somewhat higher ratings than older children using the same super good/super bad scale.

There are several factors that affect children's use of scales. Scale length is an obvious one. With fewer response choices (e.g. a 5-point hedonic scale), responses are more likely to be crowded in the upper end of the scale range (Crawford *et al.*, 2003). Crawford *et al.* (2005) investigated other scale factors which may affect scale usage among 8–14-year-olds. Using a 7-point hedonic scale, the authors concluded that a vertical scale orientation leads to more positive responses than a horizontal orientation, and that a horizontal scale with the positive end on the left leads to higher ratings than one with the negative end on the left. Similar scale effects have been reported for adults (Friedman and Amoo, 1999; Sauerhoff *et al.*, 2005). These findings suggest caution is needed when comparing findings across studies that have used ostensibly identical, but differently formatted hedonic scales.

The reason that children favor the positive end of the scale more than adults is not clear. Perhaps, unlike adults, children do not feel a need to 'hedge their bets,' by reserving the scale end-points for future, yet-to-be tasted products. Perhaps children lack the frame of reference that adults have developed over the years, or perhaps children are simply easier to please. Whatever the reason, the tendency for children to favor the positive end of any hedonic scale may result in a 'ceiling effect,' especially with highly liked foods. When such ceiling effects are a concern, some researchers have found that a preference question may provide better discrimination than scaled liking. In general, however, children's hedonic ratings discriminate very effectively among products. A recent unpublished review

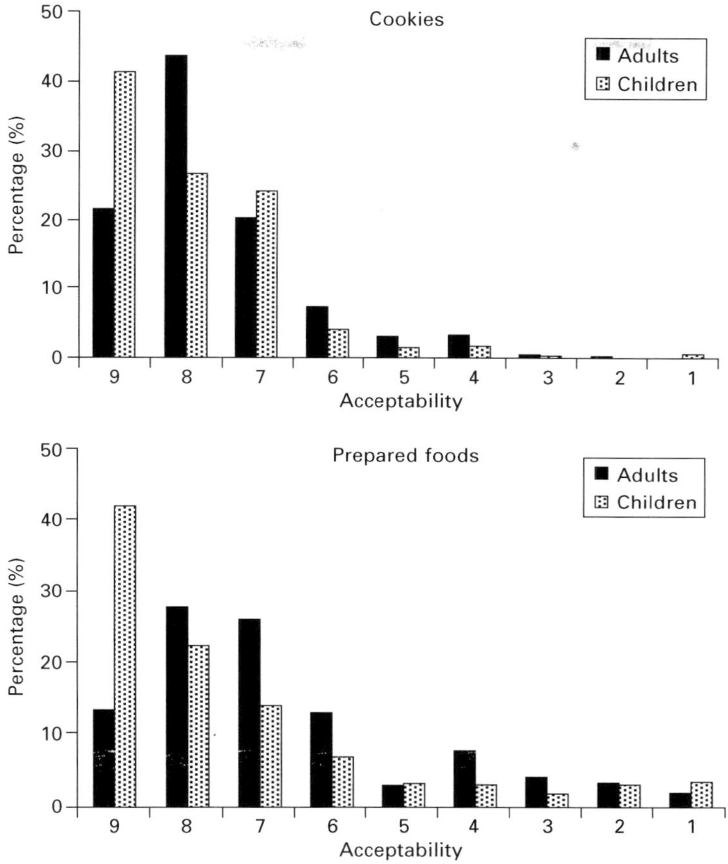

Fig. 9.2 Distribution of hedonic ratings by adults and children (8–12 years old) who evaluated acceptability on a 9-point scale. For cookies: $N = 220$ per age group, four samples. For prepared foods: $N = 125$ per age group, nine samples. For adults: 9 = like extremely; for children, 9 = super good.

by Peryam and Kroll of 14 studies involving five product categories (including such popular categories as cookies and pasta), with children and adults rating the same products, found that children's overall liking ratings (using the super good/super bad scale) were as likely to show significant differences as were the adults' ratings (albeit not always favoring the same products). In fact, in the six cases where significant differences were found with one group and not the other, it was the children who showed significant differences, not the adults.

9.6.2 Hedonic scale structure

One potential concern with any verbally anchored hedonic scale is how the choice of verbal scale anchors affects the psychological spacing between the scale points. The development of the standard 9-point hedonic scale was supported by extensive psychometric research (Peryam and Girardot, 1952; Jones *et al.*, 1955), which provided the basis for the selection of the phrases used to anchor the nine scale points. On the basis of an analysis of the ratings of different words or phrases, these early investigators were able to select phrases for anchoring the nine scale points that were approximately equally spaced psychologically. As Lawless and Heymann (1998) point out, the equal interval property is important, since the analysis of hedonic scale data almost always involves the assignment of numerical values to the responses and the application of parametric statistics, which assume equal interval spacing. Crawford *et al.* (2005) used a semantic analysis approach with children similar to the one Jones *et al.* used with adults, in order to investigate the psychological spacing of hedonic phrases, including six of the phrases from the standard adult scale. While the authors do not compare children's perceptions to those of adults, the agreement between the children's perceptual scale values and those reported by Jones *et al.* for the corresponding six phrases is very high (linear correlation $r = 0.98$), indicating similar semantic spacing of those phrases by children and adults.

Studies such as Jones *et al.* base their conclusion about the equal interval properties of the scale on studies of word perception. These studies leave open the question of whether the equal interval nature of the scale is preserved when respondents actually use the scale to rate stimuli (such as foods).

To investigate this question and to compare scale usage by children and adults, an analysis was conducted for the purposes of this chapter using a modified correspondence analysis approach. The data comprised ratings of 15 crackers, collected over the course of three test sessions. Overall liking ratings were collected from adults ($N = 200$) using the standard nine-point liking scale. Children (aged 9–12, $N = 200$) rated overall liking using the 9-point P&K (super good/super bad) scale. In addition to rating overall liking, both adults and children rated the products on a number of other liking dimensions (e.g. appearance, flavor) and rated several sensory attributes using intensity scales.

Multivariate mapping techniques are often used in sensory analysis and consumer research to map products spanned by 'attributes' (hedonic or intensity scales). In the present case, the perceptual mapping techniques are used to learn about differences between children and adults in scale usage, in particular in their use of an overall liking scale.

Greenacre (1984, pp. 169–184) describes how correspondence analysis can be used to analyze rating data, as opposed to frequencies (the typical domain of correspondence analysis). A related technique, dual scaling, has been described by Nishisato (1980). Only recently has this approach been applied to sensory and market research data (Abdi and Valentin, 2007; Chrea *et al.*, 2004, 2005; Torres and van de Velden, 2007). The technique is well suited for the present purpose, because it allows for the determination of the perceptual distance between scale points.

The correspondence analysis included all rating scale results (liking and intensity), though only the results for overall liking are reported here. Figure 9.3a shows the product map, in which products that are perceived similarly are positioned close together and products that are perceived very differently are far apart. The map shows product projections for the children, the adults, and for the consensus between the two, which represents a weighted average of the ratings of adults and children. The consensus projections of the scale points for overall liking are also shown.

Children and adults appear to rate the liking of products similarly in some cases, but not others (the interpretation of the map in terms of product attributes is beyond the scope of this chapter). Adults rated all products somewhat lower than the children (in the map, liking increases from left to right and the adult means are positioned to the left of those for the children), consistent with the age effect on liking ratings discussed above. In addition to this systematic shift, there are some differences between adults and children

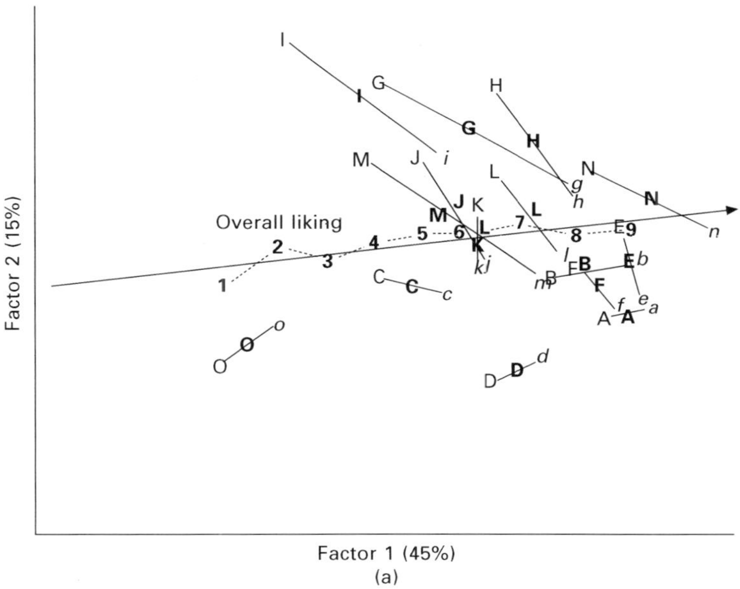

Fig. 9.3 Hedonic scale structure for children and adults as determined by correspondence analysis. (a) Products (letters) are projected in the map according to the adults' (upper case) or children's (lower case) ratings of overall liking and other hedonic and sensory attributes (only overall liking is shown). The consensus of the children and the adults (bold capital letters) is located between each pair of projections. The numbers represent the consensus projections of the nine scale points on the overall liking scale. (b) Separate projections of the overall liking scale points for adults (dashed line, traditional nine point hedonic scale) and children (solid line, P&K hedonic scale for children), indicating similar scale structure for both age groups.

(Continued overleaf)

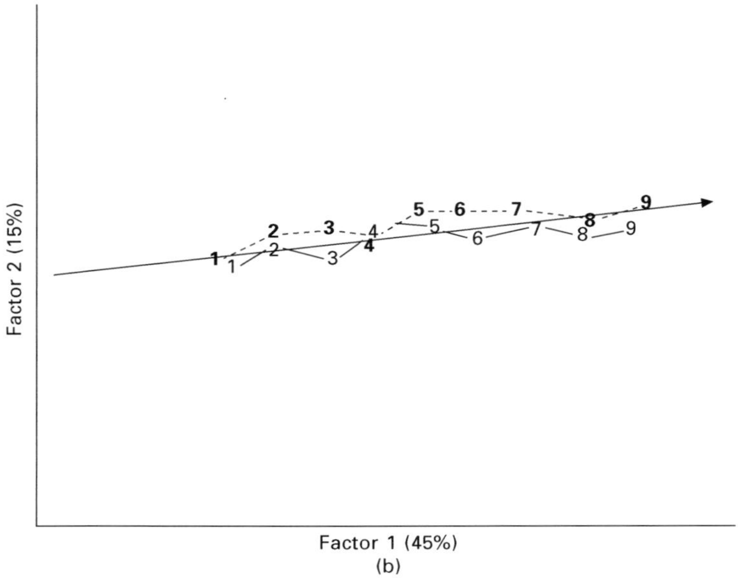

Fig. 9.3 Continued

in the relative liking of certain products (such as M, N, and G). For example, product N is the best liked product for children, but not for adults.

Figure 9.3b shows the separate projections of the overall liking scale points for adults and children. The scale points for the standard adult liking scale and the P&K super good/super bad scale project very similarly, and are spaced at approximately equal intervals, except for some slight compression in the middle of the scale. These results provide strong evidence that the two overall liking scales are highly similar measurement instruments and are both approximately equal interval scales.

9.6.3 Hedonic testing with pre-school-age children

The hedonic scales described so far are appropriate for testing children 5–12 years of age. Within that range, younger children (aged 5–7) will require assistance in completing the test, if for no reason other than that their reading ability is limited. As an alternative to one-on-one interviews (which are costly and time-consuming to conduct), it is sometimes possible to test 5–7-year-old children using a classroom-style group administration, provided the questionnaire is short and the test moderator guides the children through the questionnaire one question at a time.

But what methods are suitable for determining liking among children aged 3–5? Birch (1979, 1980) has successfully used a 'ranking by elimination' procedure, a variation of the traditional ranking procedure. According to this procedure, children first taste a number of samples and then choose their favorite. This sample is then set aside, and children re-taste the remaining samples, once again indicating their favorite. This process continues until all samples have been ranked. While used extensively in academic research by Birch and others, the use of this method in industrial applications appears to be rare.

Kimmel *et al.* (1994) concluded that 4–5-year-olds were able to use a 7-point face scale. Chen *et al.* (1996) found that 3-year-old children were able to use a 3-point scale, 4-year-olds a 5-point scale, and children 5 years old a 7-point scale. On the other hand, Léon *et al.* (1999) found low repeatability among 4–5-year-olds using three different methods, including a simple binary classification (like and dislike).

Popper *et al.* (2002) compared two different methods for measuring liking among pre-schoolers, the ranking by elimination procedure and a 5-point bifurcated scale. In the latter procedure, the child was first asked if the sample was 'good' or 'bad,' and, depending on the answer, was then asked whether the sample was 'really good' (or 'really bad') or 'just a little good' (or 'just a little bad'). If the child had trouble committing to whether the sample was good or bad, the answer was recorded as 'neither.'

Pre-school-age children are pre-literate and must by necessity be interviewed one-on-one. Typically, research personnel (usually female) serve as interviewers. Popper *et al.* included two interviewer conditions: in one condition, the child's mother was the interviewer, in the other condition, the interview was conducted by a female researcher (P&K staff person) unfamiliar to the child. When interviewed by the researcher, Mom was not present in the room with her child.

Both the ranking procedure and the bifurcated scale resulted in significant differences among the samples tested. Greater discrimination, using either procedure, was obtained when the child was interviewed by the mother than by the unfamiliar researcher (see Fig. 9.4). When Mom did the interviewing, the average ratings for the three formulations spanned a larger range than when the researcher did the interviewing, and the differences were more likely to be statistically significant. This effect varied by age – the benefit of Mom as interviewer was evident at ages 3 and 4, but was largely absent by age 5, where Mom and the P&K interviewer gave very similar results. The authors caution that using the mother as interviewer may not be preferable in all situations, especially when there is a risk that the mother could introduce her own biases about the products. In the study, the samples the child evaluated all looked the same (and the mother did not taste them). In situations when the appearance of the samples might suggest differences in nutrient content or when brand information is provided as part of the test, the mother's role as the interviewer would need to be carefully assessed.

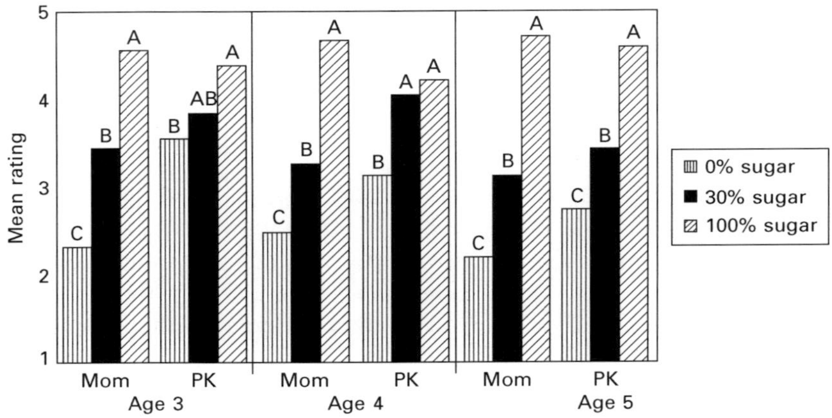

Fig. 9.4 Effect of interviewer (Mother vs. Peryam & Kroll researcher) on children's liking ratings (5 = 'really good') for powdered orange drinks differing in sugar concentration. Means sharing a common letter are not significantly different from one another ($p < 0.05$). From Popper *et al.* (2002).

9.7 Use of intensity and just-about-right scales

The research cited in Section 9.2 on intensity scaling with children demonstrates that children are capable of using intensity scales, although their ratings may differ from those of adults. In these studies, children typically become familiar with the scales using some practice tasks (e.g. scaling visual stimuli) prior to using them to rate foods. Also, these studies usually focus only on one or at most a few sensory attributes at a time.

Swaney-Stueve (2002) undertook the challenge of attempting to train children in descriptive analysis. Using six brands of peanut butter and a ballot including 14 or more attributes, she demonstrated that it is possible to train children as young as 9 years old to reliably discriminate among products using intensity ratings. The results of the 9-year-olds did not differ much from those obtained with children aged 13–14 and 16–18, although the results from the children and teen panels did differ somewhat from those obtained with two adult panels. In another example of the use of descriptive analysis with children, Narain (2005) showed that even 4-year-olds could be trained to use texture attributes to distinguish among breads. These studies demonstrate that children are capable, given appropriate training, to perform sensory tasks that are cognitively quite demanding.

In consumer tests with children, intensity scales are sometimes included in addition to hedonic scales. Intensity scales can help provide product developers information on how children perceive the differences among the products included in the test. By comparing their ratings with those of adults, these scales may also provide some insight into how children use terms such as 'sweet,' 'crunchy,' etc. In most consumer tests, children receive no or only minimal explanation of the sensory terms. For some attributes, such as sweetness, the assumption that children (typically aged 8–12) understand the meaning of the sensory characteristic they are being asked to scale is probably warranted. For other attributes, this assumption may be tenuous. The research on odor recognition and identification cited in Section 9.2 suggests that flavor concept formation and flavor naming is a learning process that extends into adulthood. Little research has been published that would tell product developers for which sensory attributes (and for which types of products) children are capable of generating meaningful intensity scaling results (in the absence of training), or what words to use to refer to different sensory characteristics (e.g. do children understand the meaning of 'mouth coating'?). Examples from Peryam and Kroll's research suggests that some attributes can indeed be scaled quite successfully, as was shown in the study on crackers described earlier. Figure 9.5 shows the correlation between children and adult ratings on three attribute intensity questions, using 9-point intensity scales. The agreement between children and adults was quite high.

Information regarding the preferred level of a sensory attribute (e.g. sweetness) is often obtained from children using just-about-right scales, following the common practice of using such scales in research with adults. The adult version of the just-about-right scale is usually a 5-point scale, in which the middle category is labeled 'just about right' and other scale points are labeled, for example, 'too weak' and 'much too weak' on one side and 'too strong' and 'much too strong' on the other. For use with children, many researchers shorten the scale to three points, 'too weak', 'just about right,' and 'too strong'. Again, little research has been published on children's use of such scales, or their benefits and limitations. In Peryam and Kroll's experience, just-about-right scales can provide meaningful results with children, although as in the case of intensity scales, careful consideration must be given to the types of attributes children are asked to evaluate. For example, children appear to be able to use just-about-right scales to flag product issues regarding appearance, size, or visual amount of an ingredient, as well as for basic tastes and simple texture attributes. In the case of flavor (other than basic tastes) and more complex appearance and texture terms, just-about-right scales tend to be less informative with children, most likely because of the difficulty children have understanding these attributes. Scaling these attributes often results in a high percentage of 'just right' responses, especially among younger children (aged 6–7), compared with adults using the same 3-point scale.

9.8 Future trends

Given the importance to the food industry of conducting research with children there is need for more research in several areas. At the level of basic science, much still needs to be learned about children's chemosensory

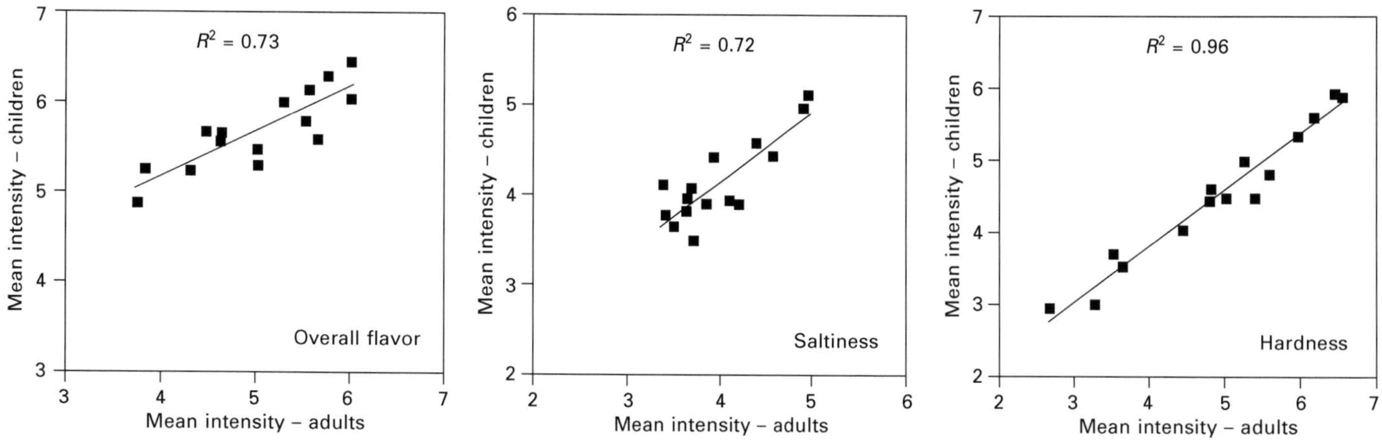

Fig. 9.5 Ratings of sensory intensity of 15 crackers by adults and 9–12-year-old children.

abilities and perceptions. The basic tastes and olfaction have been more extensively studied than other sense modalities, such as texture, yet even in the area of basic tastes, too few studies have involved complex foods, as opposed to test solutions or simple beverages.

For applied testing, the scaling methods most appropriate for children will continue to require investigation, especially as testing technology evolves to various forms of computerized testing. The potential of leveraging technology to improve children's comprehension and use of scales in consumer tests remains to be explored. The use of the Internet for research with children is also likely to grow. Cooper (2005) has reported on the use of a children's Internet panel for qualitative research.

While methods for hedonic scaling have been widely investigated, the benefits and limitations of using intensity and just-about-right scales with children in the context of consumer research requires more investigation, leading to guidelines for when to use such scales and how to refer to different sensory characteristics in a way easily understood by children.

Several other testing parameters are in need of further study, such as time of day. According to Gollick (2002), depending on the time of day, a child's IQ score on a standardized test can vary by as much as 30 points. Urbick (2002) advocates conducting consumer tests with children in the morning, when kids are most alert, and avoiding after-school hours, when children are mentally tired and need unstructured playtime and a chance to be physically active. Time of day may also affect children's reactions for other reasons. Some foods are more appropriate at some times of the day than others. Children at an early age have acquired a sense of time appropriateness for different foods (Birch *et al.*, 1984) and the effect of this awareness on test results remains to be better understood.

Food products developed for children are unique in many respects – their formulation, their packaging, and their messaging. Sensory researchers are prone to think about the product itself, but for children the success of a new product may depend not just on its taste and texture, but on how it handles, its play value, the image it projects, and how successfully all these aspects are integrated. It is likely that food developers will need to pay increasing attention to the overall 'product concept fit,' which may mean introducing advertising language and brand information into product research with children more often than is done today (if it is included at all). Little research has been conducted to understand how children process such information in the context of evaluating food and how such information impacts their liking ratings (Bahn, 1989; Allison *et al.*, 2004).

9.9 Sources of further information and advice

Birch (1999) provides a comprehensive review of research on the development of food preferences in children and the differences between children and adults in sensory sensitivity. Sensory research methods for use with children are reviewed by Popper and Kroll (2005), Guinard (2001) and Resurreccion (1998). A guide on testing with children, developed in 2003 by ASTM Committee E-18 (ASTM E-2299-03), provides a great deal of practical advice on how to conduct effective testing with children and includes recommendations regarding the age appropriateness of various sensory research methods. Journals such as *Food Quality and Preference, Appetite,* the *Journal of Sensory Studies*, and *Chemical Senses* are good sources for information and the latest research findings on children's sensory perception, food preferences, and the associated research methods. The biannual Pangborn Sensory Science Symposium provides an important forum for researchers from academia and industry to share findings regarding conducting research with children.

9.10 References

Abdi H and Valentin, D (2007), 'Multiple correspondence analysis', in Salkind N *Encyclopedia of Measurement and Statistics*. Thousand Oaks, CA, Sage.

Allison A-M A, Gualtieri T and Craig-Petsinger D (2004), 'Are young teens influenced by increased product description detail and branding during consumer testing?', *Food Qual Preference*, **15**(7/8), 819–829.

ASTM (2003), *ASTM Standard Guide for Sensory Evaluation of Products by Children*, E2299-03, West Conshohocken, PA, ASTM International.

Bahn K D (1989), 'Cognitively and perceptually based judgments in children's brand discriminations and preferences', *J Bus Psych*, **4**(2), 183–197.

Beauchamp G K and Cowart B J (1990), 'Preference for high salt concentrations among children', *Dev Psychol*, **26**(4), 539–545.

Beauchamp G K and Moran M (1984), 'Acceptance of sweet and salty tastes in 2-year-old children', *Appetite*, **5**, 291–305.

Beauchamp G K, Cowart B J and Moran M (1986), 'Developmental changes in salt acceptability in humans', *Dev Psychobiol*, **19**, 75–83.

Birch L L (1979), 'Dimensions of preschool children's food preference', *J Nutr Educ*, **11**(2), 77–80.

Birch L L (1980), 'Effect of peer models' food choices and eating behaviors on preschoolers' food preferences', *Child Develop*, **51**, 489-496.

Birch L L (1999), 'Development of food preferences', *Annu. Rev Nutr*, **19**, 41–62.

Birch L L and Marlin D W (1982), 'I don't like it; I never tried it: effects of exposure on two year-old children's food preferences', *Appetite*, **3**, 353–360.

Birch L L, Billman J and Richards S S (1984), 'Time of day influences food acceptability', *Appetite*, **5**, 109–116.

Birch L L, Fisher J O and Grimm-Thomas K (1999), 'Children and food', in Siegal M and Peterson C, *Children's Understanding of Biology and Health*, Cambridge, Cambridge University Press.

Cain W S, Stevens J C, Nickou C M, Giles A, Johnston I and Garcia-Medina M R (1995), 'Life-span development of odor identification, learning, and olfactory sensitivity', *Perception*, **24**, 1457–1472.

Chambers E (2005), 'Commentary: sensory research with children', *J Sensory Studies*, **20**, 90–92.

Chambers E and Bowers J R (1993), 'Consumer perception of sensory qualities in muscle foods', *Food Technol*, **47**, 116–134.

Chen A W, Resurreccion A V A and Paguio L P (1996), 'Age appropriate hedonic scales to measure food preferences of young children', *J Sensory Studies*, **11**, 141–163.
Chrea C, Valentin D, Sulmont-Rossé C, Ly Mai H, Hoang Nguyen D and Abdi H (2004), 'Culture and odor categorization: agreement between cultures depends upon the odors', *Food Qual Pref*, **15**, 669–679.
Chrea C, Valentin D, Sulmont-Rossé, Nguyen-Hoan D and Abdi, H (2005), 'Semantic, typicality, and odor representation: a cross-cultural study', *Chem Senses*, **30**, 37–49.
Cooper H (2002), 'Designing successful diagnostic scales for children', presented at Ann. Mtg., Inst. of Food Technologists, Anaheim, Calif., 15–19 June.
Cooper H R (2005), 'Taking directional sensory research on-line – experiences with the creative kids panel', presented at the 6th Pangborn Sensory Science Symposium, Harrogate, UK, 7–11 Aug.
Crawford C, Ward C and Simpson N (2003), 'Do scales grow with children?', presented at the 5th Pangborn Sensory Science Symposium, Boston, 20–23 July.
Crawford C, Simons C and Ward C (2005), 'When kids don't like "dislike"; creating a new hedonic scale for children', presented at the 6th Pangborn Sensory Science Symposium, Harrogate, UK, 7–11 Aug.
De Graaf C and Zandstra E H (1999), 'Sweetness intensity and pleasantness in children, adolescents, and adults', *Physiol Behav*, **67**(4), 513–520.
Desor J A and Beauchamp G K (1986), 'Longitudinal changes in sweet preferences in humans', *Physiol Behav*, **39**(5), 639–641.
Desor J, Greene L and Maller O (1975), 'Preferences for sweet and salty in 9-to 15-yearold and adult humans', *Science*, **190**, 686–687.
Friedman H H and Amoo T (1999), 'Rating the rating scales', *J Marketing Mgt*, **9**(3), 114–123.
Gollick M (2002), 'Asking kids questions: possible pitfalls', presented at Ann. Mtg., Inst. of Food Technologists, Anaheim, Calif., 15–19 June.
Greenacre M (1984), *Theory and Applications of Correspondence Analysis*, London, Academic Press.
Guinard J X (2001), 'Sensory and consumer testing with children', *Trends Food Sci Technol*, **11**, 273–283.
James C E, Laing D G and Oram N (1997), 'A comparison of the ability of 8–9-year-old children and adults to detect taste stimuli', *Physiol Behav*, **62**(1), 193–197.
James C E, Laing D G, Oram N and Hutchinson I (1999), 'Perception of sweetness in simple and complex taste stimuli by adults and children', *Chem Senses*, **24**, 281–287.
James C E, Laing D G, Jinks A L, Oram N and Hutchinson I (2003), 'Taste response functions of adults and children using different rating scales', *Food Qual Preference*, **15**, 77–82.
Jones L V, Peryam D R and Thurstone L L (1955), 'Development of a scale for measuring soldiers' food preferences', *Food Res*, **20**, 512–520.
Kimmel S A, Sigman-Grant M and Guinard J X (1994), 'Sensory testing with young children', *Food Technol*, **48**(3), 92–99.
Kroll B J (1990), 'Evaluating rating scales for sensory testing with children', *Food Technol*, **44**(11), 78–80, 82, 84, 86.
Lawless H T and HEYMANN H (1998), *Sensory Evaluation of Food*, New York, Chapman and Hall.
Lehrner J and Walla P (2002), 'Development of odor naming and odor memory from childhood to young adulthood', in Rouby C, Schaal B, Dubois D, Gervais R and Holley A, *Olfaction, Taste and Cognition*, Cambridge, Cambridge University Press, pp. 278–289.
Lehrner J P, Glück J and Laska M (1999), 'Odor identification, consistency of label use, olfactory threshold and their relationships to odor memory over the human lifespan', *Chem Senses*, **24**, 337–346.

Lee On F, Couronne T, Marcuz M C and Köster E P (1999), 'Measuring food liking in children: a comparison of non-verbal methods', *Food Qual Preference*, **10**, 93–100.
Liem D G and Mennella J A (2002), 'Sweet and sour preferences during childhood: role of early experiences', *Dev Psychobiol*, **41**, 388–395.
Liem D G and Mennella J A (2003), 'Heightened sour preferences during childhood', *Chem Senses*, **28**, 173–180
Liem D G, Mars M and De Graaf C (2004a), 'Consistency of sensory testing with 4-and 5-year-old children', *Food Qual Preference*, **15**, 541–548.
Liem D G, Westerbeek A, Wolterink S, Kok F J and De Graaf C (2004b), 'Sour taste preferences of children relate to preference for novel and intense stimuli', *Chem Senses*, **29**(8), 713–720.
Loewen R and Pliner P (2000), 'The Food Situations Questionnaire: a measure of children's willingness to try novel foods in stimulating and non-stimulating situations', *Appetite*, **35**, 239–250.
Lumeng J C, Zuckerman M D, Cardinal T and Kaciroti N (2005), 'The association between flavor labeling and flavor recall ability in children', *Chem Senses*, **30**(7), 565–574.
Mennella J A and Beauchamp G K (2005), 'Understanding the origin of flavor preferences', *Chem Senses*, **30** (suppl 1), i242–i243.
Moncrieff R W (1966), *Odour Preferences*, New York, Wiley.
Moskowitz H R (1994), *Food Concepts and Products: Just-in-time Development*, Trumbull, CT, Food and Nutrition Press.
Narain C (2005), 'Texture preference in children', presented at the 6th Pangborn Sensory Science Symposium, Harrogate, UK, 7–11 Aug.
Nishisato S (1980), *Analysis of Categorical Data: Duel Scaling and its Applications*, Toronto, University of Toronto Press.
Oram N (1998), 'Association of perceptual feel and general descriptors with food categories by 8–11 year olds and adults', *J Texture Studies*, 29, 669–680.
Oram N, Laing D G, Freeman M H and Hutchinson I (2001), 'Analysis of taste mixtures by adults and children', *Dev Psychobiol*, **38**, 67–77.
Peryam D and Girardot N F (1952), 'Advanced taste test methods', *Food Eng*, **24**(7), 58–61, 194.
Pliner P and Stallberg-White C (2000), 'Pass the ketchup, please: familiar flavors increase children's willingness to taste novel foods', *Appetite*, **34**, 95–103.
Popper R and Kroll J J (2005), 'Conducting sensory research with children', *J Sensory Studies*, **20**, 75–87.
Popper R, Schraidt M and Kroll B J (2002), 'Testing with pre-school children: the effect of the interviewer', presented at Ann. Mtg., Inst. of Food Technologists, Anaheim, CA, 15–19 June.
Rabin M D and Cain W S (1984), 'Odor recognition: familiarity, identifiability, and encoding consistency', *J Exp Psychol: Learning, Memory Cognition*, **10**, 316–325.
Resurreccion A V A (1998), *Consumer Sensory Testing for Product Development*, Gaithersburg, MD, Aspen.
Ringel C (2005), 'The change of the optimal complexity level after extended exposure – comparison of elderly people, young adults and children', presented at the 6th Pangborn Sensory Science Symposium, Harrogate, UK, 7–11 Aug.
Rose G, Laing D G, Oram N and Hutchinson I (2004a), 'Sensory profiling by children aged 6–7 and 10–11 years. Part 1: a descriptor approach', *Food Qual Preference*, **15**, 585–596.
Rose G, Laing D G, Oram N and Hutchinson I (2004b), 'Sensory profiling by children aged 6–7 and 10–11 years. Part 2: a modality approach', *Food Qual Preference*, **15**, 597–606.
Rozin P (1984), 'The acquisition of food habits and preferences', in J D Matarazzo, S M Weiss, J A Herd and N E Miller, *A Handbook of Health Enhancement and Disease Prevention*, New York, Wiley, pp. 590–607.

Sauerhoff K, Degnan D and Craig-Petsinger D (2005), 'The impact of scale orientation and labels on consumer response in an online environment', presented at the 6th Pangborn Sensory Science Symposium, Harrogate, UK, 7–11 Aug.

Spaeth E E, Chambers E C IV and Schwenke J R (1992), 'A comparison of acceptability scaling methods for use with children', in Wu L S and Gelinas A D, *Product Testing with Consumers for Research Guidance: Special Consumer Groups, Second Volume ASTM STP 1155*, Philadelphia, Am Soc Testing Materials, 65–77.

Swaney-Stueve M (2002), 'Can children perform descriptive analysis?', presented at Ann. Mtg., Inst. of Food Technologists, Anaheim, CA, 15–19 June.

Szczesniak A S (1972), 'Consumer awareness of and attitudes to food texture', *J Texture Studies*, **3**, 206–217.

Temple E C, Laing D G, Hutchinson I and Jinks A L (2002), 'Temporal perception of sweetness by adults and children using computerized time-intensity measures', *Chem Senses*, **27**, 729–737.

Torres, A and Van De Velden M (2007), 'Perceptual mapping of multiple variable batteries by plotting supplementary variables in correspondence analysis of rating data', *Food Qual Preference*, **18**(1), 121–129.

Tuorila-Ollikainen H, Mahlamaki-Dultanen S and Kurkela R (1984), 'Relative importance of color, fruity flavor, and sweetness in the overall liking of soft drinks', *J Food Sci*, **49**, 1598–1600.

Urbick B (2002), 'Kids have great taste: an update to sensory workwith children', presented at Ann. Mtg., Inst. of Food Technologists, Anaheim, CA, 15–19 June.

Zandstra E H and De Graaf C (1998), 'Sensory perception and pleasantness of orange beverages from childhood to old age', *Food Qual Preference*, **9**(1/2), 5–12.

Zajonc R B (1968), 'Attitudinal effects of mere exposure', *J Personality Social Psychol*, **9**(Part 2), 1–27.

10

Case studies of consumer testing of food products using children

N. J. Patterson, and C. J. M. Beeren, Leatherhead Food Research, UK

Abstract: Consumer research with children is vital for any new developments for this age-group. Children and adults have different sensorial perceptions which will also bring along their own preferences. Research with children itself can be somewhat more complicated than standard testing with adults. The Market Research Society (MRS) has produced specific guidelines to be adhered to when testing with children (those aged under 16) with key points: to get parental consent, to not ask children to carry out anything illegal for their age group, and to use appropriate language for the age group. This chapter describes some further considerations when working with children, including incentives, questionnaires and follow-ups, using two case studies.

Key words: children's research, research considerations, case studies, school research, children testing in sensory facilities.

10.1 Introduction

The core factors attracting children to foods are colourful packaging, cartoon imagery, unusual shapes and colours, and interactive play elements. However, the trends in childhood obesity mean that the role of parental supervision in children's foods has been increasing. According to the UK National Health Service report *Health Survey for England: Physical Activity and Fitness* (NHS, 2009), in 2008 around three in ten boys and girls were classed as either overweight or obese (31% and 29% respectively), and that figure continues to rise along with accompanying concerns on the quality of childhood nutrition. This makes the issue of parental appeal more relevant to marketers. Health is clearly the most important issue in appealing to parents and this takes many forms, from fat and calorie reduction to additive removal and the provision of wholegrain-rich, natural and organic foods. There are even some products with modern functional ingredients that are aimed at children.

Manufacturers face the challenge of having to combine child-friendly elements with those that will satisfy the demands of concerned parents, whilst children are also increasingly making their own demands as they become more exposed to healthy eating messages.

Testing food and drink products on children requires the permission or 'buy-in' from both the adult and the child. Children are becoming more savvy to health messages aimed at them so they, too, will also be more demanding of foods that are tasty and healthy, and potentially only willing to test products that meet their demands.

10.1.1 Market Research Society (MRS) guidelines for testing with children

The aims of the Market Research Society (MRS) guidelines (*Conducting Research with Children and Young People*, 2006) state that it is the responsibility of the researcher to keep abreast of any legislation which could affect research among children and young people and to ensure that all those involved in a project are aware of and agree to abide by the MRS Code of Conduct. 'Children' are defined as those aged under 16 years (young people are aged 16 and 17 years, adults are aged 18 years and over).

An adult must be present at the time of the research, responsible for the child's safety and welfare at the time of the research. Outside of a protected environment (e.g. a school), a responsible adult will be a parent, guardian or any other person on whom a parent or guardian has conferred responsibility for the child. When permission is given by the responsible adult to the interviewer, this allows the interviewer to approach the child, but it is not permission to interview them; the child must have the opportunity to decline to take part in the research.

It is possible to interview 14 and 15 year olds on the street or in a public place without parental permission. However, a thank-you leaflet or a letter stating what has taken place, why and by whom, must be handed to the child to pass onto their parents. Online surveys still require permission to be sought to continue with a survey. This is obtained by inserting an age screener before moving onto the questionnaire section. If a respondent is under age, then they can be asked for parental contact details to call to ask for permission to continue. This should not be done by email as personal identification is impossible.

The main aims of the MRS guidelines for conducting research with children are:

- To protect the rights of children physically, mentally, ethically and emotionally, and to ensure they are not exploited

- To reassure parents and others concerned with their welfare and safety that research conducted under these guidelines is designed to protect the interests of children and young people
- To ensure good quality research
- To promote the professionalism and value of research
- To protect the researcher and client by publishing the necessary good practice required to meet their legal and ethical responsibilities.

10.1.2 Studies with children

When carrying out studies with children, additional care should be taken and the factors to consider include the power relationship between the adult researcher and the child participant(s). The adult researcher should consider the language used, the setting of the research, appropriateness of the analysis, quality of the data, ethical factors such as the purpose and risks of the research, confidentiality of the participants, recruitment of the children, funding of the research, information given to children and parents/guardians, consent and dissemination of appropriate protocols and methods. Methods to use could include quantitative techniques such as questionnaires and qualitative approaches including 1:1 or group interviews. In some cases, drawings may be more appropriate than words for children to understand (Marshman and Hall, 2008).

There are many challenges associated with using children in food and drink research, especially when carrying out descriptive analysis (e.g. sensory profiling), with difficulties due to lower cognitive ability, lack of concentration and limited vocabulary (Kimmel *et al.*, 1994; Guinard, 2000). Popper and Kroll (2005) caution against hasty over-generalisation in the similarity between adults and children as it is known that differences do exist in children's sensory perceptions and those of adults. They also point out that children may differ from adults in the importance they place on various product dimensions. Hence, sensory attributes that children may regard as important in influencing preference may not be the same as those that adults may consider important in determining preference. These differences in adults and children raise the question of whether adults should continually be used to profile food intended for children.

Despite these challenges, various researchers have been able to use panels made up of children for descriptive analysis (for example studies by Blay and Beeren, 2007; de Penna *et al.,* 2000; Baxter *et al.*, 1998, 1999; Swaney-Stueve, 2002). Blay and Beeren (2007) describe the basic training of a children's panel to prepare for free choice profiling by using pictures of fruits to aid children in creating vocabularies. Children were also trained in the basic tastes and perception of foods and beverages.

Children are able to use magnitude estimation (Fig. 10.1) (with appropriate training) and 6 point labelled category scaling (Fig. 10.2). A labelled category scale might be easier to use for children than continuous response scales/

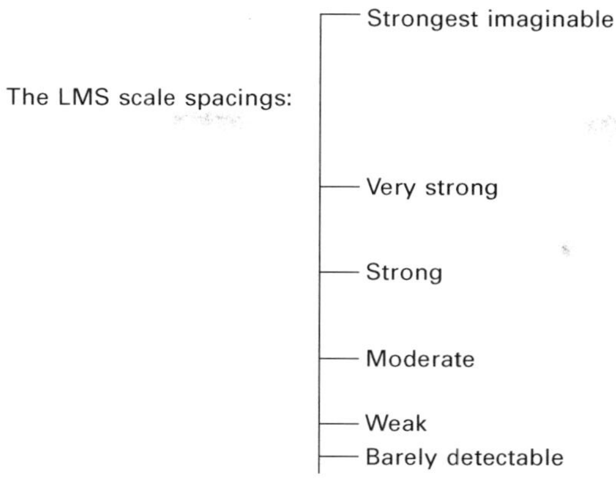

Fig. 10.1 Labelled magnitude scale (LMS) (adapted from Lawless and Heymann, 1998).

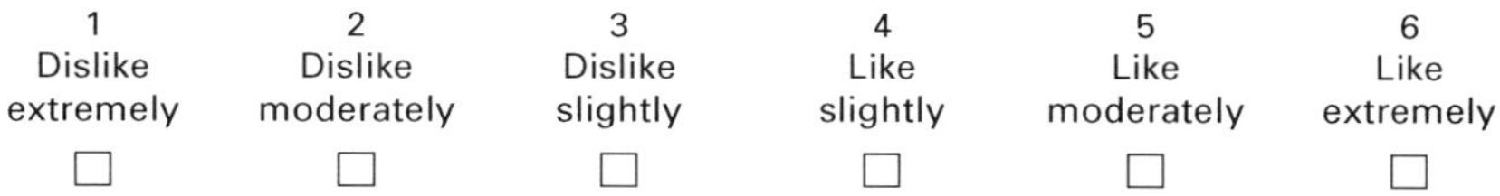

Fig. 10.2 Example of a 6-point category scale.

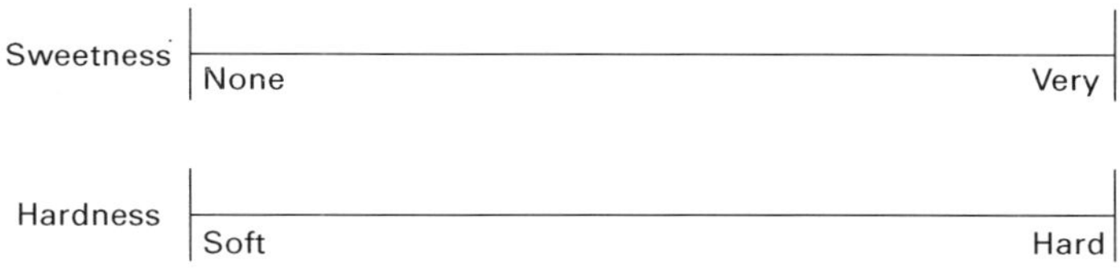

Fig. 10.3 Examples of line scales.

line scale (Fig. 10.3). The inclusion of expressive faces will help children to understand the orientation on the scale (Fig. 10.4) (Chen *et al.*, 1996; Issanchou and Nicklaus, 2006).

Incentives

In terms of incentivising the children for their participation in the research, there are many different trains of thought. Fundamentally, the incentive has to be enough to encourage the child and their guardian that it is worth their while giving up their time to test the product and to cover for any expenses of travelling to the test location. Yet, the incentive should not be so high that it becomes more than that required to motivate attendance; a large remuneration could typically skew the resultant test data (e.g. the child may feel obliged to respond more positively than honestly, to be worthy of the incentive offered).

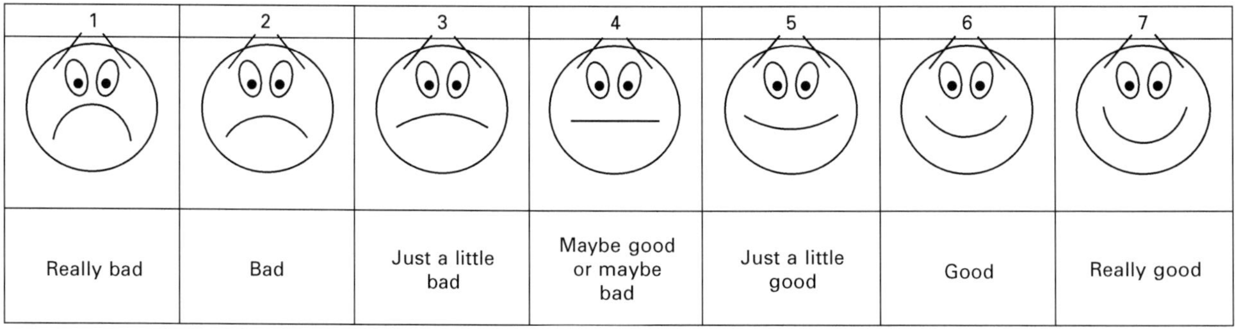
1
2
3
4
5
6
7
Really bad
Bad
Just a little bad
Maybe good or maybe bad
Just a little good
Good
Really good

Fig. 10.4 Hedonic 'facial smiles' scale, adapted from Kroll, 1990.

The provision of incentives for testing has to be considered on a project-by-project basis and there are many factors that have to be taken into account, including length of time for the testing, journey to and from the test location, type of product(s) and their acceptability, and the level of complexity of the questioning. The 'incentive' does not necessarily have to be monetary: if the product is considered particularly acceptable to the children and the test is relatively short with a fun element, the incentive can be the product under evaluation or another (food or beverage) product. It is typical for the company commissioning or carrying out the research to offer variants of the test product, or one of their products from another category, as take-away incentives. Product incentives may reduce the cost of the research whilst also marketing the company's goods.

In some cases it may be difficult to attract the particular quota of sample required, e.g. children within a limited age band, testing necessary at a time of the year when children are not so readily available such as during school time, researching less favourable products, or testing over a period of time. In cases such as these, the incentive would have to be increased accordingly. When research requires the same child to carry out testing over a period of time, the incentive is often a token at the first stage, with a more substantial offering on completion of the research to ensure continuity of sample.

Other considerations

For any research carried out with children, the staff involved and/or present should be informed that the research involves testing with children and given a briefing/training on the factors to be considered to ensure a safe and appropriate test environment for the children, parents/guardians and staff involved. The test set-up may differ from that of tests involving adults only: additional space would be allocated in each of the test area(s) to allow for the parent or guardian to be present also, and the area would need to be set up appropriately. Additional care should be taken with any hot test products and there is greater likelihood of spillage with children; therefore additional product must be available if required and tools to quickly clean the test area. During the test, the children must be monitored to ensure they refrain from speaking to other children and voicing their opinions on the product. A negative comment voiced or facial expression shown by a child could easily influence the surrounding children carrying out the testing.

The factors that influence food preference in children are numerous and include a genetic disposition for the aversion of bitter foods and liking of sweet foods (Anliker *et al.*, 1991), age differences, and parental influence (Skinner *et al.*, 2002; Benton 2004). Children have also been found to prefer simple foods with smooth texture (Rose *et al.*, 2004a,b). Popper and Kroll (2005) cited that peers also influence preference in children between ages 3–5 years and often this influence has a lasting effect.

A test briefing is imperative and would have to be pitched both at the level of the child(ren) testing and the accompanying adult. The adults will also be informed of the extent to which they can be involved in the test (i.e. constructive and unbiased guidance rather than leading the answers).

10.2 Case study 1: consumer research under standardised conditions

This case study describes a consumer research project on juice drinks, using children as the consumers. The objective of this research was to ascertain whether different storage conditions and packaging materials made a difference to the liking and other attributes related to the drinks.

A preliminary research project using trained assessors showed that differences between the drinks existed. This follow up research investigated whether the target consumers, children, did show a difference in their liking towards the four different drinks.

10.2.1 Method and scope of the research

Testing with children can be undertaken either in their supervised environment, in standardised conditions or non-supervised conditions (e.g. teenagers at home). This case study illustrates a test undertaken under standardised conditions. Case study 2 describes a test carried out in a supervised environment.

Standardised conditions could include a research or laboratory facility, hall tests and in-street testing. Factors that must be taken into consideration are:

- Permission must be sought from the parent/guardian, followed by consent by the child to take part
- Timing of the testing must be convenient for the accompanied child and the research staff (often outside typical office hours, e.g. Saturday)
- An incentive is often paid to cover expenses of travelling to the research or laboratory centre
- The environment must be made safe and appropriate for testing with the age groups.

Children assessors

One hundred and fifty-three children aged 6 to 13 years took part in the research; 77 children between 6–9 years, 76 children between 10–13 years.

Adults from Leatherhead's Consumer Database, with children in the required age groups, were pre-selected and then emailed. The email informed the adults of the research product to be tested, declared any ingredients present in the product (including possible allergens), and the requirement for an adult to be present and responsible for the child during the research test.

The email also detailed the date and time of the proposed test, and explained how the adult should respond if their child was interested in participating. Full contact details were given to enable consumer queries to be resolved as soon as possible.

One hundred and sixty children aged 6–13 years were actually recruited in total (150 were required and 153 took part in the research. It is typical to over-recruit to ensure at least the required number of responses are obtained):

- All children were prepared to taste 100% blackcurrant juice drinks and had no related food/drink allergies
- Each child was accompanied by a parent/guardian
- By quota recruitment, 50% of the sample were aged 6–9 years, and 50% of the sample were aged 10–13 years
- Through natural fallout, 58% of the sample were male and 42% were female.

Samples

The fruit juice drinks had been stored at 4° Celsius (fridge) and 21° Celsius (shelf/ambient) and were packed in two different packaging formats: glass and plastic bottles, resulting in four different samples. The objective of the test was to ascertain whether the different storage conditions made any difference to the liking and other attributes related to the drink.

Sample presentation

Each child was presented with the four samples blind (no branding), in a sequential monadic format (i.e. each sample presented one at a time, one after the other). Samples were decanted into 100 ml clear polystyrene pots, and were presented in a balanced and rotated order between children to remove any bias from order effects. Pots were coded with three digit numbers to avoid any bias with product names.

To familiarise children with the whole process, two light flavoured drinks were given to the children as a warm up exercise.

Questionnaire

The questioning covered: Overall Liking, Appearance, Taste, Strength of flavour (intensity), Sweetness, Texture and Aftertaste. For each of the four samples tested, children were asked to *Look at, Smell* and *Taste* the drinks.

To ensure the attributes were understood, the attributes were described to the younger children as follows:

- Appearance was described as 'the way this drink looks'
- Strength of flavour was described as 'flavour intensity'
- Aftertaste was described as 'the taste in your mouth after you finish drinking'

Figure 10.5 shows an illustration of the questionnaire. The facial smilies

Please **taste the sample**, how much do you like it?

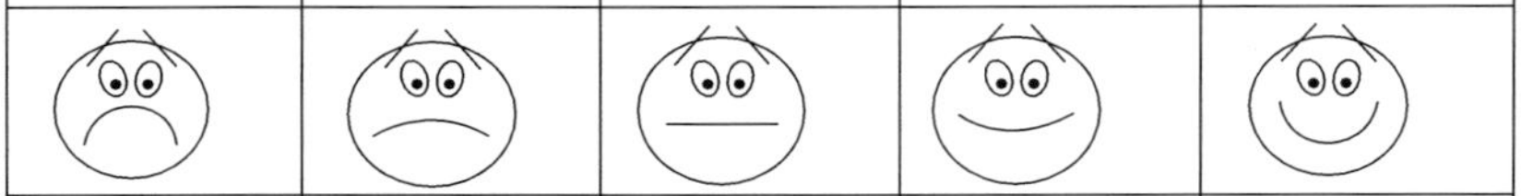

1	2	3	4	5
Really Really Yucky	Yucky	OK	Yummy	Really Really Yummy

Please **look at the sample**, how much do you like the way that this drink **looks**?

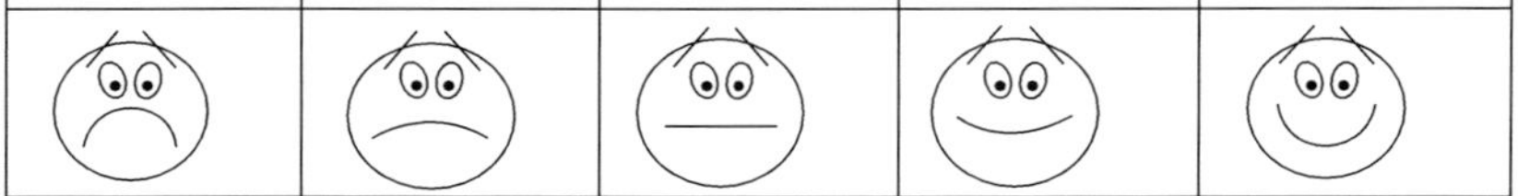

1	2	3	4	5
Really Really Yucky	Yucky	OK	Yummy	Really Really Yummy

Please **taste the sample again**, what did you think of the way this drink **tastes**?

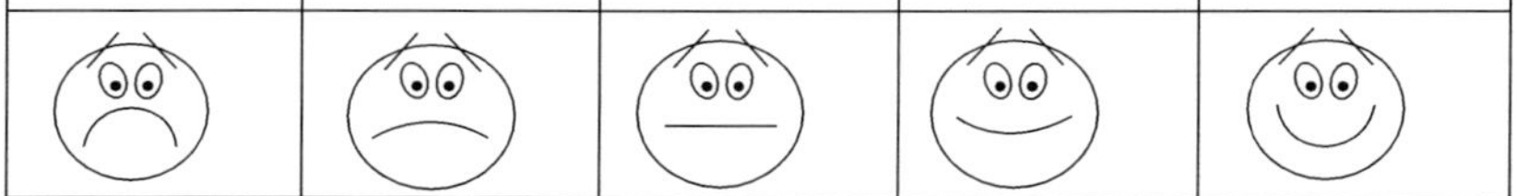

1	2	3	4	5
Really Really Yucky	Yucky	OK	Yummy	Really Really Yummy

Was the flavour intensity of the juice **too weak or to strong**?

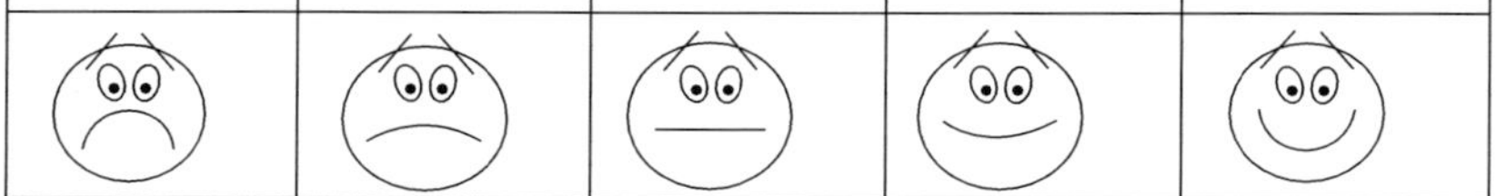

1	2	3	4	5
Much too weak	Too weak	About right	Too strong	Much too strong

Was the taste of the juice **too sweet or not sweet enough**?

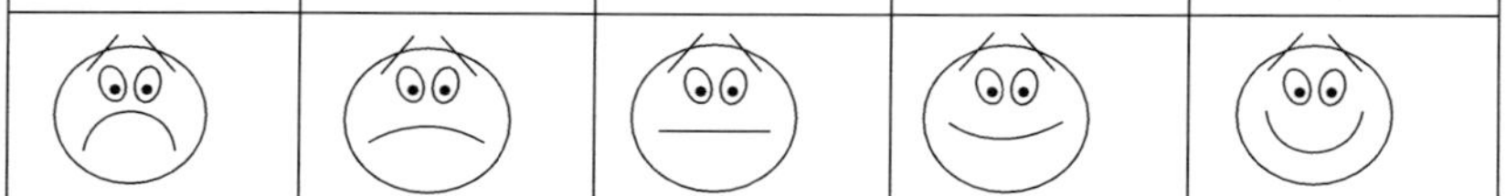

1	2	3	4	5
Not sweet enough	Not quite sweet enough	About right	A little too sweet	Too sweet

Fig. 10.5 Full hedonic 'facial smiles' scale, adapted from Kroll, 1990.

Please **taste the sample again and tell how the sample feels in your mouth**?

1	2	3	4	5
	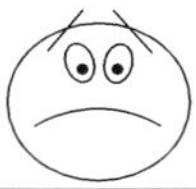	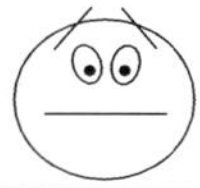	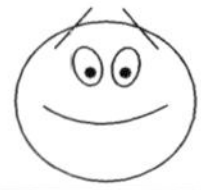	
Really Really Bad	Bad	OK	Nice	Really Really Nice

How much do you like the **taste left in your mouth**?

1	2	3	4	5
	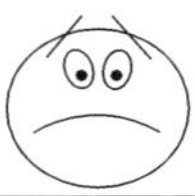		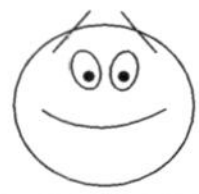	
Really Really Yucky	Yucky	OK	Yummy	Really Really Yummy

Fig. 10.5 Continued

were primarily directed towards the youngest of the sample group. It was important not to appear to patronise the teenagers in the sample group, so it was explained to them that the pictorial references were there to help the younger children, and they could merely focus on the numbers and the word descriptions if they preferred. With their maturity acknowledged, the teenagers were then enthusiastic to be involved. Incorporating both words and pictures with the number scale enabled testing across a broad spectrum of children's ages together, and then have a more robust sample size with which to analyse results.

10.2.2 Results

There was no significant difference in liking of the drinks across the different packaging formats – glass and plastic – at either storage temperature. However, there were significant differences in liking across the different storage conditions. More than twice as many children preferred the products that had been stored at 4° Celsius (fridge) compared to those stored at 21° Celsius (shelf/ambient). The attributes driving liking were Strength of flavour, Taste and Aftertaste, all of which scored statistically significantly higher at 95% confidence. When analysing the data by gender, females were even more likely to prefer the products stored at 4° Celsius than the males; and by age group, the older children had the stronger preference for the refrigerated product, notably the aftertaste was significantly preferable. There were no statistically significant variations by gender or age for the packaging formats.

10.2.3 Follow up with children

Following the completion of the testing and analysis of the results, appreciation of the children's involvement (over and above the incentive for taking part) was shown by sending them an email with a thank you, a few findings and a reminder that through participating in the research they had played a part in selecting the best product that would be launched onto the market soon. This additional follow up is likely to encourage children to take part in more research the future.

10.3 Case study 2: consumer research using children at school

Whilst Case study 1 describes a consumer study carried out under standardised conditions, this second case study looks at an example of children's research carried out at local schools. It describes carrying out consumer and profiling testing with children on familiar and novel juices, the effect of a short exposure to these products on children's acceptability levels, and the use of the profiling method.

10.3.1 Method and scope of the research

Supervised environments include school, but also home and after-school clubs. The children in this test carried out all testing at school, supervised by teachers and Leatherhead staff researchers. Factors that must be taken into consideration if the research is carried out in school time are:

- Permission must be sought from the head teacher
- The testing will be incorporated into the school day (either in an appropriate lesson such as Home Economics, or at lunch time)
- Consent will have to be sought from all parents of children taking part (issues can arise for those children who do not have parental consent and cannot then take part – extra supervision required)
- Teacher(s) will need to be fully briefed prior to the testing and involved during the testing
- Delivery and appropriate storage (e.g. chilling) of products must be organised
- The school will expect an honorarium for their involvement.

Factors that must be taken into consideration if the research is carried out at home are:

- Permission must be sought from the parent/guardian, followed by consent by the child to take part
- An element of control may be lost: there often will be no research staff present at the time of the testing and so these will be heavy reliant on

briefing notes and the active involvement of the parent/guardian
- Delivery/collection of products must be considered
- Delivery (ideally online) of questionnaire and instructions will be required.

Children assessors

Several local schools were contacted to discuss the research. Interested schools were visited to meet the head teachers and teachers of the classes involved. The research was explained and some of the teachers were asked to include the tasting session in a full lesson, starting with an explanation of human senses and how we perceive foods and beverages, and finalising by explaining the results of the research to the children.

Discussions took place on the classroom set-up that would prevent the children talking too much and, where possible, prevent spillages.

The schools honorarium was agreed at this meeting, which consisted of a payment per participating child and, in addition, a small healthy food incentive for each of the children.

Consent forms were given to teachers to be signed by children's parents or guardians. Very few parents/guardians did not sign the forms: those children without signed consent forms could, unfortunately, not take part in the tasting session.

A total of 108 children were recruited. Two panel groups were formed; a consumer panel consisting of 96 children aged 7–10 years and a profiling panel consisting of 12 children aged 9 and 10 years.

Sample presentation acceptability test

Water was given as a training sample, to help the children to work through and understand the questionnaire together. Twelve drinks were then selected for the test, six familiar drinks and six novel juices. Each child received all of the samples in a sequential monadic format (i.e. each sample presented one at a time, one after the other). All samples were given blind, coded with three digit coding. The children were told why samples had these types of codes. They had a short break after three and six samples and a longer break after nine samples.

The children were given bottles of each sample to take home to taste over a week's period. They were also given written instructions detailing the amount to consume and that they had to taste each sample three times.

After the home exposure, the children carried out the same school test as described above. Samples were presented in a similar format but different codes were applied to ensure that children would not associate certain codes with certain juices.

Sample presentation profiling test

The same 12 drinks studied on preference were also given to children assessors for sensory characterisation using Free Choice profiling principles.

Children received screening and training in basic tastes as described below.

Each child was given the 12 drinks and was asked to generate descriptors for each product based on appearance, aroma, flavour, mouth feel, after feel and aftertaste. Individual terms were discussed with each child to remove duplicated words and clarify unfamiliar terms with the researcher. Unfamiliar terms were not discarded as they were meaningful to the assessors in describing the products.

Samples were presented in sequential monadic format (i.e. each sample presented one at a time, one after the other) in duplicate (i.e. each child received each sample twice). Testing was carried out over two days, with four samples being evaluated in each session followed by 20 minute breaks between sessions to reduce fatigue.

For continued exposure to the products, the same procedure was followed as described above in the section for acceptability testing. After exposure, a new vocabulary was generated by each child and the new sets of descriptors used to profile the products. The products were re-coded to reduce bias.

Basic taste training

Child assessors in the profiling group were given 20 mL each of four of the five basic tastes: sweet, sour, salt and bitter, in labelled 30 mL clear polystyrene pots. The training concentrations used are shown in Table 10.1.

The assessors were first asked to taste the samples and familiarise themselves with each of the basic tastes. To aid recognition, the assessors were encouraged to relate the tastes they experienced to a familiar product. To test if assessors were able to recognise the basic tastes, they were given coded samples of each basic taste, at the same training concentration as before and at a lower concentration, to identify.

Vocabulary generation training

The child assessors were provided with pictures of fruits and asked to derive words that described the fruits such that another person would recognise the fruit from their words without seeing the picture. The children worked individually on their terms. Each set of descriptors was then read to the whole group to see if the other children agreed that the descriptors gave a good picture of the fruit being described. The children were taught to exclude

Table 10.1 Concentrations of basic taste solutions used

Basic taste	Chemical	Concentration of solution gL^{-1}	
		Training conc.	Low conc.
Sweet	Sucrose	10.0	5.0
Sour	Citric acid	0.8	0.4
Salt	Sodium chloride	2.0	1.0
Bitter	Caffeine	1.0	0.5

hedonic terms that described the way they felt about the products. A second session in vocabulary generation was carried out using two fruit juice samples, namely Ribena and Orange juice. In this session, the terms were discussed individually to ensure that each person understood their requirements.

Scale training
The child assessors were taught how to use an intensity scale in a trial profiling session of the two juice drinks they had previously used in the vocabulary generation training. A 7-point box intensity scale was used. The scale was labelled 'not' to 'very' at the extreme poles.

Questionnaire acceptability test
Children carrying out acceptability tests were asked to answer five acceptability test questions based on appearance, aroma, flavour, mouthfeel and overall preference of the products. A 7-point preference scale ranging from 'dislike very much' to 'like very much' was used. Child consumers used the 7-point hedonic 'facial smilies' scale with the Peryam and Kroll (Kroll, 1990) descriptors (Fig. 10.1).

Questionnaire profiling test
Children used their own generated vocabulary to score each of the samples on the intensity of these identified sensory characteristics. The method used, Free Choice Profiling, was applied to identify the sensory characteristics by using children's individual terms. The intensity was rated on a 7-point intensity scale labelled from 'not' to 'very'.

10.3.2 Results – children acceptability test

Children's acceptability score range appeared wider for children compared to a similar test carried out with adults. The six familiar products were each equally preferred by the children. The children's least preferred products were two unfamiliar products; tomato-juice and prune juice. After continued exposure, a significant decrease in liking (95% confidence) was observed for the attribute Appearance only.

10.3.3 Results – children profiling test

On average, the children generated 29 descriptors, with each child generating between 24 and 42 words to use for the evaluation. Generated words included typical characteristics for the products such as 'raspberry flavour', 'red colour' and 'sweet', but also some less conventional descriptors such as 'weird lemon', 'munky orange', 'hot dog brown colour' and 'like shiny apples'.

After repeated exposure, children agreed less with each other as their judgements became more subjective and less analytical, possibly due to loss of interest in the products or the test after continued exposure.

10.3.4 Follow up with children

After finalising the experiments, all schools were sent a thank you letter. In addition, researchers went into the school explaining how the data was analysed from completed questionnaires, and several graphs were shown displaying the children's results. Showing results to assessors is known to work motivationally, and for the schools it was taken as additional learning for the children.

10.4 Conclusions

It is the responsibility of the researcher to keep abreast of any legislation relating to research with children, and the MRS website would typically be the reference for this. Definitions of words will change with each younger generation – e.g. convenience is taken for granted and the 'new convenience' of the next generation has to meet their growing convenience-led demands. It helps if the researcher and the manufacturer can try to see things through children's eyes wherever possible and think like that through the product development and the product lifecycle. Children's research is exciting and allows for real flexibility and creativity in the methods and techniques. Every research project with children will bring with it new insights into 'children's research' and a greater understanding of their capabilities, requirements and key drivers.

10.5 References

Anliker, J. A., Bartoshuk, L., Ferris, A. M. and Hooks, L. D. (1991) Children's food preferences and genetic sensitivity to the bitter taste of 6-normal-propylthiouracil (Prop). *American Journal of Clinical Nutrition,* 54, 316–320.

Baxter, I. A., Jack, F. R. and Schroser, M. J. A. (1998) The use of repertory grid method to elicit perceptual data from primary school children. *Food Quality and Preference,* 9, 73–80.

Baxter, I. A., Schroder, M. J. A. and Bower, J. A. (1999) The influence of socio-economic background on perceptions of vegetables among Scottish primary school children. *Food Quality and Preference,* 10, 261–272.

Benton, D. (2004) Role of parents in the determination of the food preferences of children and the development of obesity. *International Journal of Obesity,* 28, 858–869.

Blay, M. Y. and Beeren, C. J. M. (2007) Adults versus children: Differences in perception of food sensory attributes, *Leatherhead Food Research Member Forum Report, 121639.*

Chen A. W, Resurreccion A. V. A. and Paguio L. P. (1996) Age appropriate hedonic scales to measure the food preferences of young children. *Journal of Sensory Studies* 11: 141–63.

De Penna, E. W., Timermann, A. B. and Valdes, L. S. (2000) Sensory training of children. *Archivos Latinoamericanos De Nutricion,* 50, 19–25.

Guinard, J. X. (2000) Sensory and consumer testing with children. *Trends in Food Science and Technology,* 11, 273–283.

Issanchou, S. and Nicklaus, S. (2006) Measuring consumers' perceptions of sweet taste. In *Optimising Sweet Taste in Foods*, (ed. W. J. Spillane) 97–131. Woodhead/CRC, Cambridge, UK.

Kimmel, S. A., Sigmangrant, M. and Guinard, J. X. (1994) Sensory testing with young children. *Food Technology*, 48, 92.

Kroll, B. (1990) Evaluating rating scales for sensory testing with children. *Food Technology,* 44, 78–86.

Marshman, Z. and Hall, M. (2008) Oral health research with children, *International Journal of Paediatric Dentistry*, Volume 18(4), p 235–242.

MRS Guidelines (2006) *Conducting research with children and young people* Web: http://www.mrs.org.uk/standards/children.htm [Accessed November 2009].

NHS Information Centre (2009) Health survey for England 2008: *Physical Activity and Fitness* Web:http://www.ic.nhs.uk/webfiles/publications/HSE/HSE08/Volume_1_Physical_activity_and_fitness_revised.pdf [Accessed Jan 2010].

Popper, R. and Kroll, J. J. (2005) Conducting sensory research with children. *Journal of Sensory Studies,* 20, 75–87.

Rose, J., Laing, D. G., Oram, N. and Hutchinson, I. (2004a) Sensory profiling by children aged 6–7 and 10–11 years. Part 1: A descriptor approach. *Food Quality and Preference,* 15, 585–596 (2002b). Part 2: A modality approach. *Food Quality and Preference,* 15, 597–606.

Skinner, J. D., Carruth, B. R., Bounds, W. and Ziegler, P. J. (2002) Children's food preferences: A longitudinal analysis. *Journal of the American Dietetic Association,* 102, 1638–1647.

Swaney-Stueve (2002) Can children perform descriptive analysis? *IFT Annual Meeting Technical Programme.* Anaheim, California, Institute of Food Technologists.

11

Working with children and adolescents for food product development

Bryan Urbick, Consumer Knowledge Centre Ltd., UK

Abstract: Winning with kids need not be a terrifying task. Firstly, it is critical to understand their physical and cognitive development. What is also important are key and underlying drivers of young people: control, aspiration, creating excitement/stretching boundaries and neophobia all drive acceptance or rejection of products. We can build on the understanding of the age and stage of the child, maintain a keen focus to deliver control, instill aspiration, create excitement/stretching boundaries, and build on ways to overcome the innate neophobia that kids have, in product development but also in research. Following straight-forward guidelines will help the product developer and marketer create winning products for children, tweens and teens, faster, with confidence, and ultimately, with increased market success.

Key words: children, aspiration, control, neophobia, child development, gender differences.

11.1 Planning and creating for the future: why consumer and industry demands will require us to unleash the power of genuine consumer connectedness in new product development

As the world becomes more connected, there is an expectation of consumers that brands and products will do the same. Even though the 'connectedness' may be artificial and contrived, this does not matter. Consumer expectations drive their choice, and as in so many aspects, truth is all about perception and expectation, even more than rationality and 'reality'.

Young people are at the forefront of this evolution. Children have never known a world without 24-hour news, the internet with all that it offers, and the youngest cannot recall when social networking did not exist. Concurrently, there is also a move to hyper-personalisation. Jones Soda in North America captured this insight in the beverage segment, though the move is deeper as scientific investigation into gene therapy drives the view to personalise medical treatment at a genetic level. Personalising the home page on MySpace and Facebook and developing their personal avatar in Club Penguin has allowed children, tweens and teens the vehicle to express their individuality, giving them a taste of a contemporary independence. This taste makes them hungry for further personalisation in other categories as well. 'Connectedness' in food and beverage development has never been more important.

11.2 Setting the scene: understanding the importance of a holistic approach to building brands and products, particularly for young customers

In order to develop truly motivating and ultimately successful products for children, tweens and teens, involving them in the new product development process is key. Though basic testing with young people is good, it may not be enough – particularly if not done in the right way. How to structure that testing is a challenging question, though thinking beyond mere testing and considering a much richer involvement of young consumers throughout the whole process may be a better approach.

11.2.1 The holistic view

Research typically tests each facet of a product idea and then brings them all together at the end. For example, we look first at the idea (concept), and then begin the process of food development, often separately testing each aspect: product, packaging, and communication. In some cases, we test separate attributes of each aspect, adding further complexity.

Where this goes wrong is that kids, tweens and teens buy into the whole product experience, not an individual part. The taste of the food is important, but eating the product out of its packaging in the context of the young person's real life gives much clearer guidance. Importantly, the sum of the parts, in product development for kids, does not always equal the whole. The whole thing has to work together. The overall objective in the research should be that no element be taken unnaturally out of context: we should see how all the elements work together toward a total solution, from the young consumer's perspective.

The reasons for difficulty in the more traditional approaches to product development are most often linked to the way in which a young consumer looks at a food or beverage product. He or she does not consider each product based on each of its individual attributes, but looks at it holistically and tends to make a judgement overall. If we drink a soft drink that is perfect in every way except for the sweetness, for example, then would we forgive that attribute or would we probably seek a product that is closer to our ideal? Granted, there is likely to be a hierarchy of attribute importance, and some attributes are more 'forgivable' than others, but the truth is, we do not think about it broken down into the various parts. We either like it, or we do not. Kids are more adamant and perhaps less forgiving.

11.2.2 Understanding young people

In order to ensure that the deeper involvement with children, tweens and teens is fruitful, it is critically important to deeply understand them. Young people are not merely adults running around in smaller bodies – they are different from adults in many ways.

A basic understanding of child development helps to provide the necessary context. This understanding should include their physical, cognitive and emotional development, the key and underlying drivers of choice, and particularly the factors involved in making their food and beverage choices. An in-depth understanding of their food and beverage choices has unique implications for development, product testing and then ultimately successful communication of the overall idea. With this solid foundational understanding, success becomes far easier, and far more likely.

Each year we work with children, tweens and teens on food and beverage projects in many countries throughout the world. On average, we qualitatively work with over 4 000 young consumers. Inevitably we see a recurring theme of what they desire: '*…give us something new and different…*' is their plea. Hearing this, companies tend to work diligently to deliver, and again and again, when these 'new and different ideas' are ultimately tested with young consumers, they frequently fail. This is because of kids' innate neophobia (fear of the 'new'). So not only do we need an understanding of their development, but we also need understanding of young people's neophobia and how to combat it. This is particularly important in innovation.

11.2.3 Innovation for young people

To kids, tweens and teens, innovation is not the primary driver to choose one product over another. The key to their choice lies in the *benefit* that the particular innovation provides, within the context of the product. This highlights another important reason to think holistically when designing products for young people. Product innovations in most recent years have focused on perceived lifestyle 'needs' – so rather than on actual traditional needs, innovative products for kids have been more about their ability to be available when and where they want them, or about providing a greater taste or eating experience. The benefits to kids in these innovations are immediate, and they provide instant gratification: yoghurt in tubes delivers a snack that doesn't interrupt kids' fun; sports tops on drinks provide better portability and give kids more control; or extreme flavoured snacks and confectionery offer an enhanced sensory experience and relieve boredom. These ideas, if tested in isolated attributes, may not have achieved the research results needed for launch. It is only in their total, holistic experience that the ideas begin to express the true potential.

In the era of fears of childhood obesity, successful innovation in more healthful foods and beverages for kids is an even tougher task. Not only do the products need to provide some nutritional benefit above and beyond what is currently offered in the mainstream, but also deliver on some immediate lifestyle needs as well. It is not as simple as solving the often very difficult technical issues surrounding the stability of products or ingredients and doing it in a way that delivers an acceptable eating experience – kids today demand more. They want it to fit in their lives, be as good an eating experience (or better) than existing products – and if it provides a functional benefit, that benefit ideally needs to be felt immediately (because of kids' need for immediate gratification). Only a holistic view would provide the needed context to truly understand what is needed to win in this scenario.

Creative methods used throughout the new product development cycle can provide a holistic view of the types of ideas that a young person sees as needed in the market place. Repeatedly, our clients have said that two to five days of creative research gives the same results as much more extensive and expensive traditional research techniques. This is not to suggest the abolishment of traditional research but simply the need to ensure that we increase our chances of testing better products by developing products that come from the consumer – either directly through ideation with them, or indirectly from observation and workshop sessions.

Similar 'non-traditional' methods have shown great success with existing products as well. Putting young people in the simulated role of brand manager or advertising executive for one to five days can provide amazing insights – insights that have been used to re-vamp a 'tired' brand or to confirm that a new brand concept will deliver to kids as intended in its positioning.

11.3 Ages and stages: the importance to new product development for kids of understanding basic child development. A brief review of key underlying drivers, including neophobia, and how these can be best utilized in connecting kids to the product development process

The first step to understanding children and young people is in understanding the basic flow of their development. Through the years of our work on new products, the utilization of this knowledge has led us to propose and conduct better projects, better research, and importantly to develop better products. This knowledge is the foundation to better understand ways in which to 'get it right' for kids.

The primary challenge for food and beverage manufacturers (and indeed all those that develop products for children, tweens and teens) is the pace of change. It can be daunting. Young people cannot be truly understood, though, without acknowledgement of the extreme pace of their change. This requires a different way of thinking about how to develop products for them.

This is evident at all ages, from newborns to older teens. '*What a difference each year makes!*' is a frequent sentiment as we work with one year and then move to the next. So much happens from birth to teens – probably the greatest natural changes that will occur in any fifteen year period in our lives (though sometimes the end of our natural lives may have a similar pace). In addition, it is important to note the direction of change: though it sounds obvious, we must remember the direction of change with kids is most often towards being older.

11.3.1 A brief overview of child development, with focus on understanding how children, tweens and teens react to and interact with their food and beverages

In the first year of life, the child spends most of his or her time sleeping, being fed and nurtured, both physically and emotionally. The baby is completely dependent upon its parents. The child's energy is focused on physical growth and within the first half year of life, the child usually doubles its size in mass.

During the early weeks, there is relatively little time when the child is awake, but when awake he or she instinctively observes the world. A key aspect to understanding child development comes from considering the impact of a child's instinctive observation and imitation. This learning by copying will continues strongly until around the age of 7 or 8 years, and importantly will become the basis for the learning of new skills all throughout life. 'Copying' is later taught to be inappropriate, though in reality, all of us continue to copy attitudes and behaviors. The benefits of understanding children's copying behaviour are many, particularly when developing marketing and communication strategies.

As the child gets a little older, he or she transforms from the helpless, observing, sleeping baby to a more awake, active, then crawling, then standing, then walking (then running!) toddler. As adults we observe these changes as big milestones.

Probably the biggest milestone, and the one most exciting to parents, is when the child learns to speak: first in single words (predominantly nouns), then in simple combinations of nouns and verbs. Eventually the child begins to use the words 'I', 'me' and 'mine' – and this awareness of self is an important sign of psychological function (the realization of the 'id' in Sigmund Freud's structural model of the psyche).

With regard to food and drink, in the first couple of years the child is able only to indicate when it wants to feed. Over time and with development, the child becomes able to decide what it wants to eat. Importantly, this is the time when the child's more active influence of food choice begins. Though the child is still completely dependent on the parent, because he or she can indicate liking (or more importantly disliking) of what is being offered, parents tend to take considerable notice.

With respect to foods and beverages, the child's copying behaviour can be incredibly important. Even if the young child does not appear to like the food being offered, the parent usually tries ways to get the child to eat the food. Perhaps the parent may eat the food her/himself in broad, over-emphasized manner, using big, happy expressions while saying 'yum, yum!'. It is desired that the child copies this behaviour and then happily eats.

In the early years, before the age of around nine, mum has much more influence in what her children eat. After this point, mum begins to lose some control of the child's diet and her strategies change, typically from the original playfulness to a new practicality. In one of her mothering roles, she acts as gatekeeper. She may allow only certain products into the home, and from these give the child a choice. In other, parallel mothering roles, occasionally conflicting with the role of gatekeeper, the mother may adopt other strategies. The study of mothering is a separate and complex subject, though in brief, she plays numerous roles providing physical and emotional nourishment. Sometimes we assume that she is driven only by 'nutrition' and 'healthy foods' – that is not the case. Sometimes she desires to reward, sometimes treat, sometimes punish, sometimes merely to show love. We need to understand these roles and provide the right products for each role.

As the child further matures, more of the world is being discovered and understood. In this process of discovery, play has a very important role. Play gives the child an opportunity to experiment with various aspects of the world, and to try to make some sense of it. Amusingly, until about the age of 4 years, the child will play with whatever is available and in reach: boxes, scraps of paper, pots and pans with spoons, and more. At this young age, up to about 4 years, the child depends on what is available and tends to express desire only for the things it can see.

From around the age of 4, play changes quite dramatically with the addition of the child's fantasy and imagination. Suddenly the child is no longer dependent on the available to generate play, but can play with ideas generated from within: Tables covered with blankets can become in the child's imagination the inside of the genie's lamp and they play with their imaginary magic powers; large boxes become rocket ships into space; a table and chairs becomes a kitchen in which meals are prepared for the imaginary children. And though fantasy may seem to the outside observer as random and chaotic, it is not. A child's imagination has a structure and pattern, with 'rules' evolving over time and repeated again and again.

Throughout the child and the teen years there is a great deal of physical change. For this whole process, the child requires a great deal of energy to evolve and develop. The child also expends a lot of energy in the physical behaviour of running around and playing. This display of energy can be frustrating for parents, but is critical for the child in order to learn about her/himself, and discover her/his place in the world.

During the ages of 4 to 7 years (depending on the region and culture), the child first goes to school and then learns more about social and intellectual aspects of life. The child then learns more about the world and continues to discover and develop her/his own capabilities, intellectual learning, and social structures.

In this period, the baby who had instinctively observed and copied, has now matured to become a child who lives in a very 'black and white world'. As most parents and people who work with children know, words like 'good' or 'bad'; 'like' or 'dislike'; 'on' or 'off'; 'yes' or 'no' are clearly understood. 'In-between' or 'grey words' like 'maybe', 'perhaps', and 'if you are good, then you can have…' are not well understood. The child does not yet have the ability or experience to relate the 'in-between' or less clear (more abstract) aspects of life.

At around the age of 8 or 9 years, though, there is a burst of brain development coinciding with a distinctive change in the child's development. The black and white world evolves, and the child will begin to draw attention to detail. It is not that these details always were not noticed previously, but the child will now more often comment on them. Those comments are most often direct, appear to be sharp and can shock or astonish adults. The child's reaction to his own comments is similar to the parent's, and these observations then disturb the child's perception of a comfortable, safe world. From these new observations, the young child at this age begins to make new rules for her/himself ('if I lay in the bed and don't stick out my arms or legs, they won't be cut off!'). Emotions now begin to be dominated, at least on occasion, by rationality.

The important thing about this stage is that the child starts to develop the 'in-between, the grey area between black and white. As a consequence the child is more able to tell us *why* she/he likes something or why not. These reasons are critical to explore when testing food and beverage products for kids, and have implications for methods and scales used.

Starting at age 5 to 6 years, usually when children go to full-time school, it becomes particularly important to distinguish between boys and girls. Though both boys and girls go through roughly the same developmental steps, girls tend to socially mature faster and physically reach puberty one or two years prior to boys. After 11 years, children then move through pre-puberty and puberty, leading them to adulthood.

In recent years, physical development in puberty has moved down toward the age of just over 12 years, with a few girls as young as eight beginning to grow breasts and menstruate. There are two major schools of thought:

one suggests the high level of oestrogen in the 'Western diet' as the cause; the other indicates that the increase of oestrogen levels in the water supply is a major contributing factor. Whatever the cause, this earlier onset of the physical elements of puberty then adds more stress to young people because it involves drastic physical and emotional changes, now operating concurrently. How each child progresses through puberty is very individual, but tends to run the wide range of 'no problems' to highly stressful. It is a period of rebuilding, most manifested in the development of the physical body. The body becomes adult much faster than the emotions can often handle. Inside there rages a struggle for independent expression, and paradoxically, social acceptance. The teen no longer feels the need for any direct attention from parents or other adults. As the child moves to increased independence, the practical control of parent over the child gets looser, although ideally the emotional bond becomes stronger as the child moves to a mature 'friend' relationship with the parent. Importantly, the child is very likely to reject some of the parents' ideals and values at this age and seeks new role models in peers, sports stars, music or movie stars, even older teens.

With regard to food and drink in the teen years, cautious experimentation creates new favourites, preferred tastes are beginning to be more complex, and simple blends (something known with something new) are enjoyed. The need for acceptance in a social group can drive the desire to like what peers like (to feel that they 'fit in'). This, combined with the increasing desire for independence creates a unique paradox, important to acknowledge and understand when developing products for young teens.

11.3.2 Correctly targeting

The rate and direction of change is very important for a number of reasons, but it is most important to understand how to best target products. The idea that products should be targeted similarly to adults, by creating the bullseye somewhere in the middle of the target age range, is unlikely to be successful. It is also a fallacy to consider that a wider target age range will provide greater opportunity. As with adults, 'targeting narrow catches wide'. As a rule of thumb, it is always wise to target the age of the young person highest in the target age band. Because of the child's aspiration to have the benefits of older children (more on this later), targeting should be towards the older age of children. For example, if the age range for the product is, say, 12–15 years, then the bullseye target is 14/15 years.

The following sections discuss some common age bands when considering products for kids, tweens and teens.

11.3.3 Age bands

The child's first 15 years is full of physical and psychological milestones, and these are realized very rapidly. Throughout these stages, children also have different needs and wants. Though the study of child development can be involved, and indeed many volumes are written about it, it is important to understand some of the highlights of this growth period in order to create better, more appropriate, more accepted foods and beverages for kids. We turn now to some basic aspects.

Based on the general development of children, in new product development we should look at kids in six different age bands. Even though we may desire a broader target age range for our products, it is wise to consider a 'bullseye' target at the older end of these bands. Various factors in different cultures drive the specific nature of these ages, such as the age children start school or the age in which they advance from a lower school. In general, the principles and order of the bands remain the same, though the ages may slightly vary.

In an ideal world, especially when considering the move to hyper-personalisation, it would be best to break down the ages in even smaller segments. (When we work with children and adolescents in schools, we see a marked difference in each year, and even significant differences with the same classes in each term.) This is not currently practical in food and beverage product targeting though, so a sense of wider bands can be helpful in determining product development aspects.

In the main, the six age bands are:

0–1 years ('babies')
1–3 years ('toddlers')
4–7 years ('young children')
8–11 years ('tweens' – i.e. between child and teen)
12–14 years ('young teens')
15+ years ('teens' – this is the age in which out-of-home consumption without parental influence significantly increases – and the products for these ages begin to align with the products selected by young adults)

Usefully, in our experience, the adage 'target narrow and catch wide' seems to ring true, though importantly, as we will discuss later in this chapter, targeting needs to be at the upper end of the broader target, with the 'bullseye target' being at the top rather than the middle.

It is important to understand the sense of difference between the age bands, and indeed the sense of movement between each. And though we have covered some aspects in the brief overview of child development, by separating the child, tween and teen consumer into age bands, we can gather useful insight into how to develop products for and to market to them.

0–1 years ('babies')

Many consider the mum as the only target for food and beverages, and so little is done in the understanding of this very important age. We know that the child instinctively observes and imitates the world – and this intuitive observation and copying is important to teach the child new skills; ways to manage in the world that is so new to them.

Recently we have begun to explore with children from six months, using Baby Sign Language – an emerging trend among some mums. Because children have cognitive ability prior to being able to speak, many babies become frustrated in trying to communicate their desires. Baby Sign Language has been developed to help babies, and those that care for babies to be able to better understand the baby.

In a recent article published in the British Psychological Society's *The Psychologist*, G. Doherty-Sneddon discussed the theory behind this movement and evaluated some of the claims made by Baby Sign Language advocates. Baby signing is not new – variations have been used by speech and language therapists with children who have speech or other challenges. Unsurprisingly, it is widely acknowledged that communication is at the core of a child's total development and the association between a child's difficulty in communication and developmental difficulties has been well documented. While Baby Sign Language advocates extol various benefits, there is little quantifiable research, though anecdotally mums tell us that Baby Sign Language has helped their babies, and that it has also benefited the child by helping it to learn to speak earlier than average (meaning that their appears to be no impairment by using this technique).

Though it is early days in our research using Baby Sign Language, we do see that it shows some promise in being able to understand, from a baby's perspective, some sensory attribute preference and liking. We are still finding our way in determining how best to conduct and use this research, though we find it fascinating and enlightening.

1–3 years ('toddlers')

In the 1 to 3 age range, children tend to be attracted to bright colours and by simple lines and images that they recognise. The marketing is, of course, mostly to the parents. The rule still holds, however, that if the child will not eat it, then the parents probably will not buy it again.

With regard to foods and beverages, in the first year, the child gets nourishment from mother's milk/formula and eventually from 'real' food, albeit blended so that the child can consume it. In time, as the child's tastes and 'will' develops, he/she wants to do things more independently, such as get the food separately on a plate rather than all mashed together. At this stage, the child starts to feed himself, while the parents desperately try to teach table-rules and manners. Note again the importance of the role of imitation with regard to table-rules. Parents teach the child to imitate what is said until the imitation has become a conscious act, and then an unconscious habit.

Products for toddlers need to have aspects of built-in imitation and then discovery. Communication needs to reinforce product usage – showing context and occasion can help – to teach the child proper product experience. A good example, though not in the food realm, is the Procter and Gamble product Pampers Kandoo (a range of toiletry products for very young children). It clearly shows on-pack (supported on-air), the iconic frog character demonstrating use of the product – the imagery is important because, of course, the target age child cannot read. Food product communication to young children can provide a fun context, but it is important that it shows how the product is consumed, and that it is desired and enjoyed.

4–7 years ('young children')

Younger children up to the age of 6 or 7 years are particularly influenced by the basic sensory attributes of foods and beverages, namely taste, colour, and texture, and in some categories the sense of smell as well. This is a carry-over from the early development stages when the child discovered the world through absorption by the senses. These sensory factors are critical to the young child's enjoyment of foods and beverages. Basic taste profiles, bright colours and importantly, *smooth* textures tend to be most popular. These aspects should be carefully considered and tested with young people on a product-by-product basis. This age group is also attracted by communication. The child can be motivated by the appearance of the package itself. However, it will be with older kids that the package appearance will become very important.

Fantasy can be very useful with regard to food and beverages for this age band. Foods and beverages that encourage children to experience different 'places' in the comfort and safety of familiar surroundings have great appeal to these young people. Observing children and the way in which they play with certain foods will give good ideas of ways in which to incorporate the 'fantasy' qualities in products. The game can be even better, in the child's mind, than regular toys, because the child gets to eat the toy afterward!

8–11 years ('tweens')

As children grow into the next phase, age 8–11 years, they are becoming more critical about the world around them, and the items with which they interact. The basic sensory attributes are still important, but added to these sensory attributes are the more abstract and less tangible aspects of products and brands. As the child matures into an understanding of these abstract concepts, he explores these new-found abilities. The exploration manifests itself in the child's increased interest in fads, promotions, TV, internet, mobile communication and video games. Interestingly, in some food and drink categories there is also an increased acceptance of more intensely flavoured products. Taste continues to be an important influencing factor – but now we see a desire for not only sweet but also the 'game' of the sour and heat sensations.

Peer group is now more important and the child's food choices will be influenced by them. It is also worthwhile to acknowledge the humour of this 'tween' group. They are increasingly attracted by humorous advertising and often repeat and discuss ads that they see. In most cultures, children begin to understand the humour in irony.

The 'tween' age is a good one to involve the child with cooking things and creating ideas. Activities that promote understanding, and making a food or beverage are excellent ones for the 'tween'. The process of gathering, mixing, pouring, baking, microwaving and even cleaning-up become very appealing, especially because they are involved with the activity of eating. Products that support this, even simple activities such as making toast or boiling the kettle for tea, benefit the child's development. With regard to foods and beverages, the complexity of the 'goal' is related to the age of the child. The goal can be as simple as pouring out their own cereal from the box to mixing up and baking their own biscuits.

'Tween' social skills are also in use when young people tell each other about products and other things in their lives. The schoolyard conversation about 'the newest...' and 'the best...' can be one of the greatest assets to a new food or beverage brand. Sharing the product, or even just talking about it, endows the product with credibility and therefore makes it desirable. This social aspect can be a powerful tool for a product's success. Brand developers should include the social aspect in their marketing plan to 'tweens'.

12–14 years ('young teens')

We move very quickly from our children laughing at humorous advertising targeted at them, to scoffing at it in the 12–14-year-old range. The world is now theirs: they own it and, from their perspective, they know everything. Tastes they like from childhood are still liked, but the child's repertoire is increasing. Peer influence is even greater, and the appeal of adult-targeted products starts to emerge. 'Health', particularly in relation to appearance and physical prowess, may start to influence choice. The obesity issue starts to emerge as a personal concern or worry. One consequence is that education about health and nutrition begins to make more sense to the child.

Peer pressure is a factor, but peer pressure is often a 'catch-all' phrase. The bottom line is that young people want to express themselves as individuals, yet still fit in. Sometimes the desire to 'fit in' becomes very strong, developing as an almost overriding factor in the behaviour, and that is when 'peer pressure' becomes most effective. Some children find it difficult to fit in with a group for any number of reasons, but importantly the desire to fit in is part of the normal process of maturation.

Music, sport, and fashion are among ways in which young people express their individuality and therefore are major influences of the young teen. Incidentally, increasing independence also brings the need to live within a budget, so price promotions exert an increasing effect on choice. Also, in order to keep the young teen interested in a product, it is important to build in elements that drive variety.

The ever-important aspect of taste still influences young teens, yet evolving to include wider choices and even products that need 'getting used to'. Rather than simply enjoying intense flavoured products, they now know that it is relatively safe to try new flavours and blends of simple flavours.

As children reach puberty and their teen years, their friends, music, sport, fashion, independence and acceptance are all very important. Again, basic sensory attributes are important, although there seems to be a renewed interest in at least being perceived as trying new things. Young people of this age say constantly that they want 'more variety', yet most often they choose products that are more basic and 'comfortable'. To reiterate, simple blends of tastes are very good for this age group, but are best perceived if the taste is predominantly familiar with a hint of a new taste.

15+ years ('teens')
The teenagers 15+ are a healthy blend of adult and child, though very much more towards the adult. Our work with teenagers would, at first glance, not seem that different from the way one would work with adult colleagues, though it does have an important difference. Teenagers find it a lot easier to talk about feelings, fears and expectations, and share their view of the world, usually quite an optimistic one. In most projects we do not seek out 'trend setter' teenagers, nor do we seek out those teens that are particularly unusual. We work with the average teenager. For the most part we have seen these average teens to be creative, articulate, engaging and very delighted to give their opinions and share their ideas.

11.3.4 Girls and boys are different

Not a surprise, though often deemed inappropriate to highlight, there are important differences between boys and girls. That is not to say that the differences cannot be bridged, and that all boys are different from all girls – but there are different behaviours that are observed across the world, and these can be influential in understanding young people.

A number of years ago, when observing children in the waiting room for a food research project, we noted that very young boys tended to play with building blocks by stacking them vertically (and then knock them over, only to start again), but very young girls tended to play with them by laying them out horizontally and 'putting them in an order'. It was merely an observation, and did not amount to anything at the time. It was only when we saw a similar behaviour in Africa, and then again in a Scandinavian country on another project that something struck home. It was at this point we began to start to actively think about tools and techniques to help us separate nature from nurture in our work with boys and girls (and ultimately with men and women). As it turns out, we can now more clearly discern innate behaviour in various groups, and then overlay that with project needs.

In the context of working with groups of children to design, test, modify and develop food and beverage products and concepts, we have found some other important differences. When speaking generally about gender differences, Drs Acuff and Reiher in their book *What Kids Buy and Why*, put best into words what we regularly see in our work with young people around the world.

Girls

Girls tend to exhibit a much higher taste and touch sensitivity. Although there are 'picky eaters' in both genders, girls seem to exhibit a higher level of pickiness overall. When it is important to refine a product's taste, we recommended that doing the fine-tuning work with girls be considered. It is important to check back with boys for taste acceptability, but we most often find that if you get the taste right for girls, you have probably got it right for boys as well – but the reciprocal is not true.

Girls tend to be only moderately competitive (though through the years we have seen a slight trend towards increased competitiveness). Girls tend to be better communicators, with higher verbal skills, and are good at mathematical calculations – though innately not as good as boys at mathematical reasoning.

The major differentiators, though, particularly with regard to behaviour, are girls' innate and early sensitivity to the social context, their stronger group orientation, and their more empathic interpersonal behaviour. They are usually better at listening to others' opinions, making sure that everyone has an opportunity to speak, and are more keenly aware of other people's (mostly other girls') feelings. This general behaviour is regularly manifested in eating and drinking experiences. We see strong, recurring patterns. Girls eat often in social settings. In our projects, they are the most likely to prepare their 'table' by spreading the napkin, and placing the food in an orderly fashion so that all can share. In fact, they seem to more enjoy sharing food with their friends than boys, and we continually find that products that support this have an advantage with girls over those that do not. Taste quality is more important than quantity, and this seems closely linked with girls' general sensitivity to tastes, textures, and smells.

With regard to 'nutritional issues', girls care more about the effects on their personal appearance (weight, skin, hair) than on the general concept of 'well-being'. In fact, there is a strong disappointment if a 'more nutritional product' does not have an immediate, recognisable effect on appearance.

Boys

Boys tend to be more aggressive in their behaviour than girls, according to Drs Acuff and Reiher, owing to higher levels of testosterone. We regularly see this aggressiveness, and it seems to be more notable the younger the boy. In our observations we have seen that boys learn to be less aggressive as they mature.

In comparison with girls, boys generally have much lower taste and touch sensitivity. Boys eat to eat, rather than merely to taste.

Again, to compare with girls directly, there is a higher competitiveness among boys, and higher math skills and reasoning. This is very different from girls' math calculation skills, which is more about the process (and structure) of doing the calculation. Boys' math reasoning is about the understanding of mathematical thinking. Boys have a later sensitivity to the social context, and often have to be forced to consider the social implications of their actions. This leads to less group orientation and less empathic interpersonal behaviour.

With regard to foods and beverages, boys' general behaviour also plays out in their eating and drinking experiences. Boys are more frequently happy to eat alone, and they are willing to do so because then they do not have to share. This is also often evident in the way they eat – large mouthfuls rapidly consumed. This could be linked to hunger and the higher caloric requirements of boys, but this author suspects that it is also linked to their innate selfishness with regard to food.

Quantity (or more accurately, the perception of quantity) is an important deciding factor in food and beverage choice for boys. This does not mean that they do not care about taste – they do – but they are more willing to sacrifice taste for quantity. Whether this is linked to their sensitivity to taste and smell, or if it is purely related to hunger and calorie requirements, this author is not sure. This author knows, though, that it is one of the big decision factors when deciding what foods and beverages to have.

If nutrition is at all interesting (and that is a bigger 'if' than with girls), it is frequently driven by boys' desire to perform better at sports or other activities (even computers and computer games). Surprisingly, they are more able to take a longer-term view when it comes to performance, and have more patience than girls (with regard to nutrition) to realise the effect of change.

There are a number of natural connections with children, tweens and teen but they can differ significantly between girls and boys. For example, with boys the emphasis should be strong on visual connections whereas with girls the connections can be more verbal. Boys respond better to specific rhythms, sounds and pitches; with girls it's words and melody. Boys tend to be more logical than emotional; girls tend to think more linearly and are frequently organised and enjoy putting things in order. Boys tend to be single-focused whereas girls are more inclined to multi-tasking. Though it may seem politically incorrect, it is essential that marketers understand the importance of these broad, gender-led differing connection points.

11.3.5 Some important key drivers of children, tweens and teens

As we now have a good understanding of the basic child development flow, as well as a brief glimpse at some differences between boys and girls, it is important to look at some key drivers of kids throughout all ages and across both genders. Though the driver may manifest itself differently depending on the age and stage, the drivers are the same.

Control

The most important driver of kids is control. Control is about the desire of young people to 'be in charge' of both themselves and of their immediate environment. There are numerous examples of products that give kids control, such as convenience products, products that fit easily in the hands, easy-access/easy-open products, products that give choice, and even simple single-serve products to name a few. Giving kids a sense of control in a new product is likely to be a key success factor. Importantly, give this control aspect a great deal of attention in product development and branding.

When children are young, they do not control much of their world, although they want to. In broad generalizations, children are told when to get up, when to go to school, what to eat, when to do homework, even when to play. The child reacts, striving to acquire control. This striving for control translates into popular food and beverage products. Selecting the flavour of ice cream in a supermarket or ice-cream shop is one example. Selecting the topping to go on ice cream gives a bit more control. Having multiple choices of inclusions for ice cream provides even more control. To use another example, even the simple act of pouring out a bowl of cereal and adding milk gives a child control. In sum, food and beverage products that enhance the target-aged child's perception that he or she is 'in control' is more likely to have appeal than those products that do not.

Aspiration

Kids aspire to the benefits of being older. They also want to enjoy themselves and say that they want to avoid 'boring' and 'the same old thing'. It is important to note, though, that control is often the overriding desire for 'new and different', and therefore tends to be the most important.

Aspiration is usually driven by the child's desire, almost obsession, with being perceived as older. Thus 3 year olds want to reach a higher shelf, 5 year olds want to stay up later like their older brother or sister, 8 year olds want to go places with their friends and without the parents, 12 year olds want to stay out late, 15 year olds want to drive cars. And so this drive of aspiration accelerates children through their childhood years. Food and beverage products need to support this drive. Products that allow children to 'feel' older or more adult have greater chance of success. In our creativity work with kids throughout the world, we always ask them to design products for 'young people their age and older' so they do not only work on ideas for 'little kids'.

Usually, food and beverage products targeted to very young kids will not appeal to older kids, even though the taste itself might appeal. Even if older kids eat those products, they will not admit that they still like them. While they may watch certain TV shows because they have a younger sibling that does like them, or eat a certain product because it is in the house for a younger sibling, children would not be seen to choose these things themselves.

Underestimating the importance of a young person's aspiration to be "older" can completely undermine the success of a product.

Creating excitement and stretching boundaries

Making things extreme enough to stretch a child's imagination while still letting them feel safe is a 'sure bet' for product success. This 'stretching' is exhibited in different ways depending upon the age of the child. It is exciting for a child to be able to interact with his/her food. And interaction, in this case, does not mean 'playing with food'. It is better explained by dipping food into sauces, or adding cereal or sprinkles to their own yogurt. Other ways to make food exciting is to provide games on the packages or to provide new and different shapes of the same product or to provide interesting dispensers or ways to get the food into one's mouth without simply spooning it there!

Humour, starting particularly in the 'tween' years, is another way that kids make their food products more interesting, and stretch the boundaries of adult acceptability. Importantly, humour begins to help them further assert their independence. Being simultaneously disgusting and funny can be a big winner with younger 'tween' boys. If something is conventionally supposed to be a certain way, isn't it funny to make it another way? Repeating the joke over and over makes it funnier every time. And if one's parents are bothered by it, or there is an adult in the room who does not appreciate the humour, all the better!

A word of caution, however. It is better not to attempt humour than to attempt it and patronise the target audience with 'childish' humour or humour that is not up-to-date, 'cool' or in any way pokes fun at the child. Making fun of adults may be fun, as long as it is not perceived to be 'mean' and hurtful. Making fun of a child is typically strongly rejected. Also, children as heroes and shown as the ones, in the end, who 'save the day' can have great appeal – and children taking on the role of adults who sometimes 'just don't quite get it'.

Neophobia

To understand about the phenomenon of neophobia, we really need to understand fear. It is important to be aware of the connection and difference between fear on the one hand and curiosity on the other. It is believed that these two states cannot be concurrent – meaning we cannot be both fearful and curious at the same time. We need to understand, therefore, drivers of fear (and 'new' is a driver of 'fear') and what generates 'curiosity'. For a new product developments to succeed, we need to reduce kids' fear and enhance their curiosity. Keep in mind the 'Neophobia Equation': *'Familiar' = 'Liking'*

The paradox of neophobia is that kids may express their desire for 'new' and 'more exciting,' yet, in practice, they continue to eat and drink the same things to which they've become accustomed. This paradox creates a challenge for all food and beverage marketers and developers. There is a strong desire, even a need, to convey a sense of novelty and uniqueness in their products, but they must also develop tastes and food or beverage forms that are familiar. Many in the food industry will find inserting the physical stimuli to generate familiarity in new products to be relatively uninspiring and less interesting, but it is important with kid's products.

Kids are *innately* afraid of new foods, and this can be evident at a very young age. This is not just about picky eaters; even kids with wider food repertoires show some aversion to new foods, and when they refuse to eat or drink something it is very often simply because it is *unfamiliar*. When asked, 'why don't you like it?' a common response is 'because I've never had it before.'

The comfort of familiarity can occasionally mislead, when research is involved. When conducting observational research and accompanied shopping interviews, children as young as 18 months often can be observed pointing to items on the shelves. When asked, the mother regularly interpreted this behaviour as meaning that the child liked the item, yet it frequently turned out to be that the child merely *recognized it* rather than was trying to communicate liking it.

Adults also exhibit neophobic behaviour and resort to familiar, trusted, known brands and products – but adults are more willing to try new things than children. As we age into our 60s and beyond, we tend to again seek more familiar and comfortable foods, reverting back to child-like behaviour with regard to food and beverage repertoire and choice.

Dealing with neophobia

If kids tend to revert to familiar flavours, familiar food forms and familiar brands, how then can we develop new kids' foods and beverages?

(i) *To increase liking for a certain food or beverage, you must increase positive exposures to it.* This poses an important challenge to food marketers. Depending on the category, it can take anywhere from 8 to 13 positive exposures for kids to be strongly familiar with a food or beverage (and therefore indicate that it is liked). Sampling, therefore, takes on a very important role, and 'trial' may continue beyond the first purchase. There are also ramifications in new product testing and sensory evaluation.

(ii) *Good experiences with new foods decreases neophobia.* This is important in a number of ways. First of all, the converse can also be true. Bad experiences with new foods can increase neophobia. This means that launching products that kids do not like can damage brands. People can understand that they may not like certain flavour variants, but repeated negative experiences with a brand are likely to make that young person avoid trying future new products with that brand name.

(iii) *Combining the new with the familiar decreases neophobia.* This is probably the best advice of all. Taking something familiar and adding something new seems to be highly successful in developing new food trends with kids. Change the format or the food, but be careful about doing both at once. Too drastic a change, is more likely to cause rejection.

(iv) *Liking of a product by peers increases liking*. Mums have been saying for years about kids. 'I have tried for ages to get my child to eat (insert food or beverage) and he refused. Suddenly he goes to a friend's house and has it. Now he wants it all the time!' The same can also be true for adults – we learn by seeing people we know/respect try something, and we think we will too. This is why 'word of mouth' is so powerful with kids, and arguably, powerful with all consumers. It is all about reassurance and comfort, reduction of fear, and the increasing of curiosity. This helps to create a willingness in the child to try something new and makes him or her less afraid of it.

(v) *Be careful of health and nutrition claims, because they have no effect with many kids, and may decrease liking*. Though more and more information is available about nutrition and healthy eating, the results, to get kids to eat better, have not been so encouraging. Being told 'it's good for you' will not make kids like your product. Sometimes they may use nutritional elements as a negotiating tool to be able to rationalize or justify what they want: 'Mum, please get it for me. It's got vitamins and minerals!'. But in the end, we are not usually willing to eat things we don't like purely because 'it's good for you.'

Once we understand the meaning of neophobia, the kids' stated desire for 'something new and different' or 'something less boring' takes on a completely different meaning. We certainly need to deliver to them the perception of 'something new,' but in a familiar way, or with a familiar taste. We need to build new products and flavours from their existing experience, and to move step-by-step, rather than in leaps and bounds. We need to clearly communicate in a familiar way what the product is so that kids can feel more in control, and feel as if they know what they'll be getting. We need to remember as our mantra the equation 'familiar = liking' and not be ashamed to use this to power our new product development.

Much of the basic understanding about neophobia was gleaned from work by and listening to Prof. P Pliner, University of Toronto, and Dr D Mennella, The Monell Institute. It is strongly recommended to search for and read their work. The specific experiences related in this section are based on several years' worth of projects carried out by the Consumer Knowledge Centre, all throughout the world.

11.4 Implications for testing: some thoughts on taking sensory evaluation and other aspects of product testing to the next level with kids

Not only for actual marketing and product development, but the understanding of children, tweens and teens is also critical in the *testing* of new ideas and marketing activities. Though basing research with kids on adult models can, on some occasions, be successful, more often testing with young people requires a modified approach. Though each situation requires consideration, below follows some thoughts on ways to better engage young people in the food and beverage evaluation process: engagement is critical. With testing of products for young people, an understanding of the test is equally important.

Engagement with children, tweens and teens can be done in a myriad of ways. Familiar fairy tales, such as *Goldilocks and the Three Bears* as a basis of a sensory test for very young children, or mimicking playing computer games with older children are just a couple of examples. A key measure, beyond the testing parameters is to see kids' enthusiasm and involvement in the process of the test. Good facilitation is key and can be the difference between an accurate result and one that is doubtful and not duplicate-able. Likewise, the young participants understanding of what is expected of them and the evaluation process is also important. Understanding of scales and evaluative aspects takes time, and the test should not be rushed. Adults are more familiar with scales and scoring, so time taken explaining the scales can be much less than with kids. The younger the child, the more explanation of scale is required.

11.4.1 As you are working through the new product development process, remember some important dos and don'ts

There are some general dos and don'ts to keep in mind when working with children, tweens and teens:

Do be absolutely clear about who you are talking to. It is important to learn about kids and understand their development and key drivers (as discussed in previous sections of this chapter). Kids are different as they evolve through the various ages and stages, and there are important physiological and cognitive issues to consider.

Do understand kids' key drivers of control, aspiration, and their stated desire to create excitement and stretch boundaries in the context of the age and stage of child with which you are working. Remember that their desire for control is the most important driver, and you should strongly consider ways to make kids feel more in control – especially with regards to packaging (suitable for the size of the target-aged hands, fits in with their lives, easy-opening and access, etc.) and product (flavour, portion size/bite sizes). When testing, giving young people a sense that they have more control is also a driving engagement in the testing process. Aspiration, creating excitement, and stretching boundaries should be more in the tonality and personality of the brand, and in testing always remember to talk to kids in a way that is not perceived by them to be patronising.

Do accept that boys and girls are different, and find ways to either target a specific gender or ensure that both are satisfied. When you must target both, always skew the positioning to boys. Girls are more accepting of 'boy' products, yet boys are more likely to reject something that is 'too girly'. In testing, understand that the way boys and girls evaluate products can be quite different – girls tend to be more discerning about context and nuance, boys about imagery and sense of energy.

Do see the market and category through kids' eyes. Sometimes we are so involved in the language and definitions promulgated by the food and beverage industry, we forget that consumers do not see things the same way. Young people do not think of foods and beverages in the same categories we do – they do not say 'I want a carbonated beverage' or 'I want a dairy drink', rather they say 'I want a drink' (implicitly, that tastes good). In some situations they may only say 'I want something that tastes good', without certainty that it is a drink at all.

Do involve kids in all aspects of product development and testing, and learn from their creativity. To design kids' products without involvement of kids at various stages is folly. The way you work with kids is important (they are not just little adults, and have different ways of expressing themselves), but most important is that you work with them! When you do, use humour and have fun, and where possible, work in environments in which they are most comfortable.

Do be holistic in all that you do. Though it may seem logical to work on various aspects of the product, or even the marketing mix separately, with kids (and perhaps most consumers) it is best to develop and test the product holistically. A child has a difficult time to separate product attributes, for example, and younger children often take things very literally.

11.4.2 Increase time spent with the same group

In traditional research, we spend small amounts of time with multiple groups of consumers. This reduces the chance of getting accurate information. In our experience, kids do not really 'warm up' to the moderator for at least an hour. The experience is new and they are trying to find the 'right answers' as their only framework for something like this is school, and in school they are expected to come up with the 'right answers'. It is not unusual on our projects to spend at least two or three hours with the same group, with frequent projects spending a full day. On occasion, depending on project needs, we would even work with the same group of kids for several days. It is not worrying that kids have short attention spans, the worry is to develop a process, with appropriate activities, that engage the young people and *keep* them engaged.

11.4.3 Schedule the time when it is best for kids

So often we schedule groups based around our convenience, and this usually coincides with the worst time for kids. After school and early evening is the time of day when most young people are tired, irritable, and not particularly interested in sitting around and talking about things in a structured discussion group. At these times, young people should be allowed to run around, relax and have unstructured time. We recommend to our clients that group work with kids should be on a school holiday or a weekend (non-school day). Alternatively, do the work in the school – but do the discussion/thinking activities in the morning. Ask teachers. They know that young people do most of their best analytical work in the morning. We do most of our qualitative work with young people in schools, and build the work around a curricular structure. Weekends are also often better opportunities to engage with kids – especially better than the after school/early evening hours. On the occasions when it is not possible to schedule at the best time of day, the research process should be developed to deal with the young people's innate difficulties. Also, for products that target consumption for the after-school period, an exception to this 'rule' should be considered.

11.4.4 Work in the kids' environment, whenever possible (or create an environment that is reminiscent of a familiar setting)

Kids in a comfortable environment amongst their peers are extremely forthcoming. If you must use a facility, do your best to make it different from a boardroom type set-up. If possible, use other, more familiar places (schools, church halls, shopping malls, etc.) so the issues created by artificial focus group environments are avoided. If this is not possible, creating an environment that is reminiscent of a familiar locale should be done. This is particularly important the younger the child. Avoid settings that look too much like doctor's or dentist's offices – too often in our desire to minimize stimuli in a testing room, we will make the walls stark white and minimalistic, and these make kids (particularly young children) think they are going to the dentist!

11.4.5 Do not just talk and ask questions; include activities

Though imperative for work with young people, we have also built this principle into our work with adults and have found it successful. Even with the best intentions and brilliant moderating, attention wanes and peaks at different intervals for each individual. Building activity-based discussion groups helps overcome the unsynchronised 'waves'. Depending on the age of young people, a good rule of thumb is to physically move them around every 10–20 minutes, most successfully achieved by interspersing different activities in between discussion. You will be amazed at the improvement in the quality of the information.

Activities can also be developed that are consistent with the project's needs, and do not need to detract from learning for the young people. Suggesting that kids 'vote' by going to one side of the room or the other can maintain the focus on the discussion at hand, yet still move the kids around.

11.4.6 Give young people an element of control

As previously discussed, control is one of the key emotional drivers of young people. If, early in the research session, we give the young people a sense of control and 'ownership', they will more enthusiastically embrace the tasks at hand. This can be in simple ways, even by having them decide on the means by which the moderator will re-gain the group's attention to give instructions or start a new discussion. The kids often give silly tasks for the moderator to do – like jumping up and down and wildly waving his/her arms – but they get the message early in the project that what they say, matters. This makes them feel that they are in control.

11.4.7 Ideally include the holistic product including packaging, graphics and even promotional aspects

Typically, research tests each facet of a product and then brings them all together at the end. A product concept has to be comprehensive for the young consumer to understand it. This is particularly true of an innovation. Kids (and other consumers) buy into the whole product, not an individual facet. The whole thing has to work together.

11.4.8 Be involved with the young consumers

If the research is qualitative, then why are the clients kept at arm's length? For real insight, consider interacting with your consumer, rather than just view them from behind a one-way mirror. We enjoy inviting our clients into the room with the young people – admittedly a bit daunting at first, but the feedback is always positive. Frequently, this direct engagement is key to a deeper insight; to the ease and speed of making future decisions that must be taken to bring the project to a successful conclusion.

11.4.9 Recognize that kids in different cultures are still kids

There is a difference between cultural and emotional drivers. Kids everywhere aspire to be older so our style of working with young people works in many regions. Young people's product ideas will reflect the cultural preferences in a given country. But the key drivers of excitement, control, testing/stretching boundaries and aspiration are everywhere.

Work with and modify traditional methods and create new methods that simulate giving kids control of the product development process or the brand management process. The end product can be anything from a new supermarket layout or restaurant to a new package or an advert for an existing product.

Winning with kids need not be a terrifying task. We can build on the understanding of the age and stage of the child, maintain a keen focus to deliver control, instill aspiration, create excitement/stretching boundaries, and build on ways to overcome the innate neophobia that kids have. Following these straight-forward guidelines will help the company, whether product developer or marketer, create winning products for kids, faster, with much confidence, and ultimately, with more market success.

11.5 Sources of further information and advice

Acuff D. S., Reiher R. H. (1997). *What Kids Buy and Why*. New York, NY, USA; The Free Press.

Birch, L. L., McPhee, L., Shoba, B. C., Pirok, E., and Steinberg, L. (1987). What kind of exposure reduces children's food neophobia? Looking vs. Tasting. *Appetite*, 9, 171–178.

Birch, L. L., and Marlin, D. W. (1982). I don't like it; I never tried it: effects of exposure on two-year-old children's food preferences. *Appetite*, 3(4), 353–360.

Cashdan, E. (1994). A sensitive period for learning about food. *Human Nature*, 5(3), 279–291.

Doherty-Sneddon, G. (2008). The great baby signing debate, *The Psychologist*, Vol. 21, Part 4, April, 300–303.

Hemingway, M. (2002). Effective techniques for consumer research in a challenging market. Presented at *Annual Mtg. Inst. of Food Technologists*, Anaheim, CA, June 15–19.

Leathwood P., Maier A. (2005). Early influences on taste preferences. *Nestlé Nutrition Workshop Ser Pediatric Program*. 56:127–141.

Lindstrom, M. and Seybold, P. B. (2003). *Brand Child: Remarkable insights into the minds of today's global kids and their relationship with brands*. Kogan Page Ltd.

Maier A. (2007). These de Doctorat de l'Universite de Bourgogne. *Influence des pratiques d'allaitement et de sevrage dur l'acceptation de flaveurs nouvelles chez le jeune enfant: Variabilité intra- et inter-régionale*.

Maier A., Chabanet C., Schaal B., Leathwood P., Issanchou S. (2007). Food-related sensory experience from birth through weaning: Contrasted patterns in two nearby European regions. *Appetite* 49(2): 429–40.

Maier A., Chabanet C., Schaal B., Issanchou S., Leathwood P. (2007). Effects of repeated exposure on acceptance of initially disliked vegetables in 7-month old infants. *Food Quality and Preference* 18: 1023–1032.

Mennella, J. A., Griffin, C. E., and Beauchamp, G. K. (2004). Flavor programming during infancy. *Pediatrics*, 113, 840–845.

Mennella, J. A., Jagnow, C. P., and Beauchamp, G. K. (2001). Prenatal and postnatal flavor learning by human infants. *Pediatrics*, 107, e88.

Mennella, J. A., and Beauchamp, G. K. (2002). Flavor experiences during formula

feeding are related to preferences during childhood. *Early Human Development*, 68, 71–82.
Pliner, P. (1982). The effects of mere exposure on liking for edible substances. *Appetite* 3: 283–290.
Pliner, P. (1983). Family resemblance in food preferences. *J. Nutr. Educ.* 15: 137–140.
Pliner, P. and Salvy, S.-J. (2006). Food neophobia in humans. In R. Shepherd and M. Raats (Eds), *The Psychology of Food Choice* (pp. 75–92). Oxfordshire, UK: CABI Head Office.
Stueve, M. (2002). Can children perform descriptive analysis? Presented at *Annual Mtg. Inst. of Food Technologists*, Anaheim, CA, June 15–19.
Urbick, B. (2000). *About Kids: Food and Beverages.* Leatherhead Press Ltd.
Urbick, B. (2002). Kids have great taste: An update to sensory work with children. Presented at *Annual Mtg. Inst. of Food Technologists*, Anaheim, CA, June 15–19.
Zandstra, E. H. and de Graaf, C. (1998). Sensory perception and pleasantness of orange beverages from childhood to old age. *Food Qual. Preference* 9: 5–12.

Index

FSC
www.fsc.org
MIX
Papier | Fördert
gute Waldnutzung
FSC® C083411

Kolibri 360 GmbH
Ferdinand-Jühlke-Straße 7
99095 Erfurt, Deutschland
produktsicherheit@kolibri360.de